AF739461

Building Better Humans?

BEYOND HUMANISM: TRANS- AND POSTHUMANISM
JENSEITS DES HUMANISMUS: TRANS- UND POSTHUMANISMUS

Edited by / Herausgegeben von Stefan Lorenz Sorgner

Editorial Board:
H. James Birx
Irina Deretic
James J. Hughes
Andy Miah
Domna Pastourmatzi
Evi Sampanikou

Vol. / Bd. 3

PETER LANG
Frankfurt am Main · Berlin · Bern · Bruxelles · New York · Oxford · Wien

Building Better Humans?

Refocusing the Debate on Transhumanism

Edited by
Hava Tirosh-Samuelson
and Kenneth L. Mossman

PETER LANG
Internationaler Verlag der Wissenschaften

Bibliographic Information published by the Deutsche Nationalbibliothek
The Deutsche Nationalbibliothek lists this publication in the Deutsche Nationalbibliografie; detailed bibliographic data is available in the internet at http://dnb.d-nb.de.

Cover Design:
© Olaf Gloeckler, Atelier Platen, Friedberg

Cover image:
Structural diagram of a robot.
Colin Anderson, 2005. (Masterfile).

ISSN 2191-0391
ISBN 978-3-631-63513-1
© Peter Lang GmbH
Internationaler Verlag der Wissenschaften
Frankfurt am Main 2012
All rights reserved.

All parts of this publication are protected by copyright. Any utilisation outside the strict limits of the copyright law, without the permission of the publisher, is forbidden and liable to prosecution. This applies in particular to reproductions, translations, microfilming, and storage and processing in electronic retrieval systems.

www.peterlang.de

Contents

Acknowledgments

The volume is the result of four years of intense deliberations on the meaning, problems, and implications of transhumanism. Titled "Facing the Challenges of Transhumanism: Religion, Science, and Technology" (www.asu.edu/transhumanism), this project was supported by a large grant from the Metanexus Institute given to the Templeton Research Lectures on the Constructive Engagement of Science and Religion (2006-9). The grant sponsored public lectures, three annual workshops, and a monthly, interdisciplinary faculty seminar, resulting in the publication of two books (Allenby and Sarewitz 2011; Mehlman 2011), several essays (Tirosh-Samuelson 2010, 2011), a special issue published first on line (www.globalspiral.com) and then in print (Hansell and Grassie 2011).

We hereby express our gratitude to William J. Grassie, the executive director of Metanexus, for his support of the project and his direct involvement in it and the issues it generates. Grassie's engagement with transhumanism concludes this volume, and these two edited volumes enrich the nascent literature on this important topic.

Most but not all the contributors to this volume participated in the faculty seminar at Arizona State University (ASU) that lasted for a total of six years (the seminar was established two years before the Templeton Research Lectures were awarded to ASU). We are most indebted to Michael Crow, the president of ASU, for his initial support of the project. An expert on science policy, President Crow's reflections on the challenges of technology to our democratic society commences the volume, charting the kind of challenges our society will face during the twentieth-first century. The faculty seminar, "Being Human: Religion, Science, and Technology," was a truly interdisciplinary project, including faculty members from the humanities, the social sciences, the natural sciences, engineering, and law. The commitment to interdisciplinarity characterizes the structure and spirit of Arizona State University as it projects the "New American University" as a model for higher education. We are most grateful to former ASU's Vice President and Dean of the College of Liberal Arts and Sciences, Quentin Wheeler, for his thoughtful essay on the scope, promise, and peril of interdisciplinarity and for the initial support the faculty seminar received from the College of Liberal Arts and Science.

The faculty seminar was carried out under the auspices of the Center for the Study of Religion and Conflict, headed by Linell E. Cady, a scholar of religious studies who specializes in the place of religion in the public sphere in the U.S. and throughout the world. We thank Professor Cady for understanding how the disputes about biotechnology are part of larger set issues that belong to the perceived conflict between religion and science. But more than any other person, it was Carolyn Forbes, the assistant director of the Center for the Study of Religion and Conflict, who made the faculty seminar success with her tireless, intelligent, and dedicated work over six years.

Editorial work is a difficult task, but two people have made it a joyful one. Mary Egel did the initial editing and indexed the volume, and her excellent work was complemented by the meticulous editing of Mary Lou Bertucci that made it possible to submit the manuscript to the press. To both of them, we are most indebted.

Finally, we would like to thank all members of the faculty seminar who devoted six years of their lives to reflect on these issues and to show how academics across the spectrum can become a vibrant learning community.

Forewords

Science, Technology, and Democracy

Michael M. Crow

As you read this foreword, your eyes no doubt focus on the text better than would have those of our fellow humans from preceding centuries because of the technological innovations on, around, or in your eyes (glasses, contact lenses, laser surgery, etc.). Your mind is processing these words in an enhanced way as well because of your advanced diet of engineered foods and special supplements and medicines. Your understanding and awareness are enhanced through elaborate learning and information tools on or near your body, not to mention that, if you are forty years or older as you read this, your very existence is the product of hundreds of years of human modification of everything around you and all you put into your body.

It would be a mistake to conjecture that building a better human is something other than the central objective of the science we do and the policies and resources that drive that science and technology. We are creatures driven to adapt and survive on a planet of powerful natural dynamics, surrounded by a universe of even greater forces. These forces and our relationship with them over time have led us to the point in human history where we have grasped the fact that we are now a species directing and guiding – in the way that beginners do and often with many fits and starts – our own physical, social, cultural, and planetary evolution. This is now occurring at the rate and speed that it is because of conscious decisions to make our understanding of nature (science) and our adaptation to nature (technology) one of a handful of the central functions of our society. We do this through our conscious decision making regarding the resources that we allocate to this very conscious and focused set of purposeful investments and decisions.

As a consequence, we have reached the point where three questions should be asked: what are we doing, why are we doing it, and is this the outcome we want? To address these questions from the perspective of science policy, I will outline the historical development of some of our core human behaviors. As manifestations of our human limitations, after all, science policy and its close partner, technology policy, replicate fundamental aspects of our core needs and desires.

Let me reiterate the central fact that human beings are, at the end of the day, an adaptive, highly evolved product of dynamic evolutionary forces. As a highly adaptive species, we have survived and prospered through three distinct evolutionary phases. These evolutionary phases are "natural evolution," during which we sought adaptation to our environment with primitive tools; "adaptive evolution," which represents our movement through intensive development and use of tools to enhance our well-being; and, most recently, "self-directed evolution," during which we have achieved the capacity to shape not only the outcomes in our environment and, thus, indirectly ourselves but also to directly shape our organisms through self-enhancement.

Throughout human history, the coevolution of humans with other species and our adaptation to those other species, as well as to the circumstances of the physical systems around us, have been a principal driver, if not *the* principal driver, of who we are. It is a defining characteristic that we work to build a better environment around us. "Better," of course, is a term that is subject to definition, but it is nevertheless the case that, as a species, we have worked to adapt so that we might survive. In fact, for at least the past 150,000 years, we have been shaping tools to better master our environment. Our tools may have been those to conquer animals for food or to allow us to stay warm when it was cold or to walk longer distances than our natural bodily systems would permit, but, in any event, we have been working for at least 150,000 years to advance every possible mechanism to help us shape and master our environment and our individual body's relationship with that environment. In this period of seemingly natural evolution, we learned to adapt more quickly than most, if not all, other species, and we learned to modify ourselves as necessary for prolonged journeys and unexpected encounters with highly diverse ecosystems. This unique characteristic of humans rests at the heart of even our present science and technology policy design.

During the past ten thousand years, we have moved from being driven more in a natural evolutionary environment to what I call an "adaptive evolutionary environment" where we have been engineering animals, plants, and environments for our benefit in every possible way. Very little that we discovered in nature has been left unaltered by us either as a result of purposeful actions, accidental encounters, random acts, or pure stupidity. In any event, we have shaped for at least ten thousand years everything around us in a way that has enhanced our capacity to survive as well as our increasingly dominant role as a species on this planet. Within this context and further back than anyone can fully understand or document, technological advance has been inextricably correlated with our social and, to some extent, even physical evolution, serving as a chief determinant and driver of our progress as a species. During these past millennia, our technological experimentation has allowed us to establish an adaptive evolutionary platform for human enhancement that has allowed us to shape our outcomes and our destinies. Our most basic technologies – one need only imagine the most primitive canoes formed from hollowed-out tree trunks – have given us speed of movement, access to food and shelter, and an ability to protect our bodies and project ourselves across seemingly impassable barriers.

For no more than the past few hundred years, a new force has projected humans into a realm of previously unimaginable adaptive evolution. This force is science. Through our progressively more sophisticated and intricate understanding of nature during these past few centuries, our increasingly successful adaptation to the natural systems in which we are embedded has intensified our capacities for further self-enhancement. Evolutionary forces driven only by natural systems have become heavily complemented by enhanced competition among humans and between human societies. Through modern science, a range of industrial, military, social, and cultural competitions has been stimulated, which have produced dramatic differences in the relative adaptive success of societies around the globe. These differences are often attributed to the advancement of science, at least before the last few decades, and are also a consequence of the fact that organized science, in its early stages prior to World War II, outlined and empowered our ability to leap from an adaptive species to a self-directed species. With progress in scientific understanding, we learned how to control microorganisms harmful to humans, for example. We developed new tools to enhance human performance, such as extensions of our body that could hurtle us through the atmosphere at high rates of speed and simulate the functions of birds in terms of our ability to move up and down from a stationary location. In this sense, science empowered our capacity for high-speed, self-directed evolution.

Unfortunately, the culmination of our awakening as a species to the potential for self-directed evolution and thus self-determinative fate, I think, can be attributed to the scientific design and technological deployment in the mid-1940s of weapons of mass destruction. The weapons themselves, the processes by which they were conceived and developed, and the outcome of their use fueled the assumption, still widely prevalent in American culture and politics, that through science we could achieve nearly anything. Science could preserve us in competition against our enemies, as well as ensure the fulfillment of anything we might conceive.

It was, in fact, at this moment nearly seventy years ago, corresponding with the publication of the report "Science: The Endless Frontier," by Vannevar Bush, and the institutionalization of a fundamental national science policy, that we observe the transition from the basic operating realm of adaptive evolution to the early stages of self-directed evolution. In this sense, the period of the past seventy years marks a unique inflection point in our trajectory as a species. During these decades, large-scale public investment in science and technology corresponds to a drift toward systematic, societal-level, self-directed evolution. The basic premise for American science policy was established in the Bush report with its implicit promise that, if science was sufficiently funded, it would provide for the health and well-being of the population, extension of life for the infirm and aged, and defense of the nation by any means necessary against all threats.

As a consequence, American democracy has produced a science policy that in the past seventy years has outlined objectives such as the following for the science-and-technology community:

(1) Enhance the quality of life for everyone.
(2) Defeat cancer, a particularly daunting challenge because it is a natural evolutionary process driven by complex behaviors and species interactions.
(3) Render soldiers less destructible and ensure military dominance.
(4) Exert force and project power without risking individuals.
(5) Transform energy and water systems to renewable and human-controlled functions, no longer reliant on the natural systems of the earth.

These objectives are, in fact, identical to those that have motivated humans for the past few thousand years. We adapt to enhance our survival and success as a species. Only now, however, humans are empowered by a rapidly moving science seemingly capable of addressing literally any challenge. It is very difficult even to characterize the scale of the impact of science on human society during the past seven decades. As we negotiate the transition from an adaptive to a self-directed evolutionary species, we are engaged in scientific activities and technological advances that can alter who we are, how we act, how we adapt, and thus how we continue to evolve.

In an effort to understand the trajectory that led us to acquire the potential for self-directed evolution, we may be inclined to retrace our footsteps in the remote past. In my estimation, however, the answers are more likely closer at hand. I would argue that our capacities for self-modification or even the creation of new life forms are natural outcomes derivative of the core driving principle of our species: adaptation. American democracy, which has among its fundamental design parameters a focus on providing for life, liberty, and the pursuit of happiness, epitomizes this imperative for adaptation. In this sense, while our collective energy and resources are necessarily heavily focused on our own continued evolutionary success through adaptation, our adaptation in a democracy inherently seeks to provide for the pursuit of happiness of all in a society of hundreds of millions of individuals.

The result of this alignment of interests is a national science enterprise focused on a cultural outcome – the pursuit of happiness – without full consideration of the impacts of science-enabled, self-directed evolution. We are already concerned about the impacts that adaptive evolution has had on our relationship with the planet, not to mention the fact that the past few hundred years of science-and-technology outcomes have produced both enormous socioeconomic benefits and challenges. We may well then consider how self-directed evolution empowered by science may produce significant social and cultural instabilities going forward.

Just as in all evolutionary dynamics, steps forward or backward require further and still-more elaborate adaptation. When pondering human transformation and enhancement in this context, one can either be chagrined or assured that science-and-technology policy in its present simplistic stage can only guarantee that our focus will be on adaptation.

Presently under consideration is a range of investments in nanotechnology, synthetic biology, geo-engineering, and other areas that will lead either to the modification of natural systems to our benefit or our own self-modification in order not to be subject to natural forces. This is the basic and fundamental purpose of the present articulation of national science-and-technology policy, at least in the United States. So, then, what is, in fact, the question regarding transhumanism and science-and-technology policy? Transhumanism as a concept is empowered by the outcome of seventy years of focused science, preceded by hundreds of years of organized science, preceded by thousands of years of purposeful adaptation and hundreds of thousands of years of natural adaptation. How is it that we have some desire now to think that, in fact, we are not who we are? We are an adaptive evolutionary species capable of modifying ourselves so as to enhance our adaptation. This said, we must begin the serious consideration of what outcomes we seek from our science-and-technology investments. What kinds of social, cultural, and economic outcomes would we like to see as a result of our scientific investments? At present, I am of the view that our outcome logic is comprised of only three or four parameters, which have not been robustly considered or designed, whereas the much broader outcome logic we require would include perhaps dozens of parameters that are robust in their character and thoughtful in their design.

As we as a species move further down the self-directed evolutionary path, guided as we are by our national science policy, which is itself necessarily and incontrovertibly a product of human nature, we must think through the consequences of our nature and what it means to be empowered with scientific capabilities that allow us to direct further change and even to contemplate transformation of the very essence of who or what we are. In a sense, I think that we are approaching the moment in our own evolution when we have to make some assessment about whether we even want the self-directed evolutionary capabilities that we now have acquired. These allow us, after all, to produce certain outcomes. Or perhaps we may wish to operate in accordance with the basic mechanisms of evolutionary change as a force for natural selection and adaptation only. These are challenging questions but ones that, because of the speed of scientific advancement, the capabilities associated with technological innovation, and their impacts on who and what we are, merit the kinds of discussions that this book intends to initiate.

As your mind processes these words on this page, please note that I am writing this surrounded by an artificial atmosphere as my body rests in a metal object traveling at more than 500 miles an hour across more than 2,500 miles while I am connected via satellite to the Internet watching the news about a group of scientists reengineering the gut of a mosquito to produce an engineered insect that can kill off mosquitoes that carry the malaria virus. In this sense, I am not exactly sure what kind of human I am or how my life has been modified, but I am certain that there is increasingly less that is similar on a day-to-day basis between me and my ancestors of fifty thousand years ago.

Recombinant Innovation
Creative Hybrid Zones in the Adaptive University

Quentin Wheeler

Alea iacta est.[1] Academia has initiated changes that will almost certainly reshape our universities in ways that were unforeseeable a generation ago. The well-rehearsed, narrow disciplines that many of us were educated within no longer seem up to the challenge of confronting many of the problems facing society. The size, complexity, and tempo of many existing, emerging, and foreseeable problems are simply beyond the capacity of business-as-usual to solve.

The twentieth century seems to have accentuated the problems attached to specialization. A multiplication of academic departments and ever more narrowly circumscribed specializations resulted in a proliferation of intellectual silos between which communication was close to nonexistent. At least in the sciences, there was a tacit assumption that this narrowing was a good thing, a harbinger of increased precision and depth of knowledge. The experimental method, drilled into every science student, stresses the virtues of controlling as many variables as possible, and the analogy at the discipline level was clear. We literally were learning more and more about less and less, and not always about the right things:

> There is absolutely no a priori reason to expect that what we can know is what we most need to know. Science uses disciplinary organization to recognize and focus on questions that can be answered. Disciplines, in turn, are separated by methodology, terminology, sociology, and disparate bodies of fact that resist synthesis. Although disciplinary specialization has been the key to scientific success, such specialization simultaneously takes us away from any knowledge of the whole. (Crow 2007, 31)

I suspect that physics played an unintended, but nevertheless leading, role in all this. Even long after physics had moved beyond reductionism and recognized the importance of emergent phenomena associated with increasing complexity, other branches of science stayed the course. It remains seductive to believe that even the most complex problem can be solved by atomizing it into its smallest parts, resolving each, and then just putting them back together again. It is seductive, but it is wrong. In many cases, the problem is greater than the sum of its parts, and it is increasingly clear that a much richer understanding of complexity will be required for success.

---

1 I thank Hava Tirosh-Samuelson and Kenneth L. Mossman for inviting me to write this paper and for Tyna Chu for typing the final draft.

In the context of scientific practice, I am using the term *reductionism* to refer to the assumption that relatively complex problems in one discipline may be ultimately understood by breaking them down into components that are the subject of study of another discipline (Sarkar 1992). In biology, for example, it is currently fashionable to suspect that molecular genetics (sequencing genes) will offer explanations for complexity in organisms, whether cancer or bird songs, and that the mechanisms of genetic information will ultimately be understood in terms of the chemistry of nucleic acids, and these, in turn, by the laws of physics. There is ample reason, of course, to suspect that this is not so. Anderson described the proposition that parts could be reassembled to explain the whole as the constructionist hypothesis that, as he explains, "breaks down when confronted with the twin difficulties of scale and complexity" (1972, 393). He continued to explain that "at each level of complexity entirely new properties appear, and the understanding of the new behaviors requires research which I think is as fundamental in its nature as any other." A similar explanation was offered for the failure of reductionism in ecology by Levins and Lewinton (1980, 76):

> The reductionist myth of simplicity leads its advocates to isolate parts as completely as possible and study these parts. It underestimates the importance of interactions in theory, and its recommendations for practice (in agricultural programs or conservation and environmental protection) are typically thwarted by the power of indirect and unanticipated causes rather than by error in the detailed description of their own objects of study.

In spite of such warnings, reductionism remains alive and well. Sequencing the human genome was an important symbolic milestone for biology. Cracking the genetic code represents one of the great advances in exploring evolutionary processes since Charles Darwin. Many of the most exciting benefits of our newfound DNA sequencing abilities, however, lie ahead, such as the promise of personalized medicine and unraveling the details of evolutionary developmental biology. Sequencing, however, is not the answer to every interesting question in biology.

In arguing against the reductionist paradigm, I do not mean to imply that phenomena are immune to the laws of nature. Schrödinger (1944) addressed such apparent contradictions between laws of physics studied in comparative simple systems and behaviors of complex living systems and, in so doing, foreshadowed later breakthroughs in molecular biology (Dronamraju 1999). Without denying that emergent phenomena are ultimately explained by known (or knowable) physical laws, it remains that different disciplines may be the right "tools" to confront different questions. To fully understand genes, for example, we could address questions of interactions of atoms within molecules using physics, bonding among nucleic acids using chemistry, or the spread of a mutation in a species using population genetics. The lesson in this simple observation is that multiple disciplines are required to fully understand a complex system at all its levels of organization and that the number and combination of disciplines needed depend on the level at which a question is asked.

Nelson (2005) has drawn a parallel between views held by many paleontologists in the 1920s and those of contemporary molecular systematists. In each case, there is an unwarranted belief that their data source is so special that it reveals the truth of evolutionary history. In each case, that belief is wrong. Every interesting question in biology cannot be reduced to its molecular level. Evidence is growing that epigenetic factors are important in the expression of many complex features in humans and other species. And it is doubtful that we will ever be able to predict complex attributes such as a rhinoceros horn or a cycad inflorescence from sequence data alone. Even if we could, it is not clear that this would be an entirely desirable thing. There is great beauty, inspiration, and wonder to be gleaned from nature in its full grandeur and complexity. Sequencing devices have the potential of driving a technological wedge between biodiversity and its admirers that could ultimately reduce the public will to conserve species (Larson 2007).

Another stunning example of reductionist thinking in biology is so-called DNA barcoding. The idea is appealing. Sequence one short segment of one arbitrarily chosen gene, about 650 base pairs, and identify any species as easily as scanning the barcode on a carton of milk. Using molecular markers to identify species is a useful technique, of course, with both scientific and practical applications (Will et al. 2005). For example, there was an exposé that revealed restaurants serving fish to diners that were not the species advertised (Hotz 2009). As it turns out, this marker method only works at a high level of dependability when the "universe" of possible species is established and a library of known DNA sequences exists against which an unknown sequence may be compared (Little and Stevenson 2007). Unfortunately, 90 percent of the species on Earth remain unknown to science, and most of the 10 percent that are known (about two million species) have yet to be sequenced. To make matters worse, impressive progress in making species-testable theories about evolutionary history is tossed out by this so-called barcoding (Wheeler 2005). It simply uses average genetic distance values to arbitrarily say whether something is a species. Such simplistic ideas about distances mirroring evolutionary relationships were tried in the 1970s for anatomical data and failed spectacularly.

Truly understanding species is a far more complicated and interesting proposition. It involves comparisons of hundreds of characters across thousands of specimens collected from every population possible. It involves detailed studies of anatomy and turning to ontogeny (development) and molecular data when necessary to interpret those structures. Behavior yields another rich source of data.

Think about katydid songs, spider webs, or termite-nest architecture. Ecological interactions add another layer of interest: is a species a predator, herbivore, or detritivore? Biochemistry opens yet another avenue of information. Think of the toxins in a bee or jellyfish sting. Even if 650 base pairs could identify species, it would be a rather anemic view of biodiversity. Our curiosity about the world dictates not that we be able to identify and count its species but that we learn about them in intimate evolutionary detail. Biodiversity is also biocomplexity, and to know it, we must creatively draw upon a great many approaches and synthesize their inputs so as to begin to reveal the whole. Biologists, unfortunately, cling so tightly to their narrow specializations that many have not admitted that historical, nonexperimental fields even have a contribution to make (Wheeler 2004).

Toward the Postreductionist University

What will the university of the future look like? There is no single answer to that question, just as there is no single mission for the university. Those seeking to specialize in undergraduate liberal arts education or advanced technology, for example, may not look exactly like a comprehensive or Research 1 university, nor should they. Similarly, the university recruiting exclusively students in the top 5 percent of their graduating class will necessarily look different from one admitting students from the top 50 percent of their class. They must each define and attain success on their own terms. That said, there is a trend that seems destined to fundamentally shake up the long-established order of disciplines and departments in many, if not most, universities of tomorrow: *transdisciplinarity*. The idea of transdisciplinarity is far from new. The intersection of what we now think of as distinct disciplines in well-educated minds was a benchmark of the Renaissance. What is new, I suggest, is a heightened appreciation for and deliberate organizational steps to encourage transdisciplinarity in the American university following on the twentieth-century compartmentalization of discovery.

For me, transdisciplinarity can be thought of in two basic forms. First is the individual who learns to think beyond her own discipline in search of connections to, and solutions from, other disciplines. Many successful examples of thinking outside the box involve this kind of reach into other, often unexpected, fields for answers. Engineers and architects in Harare, Zimbabwe, for example, looked to entomology to save energy costs in a large office building. Australian termites that maintain near-constant temperatures within their nests while the temperatures outside swing widely were studied and emulated. The result? A building that uses passive air circulation to consume 90 percent less energy than most buildings its size (Atkinson 1995). Second is a team that is transdisciplinary, drawing its members from whichever and however many disciplines are appropriate to tackle a difficult, large, or complex challenge. A conspicuous twentieth-century example is the Manhattan Project that, from 1942 to 1945, assembled nuclear physicists, mathematicians, computer scientists, chemists, metallurgists, and others to make rapid progress in confronting an extraordinarily complex set of questions. The first requires an individual to know enough about other disciplines to at least retrieve and accurately interpret information from other fields. The information age has made this radical departure from single-discipline education increasingly feasible, as the scholar is educated to take advantage of powerful search engines and the vast quantity of information available in digital form and to assemble and synthesize diverse sources of information on demand to create integrated knowledge. This unprecedented open access to information and knowledge will enable neo-Renaissance scholars in the twenty-first century to attain unprecedented transdisciplinarity. The danger, of course, exists in what I call "undisciplined thinking." Scholars who are educated superficially in several disciplines may lack the deep, nuanced understanding of someone who has specialized in one discipline and has thereby mastered its history, aims, epistemology, and practices at the highest levels in her critical thinking. I have published conjectures about the history of my discipline that I believe explain some current issues in the field (Wheeler 2008), but to a scholar educated to specially think as a historian, my claims and methods would not begin to measure up as serious history. They are more akin to informed conjecture than proper historical analysis.

The advantage of a team approach to transdisciplinarity is that you need not sacrifice the deep knowledge and excellence that comes with specialization. Instead, you bring together all the experts needed to see a problem from all relevant angles and work together to find solutions. For such transdisciplinary teams to truly function well, we need to educate students to be comfortable and adept at talking across discipline boundaries, willing to pick up jargon, and tolerant of methods, assumptions, and traditions that are unfamiliar to them and that may, at first glance, seem to violate all that they use to judge the quality of work in their own field. Using my field as an example, taxonomy stands apart from nearly all other subdisciplines of biology in that it is comparative, descriptive, historical, and nonexperimental. Over a period of 250 years, taxonomy has developed a very rigorous epistemology such that its "descriptions" are today sets of explicit, testable theories and its work in character analysis, phylogenetics, classification, and species exploration are all hypothesis-driven (Nelson and Platnick 1981). All the same, many contemporary biologists see taxonomy as voodoo science only because it is nonexperimental. As a result, conservation biology, our understanding of ecosystems, and our responses to the biodiversity crisis all suffer because many ecologists, behaviorists, geneticists, and molecular biologists have never bothered to learn what epistemic assumptions make good taxonomy good and, thus, exclude a critical body of knowledge from their own work (Wheeler 2004).

Transhumanism is another paradigmatic example of a massively complex challenge. What does it mean to be human? How far can we go in genetic engineering and biomechanical enhancement before we have crossed a line we may not wish to cross? The film *Avatar* offers one scenario in fantasy fiction where our consciousness and emotions are intact even while leading a virtual physical existence through a high-tech surrogate body. The ultimate in cosmetic "surgery," such technology could enable me to look like Cary Grant while keeping all my own experiences and thoughts. (On second thought, I may reconsider my objections to the idea.) The implications, however, are so far-reaching that it is difficult to grasp the questions and complications, much less the "right" answers. Exploring transhumanism will require expertise from psychology, philosophy, religious studies, history, biology, and engineering, among other fields. As chapters in this volume attest, these are not hypothetical questions. The technology is heading at us fast, and the ethical, moral, and practical ramifications are coming just as rapidly.

We are information-rich beyond the conception of any previous generation. Most of that information, not to mention data, is never incorporated into knowledge (Ackoff 1989). The same can be said of our knowledge that, while advancing in leaps and bounds, seldom leads us to wisdom. Yet many challenges facing us, including transhumanism, call for wisdom. We have ample information that ecosystems are rapidly changing in response to climate and spreading human populations, knowledge that our welfare ultimately depends on ecological services, yet we lack the wisdom to assure that environments are sustainable. We have incontrovertible information that species are going extinct faster than we are discovering and describing them, we have knowledge that Earth is probably the only planet on which we can deeply explore evolutionary history, yet we lack the wisdom to complete a simple inventory of species to assure evidence of evolution is preserved for future generations.

Creativity Hybrid Zones

Transdisciplinary teams operate in creative intellectual spaces at the overlap of two or more disciplines. The advantage of working in such "creativity hybrid zones" is that the data, information, knowledge, and wisdom of well-established disciplines are brought together, compared, synthesized, integrated, and, most importantly, challenged, while being woven into creative new solutions. Because experts are assembled from disciplines, there is no dilution of the excellence or integrity of each participant's special contributions, yet its full potential is laid open to the aims of the team.

The idea of combining discovery and teaching in the university was a part of Thomas Jefferson's vision for founding the University of Virginia, and Johns Hopkins made a leap forward in the evolution of the research university in America (Cole 2009). Disciplines developed, in part, in response to society's need for solving problems, whether it was the rise of entomology in the agriculture colleges of Land-Grant universities in the nineteenth century or physics departments caught up in the theoretical and experiment possibilities unleashed by the Manhattan Project. I agree with Rhodes (2001) that the single most important word to describe the university is "community." The fragmentation of community is as much the problem as the divergent specialization of disciplines. If faculty and students interacted routinely across the disciplines, overcoming the current barriers to complex problem solving would be much easier.

The most innovative universities will escape the academic-unit provincialism that limits their creativity today. But in so doing, they will be confronted by countless problems that are the legacy of the well-worn traditional order. Competing for grants, receiving recognition for teamwork during promotion and tenure, and accumulating a *curriculum vitae* comprised in whole or part by coauthored papers are a few examples of the challenges facing faculty. Learning to communicate across majors, cultivating a genuine tolerance of and interest in "other" approaches, recognizing the value of seeing problems from diverse perspectives, and feeling comfortable as a member of a transdisciplinary learning community are among the challenges facing students.

In one possible idealized future university, we might see faculty in near-constant motion, organizing and reorganizing themselves as interests change, discoveries are made, problems are solved, and new issues present themselves. In the real world, the very real need to value and nurture social interactions and trust, occupy and manage specialized spaces like laboratories, educate students well grounded in the knowledge and principles of a discipline, and establish administrative structures to maintain some level of order and resource flow suggests that we may require departments and institutes, even if only ephemeral ones. This is one area where cyber-infrastructure and ever more life-like means of visual and auditory communication may help bridge the gap between optimal adaptation and chaos. It seems likely that some organizational structure more or less resembling academic units will remain but can be augmented by virtual teams (perhaps, more properly, teams working in cyberspace) and flexible common spaces where temporary teams can come together where physical collaboration is called for.

Not So Fast

The potential benefits of transdisciplinarity and of collaborative teams uniting the strengths of varied approaches seem plausible, if not inevitable. What, on the other hand, are dangers associated with such holistic approaches to problem solving? A few spring immediately to mind.

Undisciplined thinking. We have already mentioned the danger of too little specialization: that the very strengths we seek to tap into from diverse disciplines are lost in a homogenization of education and scholarship. This is a very real danger. Transdisciplinarity holds promise only in proportion to the excellence of disciplines that are represented in collaborative studies.

Dominant partner. Another possibility is that each discipline retains its identity and inherent strengths but is overshadowed by one dominant disciplinary partner in a team. Instances of disdain for "other" disciplines are commonplace on campus. Scientists in particular are guilty of dismissing the humanities or social sciences as too "soft." This intolerance was famously expressed by the Nobel Prize-winning atomic physicist Ernest Rutherford who said that all science is either physics or stamp collecting.

Education. No risk is higher than that of educating the next generation of practitioners of the disciplines. During a doctoral thesis is most often not the time to aim for the breadth of transdisciplinarity. In the few short years of such a study, it is impossible to truly master more than one or possibly two disciplines. What should be stressed now is a combination of educating young experts with the best of received knowledge, epistemology, and practice of the past with an attitude and the skills associated with being a good partner and team member. We are educating today the first generation of students many of whom will be expected to be collaborative rather than simply working in isolation or with like-trained colleagues. Because we are wisely moving toward transdisciplinary departments and schools, a much greater responsibility is vested in faculty. Just as in the university of the Middle Ages, where one or two faculty in any particular field carried the responsibility of assuring that students learned their discipline to its highest levels of excellence, so in the future a specialist embedded in a diverse unit will carry the burden to mentor and teach students to the same high levels as traditional departments.

Losing balance between basic and applied scholarship and research. Even with the hope that transdisciplinary teams will prove to be more than the sum of their experts, it will remain that solutions to problems will be constrained by the availability of fundamental studies. It is the basic, curiosity-driven discovery process that opens whole new possibilities for problem solving. Industry has a self-interest in solving problems of the here and now but very little incentive to support fundamental research. Even when fundamental work is successful, any practical applications for new knowledge may take decades or longer to be found. Only the university can recharge the well of possibilities. This is a unique challenge to the university to attain a balance between curiosity-driven studies and practical solutions obviously relevant to society.

Conclusion: Recombinant Innovation through Adaptation

One promising model for the research university of the future is a dynamic, adaptive, constantly reorganizing environment of learning and discovery. Faculty members will not expect to spend their entire career in one academic unit but rather to find themselves in various departments, schools, and research centers, as challenges and opportunities dictate. Over a lengthy career, however, a faculty member will accumulate a rich set of colleagues and associations such that it becomes ever easier to know where to turn for insights from diverse perspectives. All the while, this hypothetical professor of tomorrow is attracting and educating graduate students in her specialization while at the same time demonstrating by example how to be a reliable member of a diverse team.

Faculty and whole academic or research units will combine to tackle a major problem, dissolve their association after a suitable period of time, and then recombine to meet another challenge, and so forth, over and over again. Creative hybrid zones will thus be defined, dismissed, and defined. With each new creative hybrid zone will come new emergent possibilities for the future.

This trend also challenges the liberal arts. The traditional liberal arts remain as critically important as ever, but the well-educated man or woman of the twenty-first century will be expected to have mastered additional competencies such as those of technology and effective teamwork. The narrow and petty differences often seen among disciplines across the liberal arts and sciences must give way to the greater potential for respect, tolerance, and open-mindedness among the disciplines. The urgent need to confront truly complex challenges, from transhumanism to sustainable eco- and urban-systems, will be the catalyst that drives transdisciplinarity. If universities are wise, they will seize the opportunity to become more adaptive and flexible to create and benefit from creative hybrid zones only possible with the intellectual breath of such institutions.

References

Ackoff, Russell L. 1989. From data to wisdom. *Journal of Applied Systems Analysis* 16: 3-9.

Anderson, P. W. 1972. More is different. *Science* 177: 393-96.

Atkinson, Jon. 1995. Emulating the termite. *The Zimbabwean Review* 1: 16-19.

Cole, Jonathan R. 2009. *The Great American University*. New York: Public Affairs Books.

Crow, Michael M. 2007. None dare call it hubris: The limits of knowledge. *Issues in Science and Technology* 23, no. 2 (2007): 29-32.

Dronamraju, Krishna R. 1999. Erwin Schrödinger and the origins of molecular biology. *Genetics* 153: 1071-76.

Hotz, Robert L. 2009. DNA "barcodes" surface fishy imposters on menus. *Wall Street Journal*, Dec. 4: A20.

Larson, Brendon M. H. 2007. DNA barcoding: The social frontier. *Frontiers in Ecology and the Environment* 5: 437-42.

Levins, Richard, and Richard Lewontin. 1980. Dialectics and reductionism in ecology. *Synthese* 43: 47-78.

Little, Damon, and Dennis W. Stevenson. 2007. A comparison of algorithms for the identification of specimens using DNA barcodes: Examples from gymnosperms. *Cladistics* 23: 1-21.

Nelson, Gareth. 2005. Cladistics: Its arrested development. In *Milestones in Systematics*, edited by D. M. Williams and P. L. Forey, 127-47. London: CRC Press.

Nelson, Gareth, and Norman Platnick. 1981. *Systematics and Biogeography: Cladistics and Vicariance*. New York: Columbia University Press.

Rhodes, Frank H. T. 2001. *The Creation of the Future: The Role of the American University*. Ithaca: Cornell University Press.

Sarkar, Sahotra. 1992. Models of reduction and categories of reductionism. *Synthese* 91: 167-94.

Schrödinger, Erwin. 1944. *What Is Life? The Physical Aspect of the Living Cell*. Cambridge: Cambridge University Press.

Wheeler, Quentin D. 2004. Taxonomic triage and the poverty of phylogeny. *Philosophical Transactions of the Royal Society of London* B 359: 571-83.

–. 2005. Losing the plot: DNA "barcodes" and taxonomy. *Cladistics* 21: 405-7.

–. 2008. Introductory: Toward the new taxonomy. In *The New Taxonomy*, edited by Q. D. Wheeler, 1-17. London: CRC Press.

Will, Kip W., Brent D. Mishler, and Quentin D. Wheeler. 2005. The perils of DNA barcoding and the need for integrative taxonomy. *Systematic Biology* 54: 844-51.

New Perspectives on Transhumanism

Hava Tirosh-Samuelson and Kenneth L. Mossman

Transhumanism in Historical Perspective

Technology is transforming human life at a faster pace than ever before.[1] The convergence of nanotechnology, biotechnology, robotics, information and communication technology, and applied cognitive science poses a new situation in which the human has become a design project. The new technologies allow for new kinds of cognitive tools combining artificial intelligence with interface technology, molecular biology, and nanotechnology; genetic enhancing of human mental and physical capacities; combating diseases and slowing down the process of aging; and exercising control over desires, moods, and mental states. Due to genetic engineering, humans are now able not only to redesign themselves, presumably to get rid of various limitations, but also to redesign future generations, thereby affecting the evolutionary process itself. As a result a new, *posthuman* phase in the evolution of the human species will emerge in which humans will live longer, will possess new physical and cognitive abilities, and will be liberated from suffering and pain due to aging and diseases. In the post-human age, humans will no longer be controlled by nature; instead, they will be the controllers of nature. Those who welcome the vision of the posthuman phase are known as *transhumanists*.

A full history of the concept of posthumanism and the transhumanist movement is still a desideratum notwithstanding a few attempts (Bostrom 2005; Miah 2008), and the following comments are only a rough sketch necessary to contextualize the subject of this volume. The term *transhumanism* was coined in 1957 by Julian Huxley (1887–1975), the grandson of the Victorian Darwinian Thomas Henry Huxley. For Julian Huxley, *transhumanism* was another word for what he named "evolutionary humanism," namely, the deliberate effort by humankind to "transcend itself – not just sporadically … but in its entirety, as humanity. … Man remaining man, but transcending himself, by realizing new possibilities of and for his human nature" (Huxley 1957, 17). Huxley's views were quite similar to the ideas of the psychologist Abraham Maslow, the leader of the Human Potential Movement, who coined the word *metahuman* to discuss how the self-actualizing person will be able "to go beyond the merely human" and become divine or godlike (Maslow 1971, 274).

1 A version of this section appeared in Tirosh-Samuelson (2011, 15–29).

Julian Huxley was a close friend of John Burdon Sanderson Haldane (1892-1964) and John Desmond Bernal (1901-1971) who, during the 1920s, advocated many views that would become standard features of contemporary transhumanism: the belief in the ongoing progressive evolution of the human species; the advocacy of genetic engineering (then known as *eugenics*) for the betterment of the human condition; the replacement of religion by science as the arbiter of truth; the expansion of human cognitive capacity by means of human intervention; and the unbound faith in the ability of science and technology to manufacture a perfect future. This ambitious program for the betterment of humanity, however, suffered a deep set back because of the Nazis's pernicious use of eugenics and the horrors of World War II. The goal of creating a new and better world through a centrally imposed vision was invalidated, and the eugenics movement of the 1920s was discredited. The transhumanist impulse received a certain boost during the 1940s, especially in England, when cybernetics was developed by mathematicians and pioneering computer scientists who illustrated how cognition is possible without a subject, while problematizing the notion that the brain is an organ of representation (Pickering 1995; Mindell 2002; Husband, Holland, and Wheeler 2008). The ideal of enhancing humanity was restated due to these technological developments.

In the 1960s, new optimistic futuristic scenarios about humanity were articulated by science-fiction writers such as Arthur C. Clarke, Isaac Asimov, Robert Heinlein, Stanislaw Lem, and later Bruce Sterling, Greg Egan, and Vernor Vinge, who speculated about the new, transhuman future (Hayles 1999; Dinello 2002). From the late 1960s on, the futurist Fereidoun M. Esfandiary, who later changed his name to FM 2030 (the year denoting the date of his hundredth birthday) began to identify "transhumans" as persons who behave in a manner conducive to a posthuman future. At that time, various organizations began to advocate life extension, cryonics, space colonization, and other scenarios, while advances in biotechnology, neuroscience, and nanotechnology began to make their mark (Bostrom 2003). Marvin Minsky (1986, 2006), an eminent artificial-intelligence researcher, articulated many of the themes of the transhumanist vision, and he was joined by other famous scientific visionaries and technoutopians such as Ray Kurzweil (1990, 1999, 2005), Eric K. Drexler (1986, 1992; Drexler and Peterson 1991), Frank J. Tipler (1994, 2007), and Hans Moravec (1988, 1999). These technoenthusiasts have offered an apocalyptic view in which a rupture, referred to as "The Singularity," will bring an end to human existence, ushering instead an autonomous, artificially intelligent species that will be in competition with humanity. The new species of *Robo-sapiens* will supersede *Homo sapiens* as the next phase of evolution.

In 1999, Hans Moravec, a former director of the Mobile Robot Laboratory at Carnegie-Mellon University and developer of advanced robots for the military and NASA, predicted that "before the next century is over, human beings will no longer be the most intelligent or capable type of entity on the planet" (13). Due to the continued exponential growth of artificial intelligence, mind machines will become the next evolutionary step, with organic humans left behind. Moravec predicts that humans would pass their minds into artificially intelligent robots, their mechanical progeny. Moravec (1999, 127-62) imagines when and how the process will take place. In "the short run (early 2000s)," there will be profound changes in the way we organize labor, wealth, and government. In the "medium run (around 2050)," the transformation will be even more profound when "machines capable of policy-making, public relations, law, engineering, and research will replace telecommuters" (ibid., 137), transforming all aspects of human life as well as human values. Transhumanism belongs to this middle range, and it is presented as a "good compromise" to the inevitable confrontation between machines and biological humans. If indeed humans "make themselves healthier, more beautiful, stronger, more intelligent, and longer lived" (ibid., 143) then the inevitable conflict could perhaps be thwarted. For the "long term (2100 and beyond)," Moravec offers a much more fantastic scenario in which enhanced humans will leave Earth behind and move into outer space where they will be eventually replaced by postbiological "Exes." In this narrative, transhumanism is no more than a middle-range compromise to an inevitable process in which robots will replace humans.

In the 1980s, philosopher Max More (whose given name was Max O'Conner) formalized a transhumanist doctrine, advocating the "Principles of Extropy" for continuously improving the human condition.[2] According to More, humans are but a "transitional stage standing between our animal heritage and our posthuman future," which will be reached through "genetic engineering, life-extending biosciences, intelligence intensifiers, smarter interfaces to swifter computers, neural-computer integration, world-wide data networks, virtual reality, intelligent agents, swift electronic communication, artificial intelligence, neuroscience, neural networks, artificial life, off-planet migration, and molecular nanotechnology" (More 2004). For More and other technoenthusiasts (Silver 2002 [1997]; Stock 1993, 2000, 2002; Clark 2003; Bailey 2005), genetic engineering, cloning, and eugenics will reconfigure select humans into a superior transhuman species and then, using robotics, bionics, and nanotechnology, will invent a new posthuman

2 The term *extropy* was coined by Max More as a substitute for the more technical term *negentropy*, to denote negative entropy. Another spelling of More's neologism is *exotropy*, which Kevin Kelly defines as "the absence of the absence of order" or "the reversal of disorder" (2010, 63).

species no longer dependent on nature. Humans will, thus, transform themselves into posthumans, namely, "persons of unprecedented physical, intellectual and psychological capacity, self-programming, potentially immortal, unlimited individuals" (More 2004).

In the late 1990s, a group of transhumanist activists authored the "Transhumanist Declaration," stating various ethical positions related to the use of and planning for technological advances (Bostrom 2003). In 1998, the World Transhumanist Association (WTA) was founded by philosophers Nick Bostrom and David Pearce; its membership today is about five thousand people worldwide with several geographically divided chapters and special-interest affiliates. Other contemporary organizations also play a role in the transhumanist movement – for example, the Extropy Institute, the Foresight Institute, the Immortality Institute, the Institute for Ethics and Emerging Technologies, and the Singularity Institute for Artificial Intelligence, all of which take part in the emergence of a new academic discipline: Future Studies (Pessig 2008). These organizations and many others were greatly helped by the communication revolution of the 1980s and 1990s with instant communication worldwide. Indeed, cyberspace is not just a means to disseminate transhumanist ideas but part and parcel of the transhumanist eschatological and utopian vision.

Transhumanism, however, is not merely a utopian vision by techno-optimists; rather, the program receives a substantial amount of funding and scientific legitimacy from the National Science Foundation by people such as Mihail C. Roco and William Sims Bainbridge who promote the transhumanist vision under the banner of "converging technologies" (Roco and Bainbridge 2002). Futuristic ideas about human physical and cognitive enhancements through human-machine fusion have been of special interest to the Defense Advanced Research Projects Agency (DARPA) that has been "working on changing what it means to be human," as Joel Garreau (2004, 42) succinctly put it. The technoenthusiasts who promote transhumanism have considerable control over the decision of how to spend national financial resources, one reason that they are upset by critics of transhumanism who challenge these decisions, calling them derogatorily "bio-Luddites" or "bio-Conservatives" (J. Hughes, 2004, 2011; Agar 2007). The conflict between transhumanists and their critics is not just between two temperaments of technoenthusiasts and technophobes, but a conflict about how to use scarce resources to bring about a certain vision for and of humanity (Hansell and Grassie 2011).

By the first decade of the twenty-first century, established religions too have begun to engage transhumanism more seriously, as scholars began to note that the transhumanist vision of heaven on earth followed by posthuman immortality has a strong religious dimension, even though transhumanist leaders despise traditional religions or religious institutions (Noble 1997). Indeed for the technological visionary Eric K. Drexler, technology itself is divine, and scientists have godlike power to structure matter and recreate nature. Whereas some Christian theologians have been very critical of transhumanism (Waters 2006), others have been more willing to accept certain aspects of the transhumanist project for which they proceed to give theological justification (Hefner 2003; Peters 1996, 1997, 2003). The Lutheran theologian Philip Hefner offers a very useful clarification about transhumanism when he distinguishes between "upper-case Transhumanism" and "lower-case transhumanism" (Hefner 2009). The former concerns what he considers the fantastic and rather dubious scenarios about the radical transformation of the human species, whereas the latter denotes the more ubiquitous and ambiguous use of biotechnology in everyday life. The latter is based on the belief that "it is natural and good to enhance human mental and physical abilities, and ameliorate undesirable aspects of the human condition" as well as the claim that "we need not accept as our destiny the human nature ... with which we grew in our mother's womb" (ibid., 166). In 2008, the American Academy of Religion accorded formal status to deliberations about transhumanism, even though transhumanism does not define itself as a religion (Maher and Mercer 2009). At least one established religion – The Church of Jesus Christ of Latter-day Saints – not only endorses transhumanism but has its own transhumanist variant. In 2006, the World Transhumanist Association voted to recognize the Mormon Transhumanist Association as its first religious special-interest affiliate.

While the vision of the posthuman ideal state of affairs is generally clear, the precise meaning of the term *transhuman* is somewhat vague. For some, the term is short for "transitional human," a phase in human evolution from the ordinary human today to the posthuman of the remote future. Thus, the "transhuman" is a more evolved being than an ordinary human due to the use of genetic engineering, psychopharmacology, antiaging therapies, neural interfaces, advanced information-management tools, memory-enhancing drugs, wearable computers and cognitive techniques. Since the "transhuman" is an enhanced human, the advocates of transhumanism like to refer to their vision of humanity as *H+* (that is, enhanced humanity). For others, the "transhuman" does not denote a technologically enhanced person but an ordinary person who supports activities that promote the eventual evolvement of the posthuman. Echoing Julian Huxley, Nick Bostrom, the leading philosopher of transhumanism, defines *transhumanism* as follows: "a *way of thinking* about the future that is based on the premise that the human species in its current form does not represent the end of our development but rather a comparatively early phase" (Bostrom 2003). In this definition, to be a transhumanist one does not have to be physically enhanced by new biotechnologies but only share the outlook that affirms the possibility and desirability of fundamentally improving the human condition through the use of converging technologies.

Transhumanism is yet to generate systematic philosophy, although a few attempts in this direction do exist. Simon Young (2005) presents transhumanism as a unification of science and ethics and positions it as an alternative to academic postmodernism, religious theism, and radical environmentalism. Against postmodernists of the academic Left, Young presents transhumanism as a critique of cognitive skepticism, social constructivism, and cultural relativism. Objective reality does exist and is independent of human perception, cognition, and apprehension; science generates knowledge about objective reality, namely, accurate and true descriptions of reality outside the human mind that provide humans with specific courses of action, including those that change objective reality. The facts about the human condition are indeed real and painful but need not be definitive. Biology is *not* destiny because the evolutionary process has given rise to the complex human brain that now enables humans to intervene in the evolutionary process and replace it with "designer evolution," or "controlled evolution." Young argues that human consciousness is an "inevitable product of the evolutionary process" (Young 2005, 212) and the predictable outcome of "evolutionary complexification" (ibid., 209). Therefore, human beings not only can intervene and alter the biological facts through designer genes, designer drugs, and a whole range of enhancement technologies, but humans should do so to improve the human species.

A different philosophical presentation of transhumanism is articulated by Robert Pepperell (2003) who defines the "posthuman condition" as an "end of 'man-centered' universe," an "energetic theory of mind in which human thought, meaning and memory is understood in terms of the activity of an energy regulating system" (Pepperell 2003, 100). For Pepperell, transhumanism means the end of humanism, namely, the "long-held belief in the infallibility of human power and the arrogant belief in our superiority and uniqueness" (ibid., 171). Although he concedes that this belief will continue to exist well into the future, he predicts that humanism will eventually collapse because of its inherent moral weakness, as noted by feminism, the animal-rights movement, and the antislavery movement. While transhumanism moves beyond the limitation of humanism, its evolutionary perspective is "not limited to genetics, but includes all the paraphernalia of cultural and technological existence" (ibid., 152). In the posthuman future, humans will acquire machine-like enhancements and will be able to exist more effectively by recognizing "that none of us are actually distinct from each other, or the world" and that "to harm anything is to harm oneself." Pepperell's exposition of the posthuman condition sees the biomechanical technologies that blur the distinction between humans and machines as the core of the posthuman age and its philosophical implications. Whereas "humanists saw themselves as distinct beings in an antagonistic relationship with their surroundings, posthumans regard their own being as embodied in an extended technological world" (ibid.).

Pepperell's postmodern critique of humanism is shared by other so-called cultural posthumanists such as Neil Badmington (2000, 2003), Elaine L. Graham (2002), Cary Wolfe (2010), and Andy Miah (2008), who reflect on the interplay between scientific theorizing and cultural imagination against the background of several postmodern discourses. These cultural critics do not agree on the meaning of *humanism* or *transhumanism*. Whereas for some, *humanism* means the promulgation of secularism and scientific rationality, for others, the term denotes a reactionary notion that "appeals (positively) to the notion of a core humanity or a common essential feature in terms of which human beings can be defined and understood" (Soper 1987, 11-12). This notion of humanity has been under severe assault at least since the mid-nineteenth century with the critiques of Karl Marx, Sigmund Freud, and Friedrich Nietzsche and the postmodernist philosophers Jean-François Lyotard, Jacques Derrida, Michel Foucault, Roland Barthes, and Jean Baudrillard, among others. As a result, in the second half of the twentieth century in literature, cinema, politics, anthropology, feminist discourse, and technology studies, the reign of universal human has been called into question and dismantled philosophically. Searching for a new vision of humanity, the theorist Donna Haraway has issued the "Cyborg Manifesto" as a postgender, posthumanist, postmodern, postfamilial, and postnatural reality, blurring traditional distinctions between humans and animals and between humans and machines (Haraway 1991; Cf. Dinello 2002, 115, 118). Philosophical reflection about the "posthuman condition" thus takes place among literary critics, especially those who study the genre of science fiction in film, literature, television, and computer games, since science fiction serves as social criticism and popular philosophy.

The above overview of transhumanism indicates that it is not easy to engage the subject. Transhumanists do not speak in one voice, and the movement expresses a variety of impulses, which are often at odds with each other. Nonetheless, several themes are common to transhumanist discourse: the view of evolving human nature, the focus on biotechnological enhancement that will exceed ordinary human physical and cognitive traits, a preoccupation with human happiness that can be perpetuated indefinitely, a deep concern for longevity and radical life extension, and a technoutopia of human-machine fusion that constitutes practical immortality. Each of these themes has generated considerable debates, as indicated by the essays in this volume. This anthology takes transhumanism seriously not because it is a significant social movement, which it is not, but because the transhumanist vision compels us to think about ourselves in light of current technological and scientific advances and to reflect on the society in which we wish to live. The essays in the volume are largely critical of various aspects of transhumanism, while admitting that biotechnology is an important social force that will continue to transform our lives. The goal of this volume is to inspire conversation and debate about changes envisioned by advocates of transhumanism so that we will at least be aware of what is at stake in the processes ahead.

Transhumanism and World Religions

The desire to improve humanity has characterized the religious impulse of humanity: all world religions call on humans to be "better" in light of some ideal dictated by a certain conception of God. Transhumanism defines itself as a secular movement, and its main spokespersons are often associated with the current rise of atheistic critique of religions. Yet, the transhumanist obsession with improvement of humanity by means of technology cannot be fully understood unless one appreciates how transhumanism secularizes age-old human pursuits of perfection, characteristic of all world religions. Part I of this volume engages transhumanism from the perspectives of Western monotheistic religions, especially Protestantism, Orthodox Christianity, Judaism, and Islam. In so doing, the essays of Part I expose the utopian spirit of transhumanism, while highlighting the poverty of the transhumanist imagination. Whereas in traditional religions human improvement or perfection is couched in ethical and spiritual terms, is rooted in education and the cultivation of virtues, and requires some interaction with God (Tirosh-Samuelson 2003, 2010), transhumanism defines the betterment of humanity primarily in material terms as improvement of the capacities of the human body. Even when transhumanism speaks about cognitive improvement, it is the brain rather than the mind that is subject for improvement. But in what sense do these improvements make humans "better"? The essays in this section explore how diverse religious traditions can enter a critical conversation with transhumanism.

In chapter 1, Hava Tirosh-Samuelson discusses the three "prophets" of transhumanism in England during the 1920s – Julian Huxley, J.B.S. Haldane, and J.D. Bernal. By looking at the development of their thought, their personal relations, and their most relevant writings, this chapter sheds light on the origins of transhumanist thought and explores what contemporary transhumanists owe to these thinkers and where they differ. Since the visionaries of transhumanism were either members of the Communist Party of Great Britain or sympathetic to it, their vision for the betterment of humanity concerned the material conditions of humanity and depended on the involvement of the state in the engineering of the human. Contemporary transhumanists tend to be libertarians who endorse capitalism and the free market, and they rely on funding from private corporations to implement their vision. Tirosh-Samuelson argues that most of the themes of transhumanism were fully in place in the 1920s so that contemporary transhumanism is less innovative than it may appear. As an ideology of "extreme progress," transhumanism attempts to give coherence to the rapid scientific and technological advances of the past half century.

In chapter 2, Linell E. Cady seeks to get "a handle on the perils and possibilities of transhumanism" by positioning it "within the religious/secular framework that now deeply structures our imaginative and social worlds." Examining closely the work of two leading transhumanists – Nick Bostrom and William Sims Bainbridge – from the perspective of two leading theorists of religion, Mark C. Taylor and Charles Taylor, Cady reflects upon the broader narrative framework within which the transhumanist ideology and movement are located. Cady's analysis highlights the extent to which transhumanism extends in a secularized idiom a form of transcendent religiosity that has deep roots within the Western tradition. In other words, the transhumanist impulse should be seen as a secularization of Christian sensibilities and spiritual paradigms, especially the utopian impulse of Christianity.

Utopian thinking, of course, began in Judaism and can be traced to the preaching of biblical prophets. Engaging transhumanism from a Jewish perspective is intriguing because Judaism (at least in part) defines membership in the religious tradition in biological terms and highlights embodiment in Jewish self-definition. In the premodern world, the inherently embodied nature of Jews was used by Christian theologians to justify marginalization and exclusion from Western society, and in the modern period, the supposed deficient body of Jews was used by anti-Semites as an evidence of Jewish inherent inferiority that legitimized their total annihilation. The primary response to modern anti-Semitism was Zionism, the Jewish nationalist movement that made the physical improvement of the Jewish body by means of science its major goal. Zionism endorsed the use of eugenics and implemented many policies to enhance the health of Jewish bodies. But positive attitudes toward enhancement technologies can be found not only among Zionist activists but also many Jewish legal thinkers, bioethicists, and theologians across the spectrum of modern Judaism. In chapter 3, Norbert Samuelson and Hava Tirosh-Samuelson examine Jewish religious and secular discourses on human betterment through genetic enhancement and attempt to explain the probiotechnological stance of Jews. Instead of concluding that Judaism is particularly amenable to the transhumanist project, they move on to explore three leading Jewish thinkers in the twentieth century who reflected on the utopian project: Mordecai Kaplan (1881-1983), Martin Buber (1878-1965), and Franz Rosenzweig (1886-1929). By explaining their understanding of utopia, the chapter offers a critical vantage point from which to examine transhumanism.

A similar critique of transhumanism is offered in chapter 4 by Farzad Mahootian who examines the futuristic scenarios of transhumanism from the perspective of Sufism as articulated by the Persian Sufi Shahabuddin Yahya Suhrawardi (1155-1191) and explicated by Henry Corbin (1903-1978). Focusing on the idea of "perfect human nature" and its cognates in Iranian Sufism, this chapter explains the role of the imagination in the Sufi pursuit of perfection and how symbolism functioned in Sufi metaphysics. Transhumanist claims that there is no supernatural spirit, that the mind is a product of the brain, and that machines with self-aware intelligence are possible appear particularly thin when compared with the Sufi imagination in which the pursuit of perfection is an effort of "the archetypal imagination, not that of dogged replication of historical acts and events." In light of Sufism, the transhumanist obsession with endless "progress" through biological enhancement appears particularly wrongheaded.

The poverty of the transhumanist imagination becomes even clearer when it is studied in comparison to Orthodox Christianity. So far, Anglo-American transhumanists have dismissed their Christian critics, presenting them as opponents of progress. In sharp contrast, the Russian Transhumanist Movement founded in 2003 adopted the teachings of Nikolai Fedorovich Fedorov (1829-1903) as its inspiration. In chapter 5, Eugene Clay examines the teachings of Fedorov on the destiny to humanity and Fedorov's indebtedness to the brilliant theologian Maximos the Confessor (580-662). On the basis of Maximos's ideas about human participation in cosmic redemption, Fedorov "contended that all humanity should unite in the common cause of raising the dead and regulating the universe through scientific means." Seeking to spark a constructive conversation between transhumanism and the Orthodox theological tradition, this chapter presents Orthodox understanding of human nature, spiritual development, and human destiny that could enrich the discussion of the future of the human species.

The essays of Part I reflect the discipline of religious studies that came into its own only in the second half of the twentieth century. Originally the discipline was known as "History of Religions," founded by Mircea Eliade (1907-1986), a Romanian-born, prolific author of scholarly books on religion and editor of the *Encyclopedia of Religion.* In chapter 6, Steven M. Wasserstrom exposes the transhumanist commitment of Mircea Eliade, a topic to which no attention has been given so far. In his journals, fiction, and scholarship, Eliade expressed a vision of "ideal humanity, a humankind that transcends itself by following an *avant garde* of the few, the brave, the adepts." Eliade articulated his transhumanist ideas already in 1940 in his novella *The Secret of Dr. Honigberger* and continued to nourish these ideas in private correspondence during the World War II years. In 1960, he gave full expression to his technosophic transhumanism in *Morning of the Magicians*, which would serve as the basis of his 1978 novella *Youth without Youth*. By highlighting the intellectual sources of Eliade's transhumanism – European *Naturphilosophie*, fantastic literature, Western occultism, and Eastern Yoga – Wasserstrom exposes the disturbing aspects of Eliade's vision, a person who had close ties to Fascist circles in his native Romania.

Together the essays of Part I show that, although transhumanism treats the traditionally religious with disdain, the transhumanist pursuit of perfection is a secular variant of traditional religious themes and that several world traditions offer much deeper engagements with the core issues of transhumanism: the reflection on the meaning of being human, the dream about transcending human biological limits, and the faith in science and technology to perfect the world. The essays of Part I also make clear that a proper engagement with transhumanism must not be framed simply within the discourse of bioethics, as has been the case so far (for example, Gordijn and Chadwick 2008; Bostrom and Savulescu 2009; Savulescu et al. 2009), but that it must take into consideration the humanities, especially history, religious studies, and philosophy. By looking at transhumanism from these perspectives, we gain a deeper appreciation of what is at stake in the biotechnological revolution.

Transhumanism and Medical Enhancement

Whereas the essays in Part I offer historical and cultural perspectives on transhumanism, the essays in Part II engage the more familiar debate about biotechnological "enhancement." Humans have always enhanced themselves through technological inventions in their attempt to master their physical environment. In so doing, they have also transformed every aspect of human life and shaped human culture. Thus, technologies as diverse as agriculture, writing, calculus, antibiotics, and computers have all transformed human life and have definitely "enhanced" humans, but it is important to be aware of the qualitative difference between contemporary biomedical technologies and earlier technologies. Today, humans are able not only to interfere with and transform their biological makeup but also to engineer future generations. Whether we call the process "directed evolution," "enhancement evolution," or "designer evolution," the goal is to replace chance with choice (Buchanan et al. 2000).

The proponents of biotechnological enhancement consider it a good that will improve human physical and mental capacities, extend life, and in general improve the quality of human life. Through genetic engineering, humans will eliminate deleterious genes that cause disease, pain, and suffering and will even try to postpone the ultimate threat to human life – death. The philosopher John Harris, who does not consider himself a "transhumanist" since for him transhumanism is "a program and an identity" (Harris 2007, 38-39), has articulated the most sustained philosophical arguments in favor of enhancement (1992, 2007). Similarly, Nicholas Agar (2004) has attempted to defend what he calls "liberal eugenics" (in contrast to the "authoritarian eugenics" of the Nazis) because it expands the liberal ideals of freedom, choice, and diversity. Conversely, the ameliorist agenda has had many critics including Francis Fukuyama (2002), Leon Kass (2002), Erik Parens (1998, 2006), Bill McKibben (2003), Jean Betke Elshtain (Baily and Casey 2005; Mitchell et al. 2007), and Michael Sandel (2007), to mention just a few. For over two decades the debates about enhancement have considered diverse issues such as the meaning of human nature, fairness in sports, equality in education, social justice, sex selection, cosmetics and antiaging, the institution of the family, reproductive liberty, abortion, disability, stem-cell research, human cloning, organ replacement, child welfare, and human mortality. Needless to say, no consensus has been reached on any of these issues, but the intensity of the debate indicates how important it is to reflect on the social, political, legal, and cultural implications of biotechnology.

The essays in Part II do not review the extensive literature on these topics but consider a few specific questions that have been raised by the on-going debates. Expanding the scope of the relevant disciplines, these essays consider the disciplines of history, sociology, and evolutionary psychology, as well as law and medicine. The essays offer a critical and somewhat disturbing view of genetic engineering and its social implications, while agreeing that biotechnology is here to stay and that it will be difficult, if not impossible, either to control it or regulate its use.

In chapter 7 Brian Gratton highlights the continuity of transhumanism with the eugenics movement of the 1920s by looking at the question of race and ethnicity in light of evolutionary theory and evolutionary psychology. Gratton argues that neither branch of evolutionary science provides much room for optimism for transhumanism. Evolutionary psychology implies a deep branding of human nature at odds with the movement's desire to transform it; should evolutionary biology sustain deep racial and ethnic differences, the eugenics wing of the movement will become strengthened. Gratton thus highlights the nexus between transhumanist thought and the eugenics movement that saw race as a fundamental, differentiating characteristic of human beings. He challenges the proponents of transhumanism to consider how much their agenda contributes to racial prejudices, notwithstanding their protestation to the contrary.

Much of the debate about enhancement technologies revolves around the difference between "enhancement" and "therapy" (Juengst 1998; Frankford 1998). Unlike Eric Juengst, who has analyzed enhancement as a "boundary concept …

that plays both descriptive and normative role" (Juengst 1998, 30), Kenneth L. Mossman engages this question from the perspective of the history of medicine, namely, how enhancement technologies become established in society, showing that almost all enhancements emerged from medical interventions for disease therapy. In chapter 8, Mossman argues that the transition of medical interventions from the medical to the public arena is linked to how well "disease" can be distinguished from "normal." He raises fundamental questions about the meaning of *disease*, the parameters of normal variations in human anatomy and performance, and the safety and efficacy of enhancement technologies. He suggests that, because the concepts of therapy and enhancement are difficult to separate, the justification and acceptability of enhancement cannot be easily uncoupled from concepts of health and therapy.

It is reasonable to assume that biotechnology will continue to shape many aspects of human life, as humans will seek to enhance themselves in terms of physical performance, appearance, cognition, mood and creative abilities, military effectiveness, reproduction, and life expectancy (Mehlman 2009, 6-34). What should be our social response to the preoccupation with enhancement technologies? In chapter 9, Gary E. Marchant and Alexandra López explore the question of whether we can stop human enhancement even if we wanted to and examine the feasibility of using law to restrict the availability and use of human-enhancement technologies. Analyzing the limitation of legal control, Marchant and López conclude that law will only be effective in blocking enhancement technologies that are either unsafe or ineffective. Ironically, by ensuring the safety and effectiveness of enhancement technologies, legal regulation will have the (unintended) effect of assisting and accelerating the widespread use of enhancement technologies.

Transhumanism and the Human Person

Biomedical innovations have expanded human ability to intervene in the evolutionary process itself in an attempt to select desirable traits. These interventions include not only the selection and enhancement of certain physical traits but also the modification and enhancement of mental and cognitive capacities. Today, a growing arsenal of interventionist techniques for modification and control of the brain is now available, many of which raise a host of ethical, legal, and policy issues (Blank 1999). Because of advances in neuroscience the possibility for enhancement of human capacities has risen to new levels. IQ, memory, cognitive performance, and intelligence are all enhanced by means of medications, drugs, or Transcranial Magnetic Stimulation (TMS), and future technologies will include conversion of stem cells in specific areas of the brain where enhancement of particular traits can be achieved or even transplantation of stem cells from external sources. Gene therapy, in which "DNA that is known to be associated with specific learning could be introduced into brain cells to modify and enhance a person's ability to perform a specific function" (Tancredi 2004, 102), will undoubtedly extend the human capacity to modify and control the brain and will accelerate attempts to find genetic bases of mental and behavioral traits.

Enhancement of human mental and cognitive capacities is one of central features of transhumanism that calls us not only to understand how the brain works or how to improve its capabilities but also "to reverse engineer the human brain, and essentially copy its design" (Kurzweil 2002, 32). The essays in Part III reflect on various philosophical issues raised by the new brain sciences that undergird much of the optimism of transhumanism in regard to cognitive enhancement. Again, the essays do not represent a single critique of transhumanism, but they challenge the dualism of mind and body characteristic of transhumanist discourse.

In chapter 10, Steven A. Hoffman considers the aspect of transhumanism that focuses on nanotechnology, biotechnology (including genetic engineering), neurocognitive technologies, and artificial intelligence to enhance human attributes, leading to the presumed emergence of the posthuman. Hoffman argues that the transhumanist approach does not do justice to the full spectrum of human capacities. In response to transhumanism, Hoffman suggests that the emerging field of immunoneuropsychology (INP) shows a new approach to integrate the physiological, mental, emotional, and social dimensions of being human, thereby overcoming the materialism presupposed by transhumanist literature. He illustrates the holistic understanding of the human in regard to the concept of human happiness and the concept of the Self and concludes that, even though improvement of humanity is a laudable goal, biotechnology alone cannot accomplish the betterment of humanity.

Another attempt to offer a holistic approach to human beings is illustrated in chapter 11, which focuses on the nature of personhood and the related concept of identity. Combining psychology and gender studies, Craig Nagoshi and Julie Nagoshi critique the Cartesian dualism that undergirds the proposal to upload human minds into artificially intelligent machines. This approach assumes a mind-body dualism in which the body is merely an imperfect, burdensome machine to be tinkered with by a separate, personal, free-willed consciousness. In contrast, the Nagoshis argue that the experience of being conscious and having free will is the essence of being human and that personhood is inextricably linked with the experience of the body on its journey throughout life. Personhood is inseparable both from lived experience, as well as from the interpretation and narration of the experience. They illustrate their nondualistic understanding of the human self by looking at the experience of suffering in medical treatment and considering the identity of individuals who are bi- or transsexual or who have had sex-reassignment surgery. Their analysis of ambiguous and ambivalent narratives makes clear that the transhumanist understanding of the human Self is much too simplistic and superficial, similar to Hoffman's critique.

The decision to undergo sex change is the ultimate example of human free will, which, in turn, raises the issue of human responsibility. In chapter 12, Michael J. White considers transhumanism in the context of Western philosophical reflections on the freedom of the will and the concept of responsibility, analyzing the history of the problem of responsibility and determinism that has been focused on what constitutes *force majeure*. In discussing responsibility, White offers two principal claims. First, our conception of persons' responsibility depends on the assumption of normalcy with respect to human nature. Were enhancements to provide sufficient grounds for substantial alteration of certain of these assumptions about normalcy, then it is likely our current norms of responsibility attribution would fail to apply to persons whose natures thus "diverge from the norm." Second, it seems likely that there will arise novel legal issues of responsibility in connection with prenatal enhancements that turn out to be unwanted by those who receive them. White reviews some recent discussions of conceptual problems that could arise with tort actions for "diminishments," discussions that connect such action with "wrongful-life" suits.

Human free will has been a major area in which the new brain sciences have interacted with philosophy. Walter Glannon, who has written extensively on the topic (2002, 2007), ponders the following questions: Do brain interventions and other neural transitions from human to posthuman threaten free will? Can free will be lost in becoming posthuman? In the last chapter of Part III, Glannon carefully argues that free will is not an illusion born out of the mechanistic view of brain and mind. He claims that neuroscience does not undermine free will, since there is little convincing evidence that to show that deterministic or mechanistic neural processes completely explain human behavior. In Glannon's view, any satisfactory account of human agency must include both unconscious physical and conscious mental states and events as causes of our actions because the brain generates and sustains the mind and reciprocally the mind can influence the brain. After examining the possibility that future advances in neuroscience may lead to a radical revision of the notion of free will and interpretation of the Self, Glannon concludes that, at present, neuroscience arguments against free will do not support the claim that we are evolving from a human to a transhuman world.

Transhumanism as a Futuristic Vision: The Interplay of Technology and Culture

As a futuristic vision, transhumanism is rooted in the assumption that science and technology will enable humanity to transcend biological and physical limitations, be it stupidity, disease, pain, aging, or death. The transhumanist trust in technology has to be assessed in its proper cultural context, acknowledging the degree to which contemporary culture "seeks its authorization in technology, finds satisfaction in technology, and takes its order from technology" (Postman [1993] 1992, 71). *Technology*, of course, is an ambiguous term that covers all forms of human creativity and ingenuity and is closely related to a wide range of productive activities (T. Hughes 2004). The new disciplines of science studies and technology studies have shown the degree to which technology permeates or inheres in all human practices and ideologies and that the technological is not easily distinguished from "the human" (Aronowitz 1996). Technologies are always mixed with science, nature, and culture; they shape how humans function; and they affect human experience in ways that go beyond any specific function. This insight applies to transhumanism as well: we can understand how technology functions in the transhumanist vision only if we consider it in its proper cultural context. The essays in Part IV critically engage various aspects of transhumanism's celebration of technology and challenge some of the optimistic futuristic scenarios.

In chapter 14, Barry G. Ritchie considers the most expansive technical goal of the transhumanist project: the attainment of an unlimited lifespan. The repair, replacement, and rejuvenation of many components of the body are already at hand, and medical advances will expand the realm of components for which repair and replacement are feasible. Ritchie argues that the real target for the immortality goal necessarily must lie in addressing how the brain can be made immortal and that successfully achieving that goal is unlikely unless one grants "the Fundamental Principle of Futurism": at some time in the future, we will be so clever that we will be able to do anything. After a review of the "failure modes" that lead to death, Ritchie focuses on a series of possible scenarios that have been suggested for giving the brain an indefinite lifespan. He discusses the daunting and most likely insurmountable challenges presented for strategies to repair all forms of the pervasive age-associated DNA damage in brain cells via gene therapy. His essay then assesses the use of cryogenic-preservation technique designed to preserve the brain (with or without the body), where the considerable damage done to the brain during the vitrification process makes the likelihood of successful revival appear to be negligible. After critiquing the notion of "Brain uploading," he concludes that none of the five "R's" – repair, replacement, rejuvenation, refrigeration, and replication – appears to provide any realistic hope of a high-tech path to immortality.

A similar skeptical assessment is offered by Daniel Barben in chapter 15 that begins by noting that the basic ideas of transhumanism are not new. Yet the emergence of the so-called converging technologies has helped revitalize the pursuit of transhumanist ideas, as well as make their realization seem more plausible. Since the relationship between converging technologies and transhumanism is not self-evident – and the future impact of each of them on society is uncertain – Barben aims at elucidating some key issues pertaining to the ways in which interdependent technological and societal changes are being shaped. He empirically explores the notion of converging technologies – that is, the technologies rooted in the nano-, bio-, info-, and cogno-sciences that are expected by many to combine and multiply their scientific and technical potentials. He offers criticism from the perspective of the social sciences about the way in which transhumanists inadequately conceive of the relationship between human nature, technology, and society, neglecting the fact that the predominant dimension of human development is constituted by social relationships and institutions, not biology, and concludes that comparative perspectives are needed if we assume considerable cross-national differences in how converging technologies and transhumanist visions are conceptualized and practically pursued. Even more, while the significance of converging technologies is shaped by numerous factors concerning their generation, regulation, and enculturation, the impact of transhumanism will depend on its societal resonance and its ability to effectively relate to various institutional and cultural contexts.

The transhumanist celebration of technology has serious ecological ramifications because the dreams of transhumanism require the exploitation of limited natural resources. To a great extent, the transhumanist determination to transcend biology, or nature, pertains to the physical environment no less than to the human body. In chapter 16, Joan L. McGregor considers transhumanism in light of the discourse on sustainability, even though there is little consensus about the meaning of the concept and its implications. The minimum assumption is that sustainability concerns our preserving resources and the welfare of future generations. The normative claim is that the current generation owes future generations a world that is not fundamentally depleted of natural resources, where they are capable of living satisfying human lives, freeing humans from diseases and drudgery; but the current generation has also produced devastating environmental harms that will continue into the future and will threaten to fundamentally change and even destroy human life as we know it. Technology's ability to enhance humans and possibly transform them into entities that only resemble current humans raises challenging moral questions about what we owe future generations. Do future generations have a right to the genetic and biological heritage? If there is a human nature, will attempts to change violate the rights of future generations? Is human enhancement consistent with the goals of sustainability? Inspired especially by Hans Jonas's critique of technology, McGregor considers weak and strong versions of the concept of sustainability and concludes that it would be reckless to proceed with enhancement technologies without further knowledge of the risks they pose.

Technological advances are indeed an inherent feature of the human story, but the twentieth century has witnessed the acceleration of technological innovation, and the pace of this innovation will most likely be accelerated in the twenty-first century. But it is a mistake to think that there is a necessary progression here, as transhumanists urge us to think. In chapter 17, Jerry Coursen argues that all futuristic visions are imaginative scenarios, disseminated through popular culture, reflecting prevalent cultural values, and requiring human decisions. Since descriptions of the future are fictional, technology alters the trajectory of social evolution. Coursen encourages us to debate technoculture and not take its fictional accounts for granted as inevitable outcomes, as previous optimistic scenarios about the liberation of humanity by technology have been proven illusory.

The essays of Part IV acknowledge the accelerating evolution of emerging technologies, especially the so-called Five Horsemen – nanotechnology, biotechnology, robotics, information and communication technologies, and applied cognitive science. Together they create a situation in which many core constructs of Western thought previously assumed to be stable are becoming radically contingent and thus subject to renegotiation. In chapter 18, Braden Allenby, one of the Templeton Fellows in the project that gave rise to this volume, argues for the novelty of the current situation: the evolution of emerging technologies makes both institutional and individual characteristics contingent and unpredictable to the point where even the human becomes a design space. The challenges this poses to existing intellectual framework and indeed to the assumption of the Enlightenment itself are deep, difficult, and, for the most part, not yet recognized, much less addressed, by the current debate surrounding transhumanism. This chapter inquires whether the transhumanism debate is obsolete and, if so, what it tells us about the nature of the "human" and about technology and the human condition.

The volume concludes with a closer consideration of the most fantastic feature of transhumanism, the downloading of human mind into a superintelligent machine. In chapter 19, William J. Grassie attempts to distinguish between what is probably no more than silly futurism and what is definitely worthy of serious consideration. Grassie discusses the challenges of computational finitude, complexity, the limits of exponential logic, the misuse of metaphors, and the dangers of category mistakes. He shows the Singularity Movement, associated mainly with the name of Ray Kurzweil to be a quasi-religious endeavor with its own secular salvation story, torn between premillennialist and postmillennialist interpretations of evolution and the human prospect comparable to Jewish and Christian chiliastic movements through history. Grassie argues that, as we consider transhumanism from an evolutionary perspective, it is better to apply the term to our current hominid condition rather than to some futuristic age: "perhaps by calling ourselves posthumans, we can begin to see the many ways that our human nature is a moving target in an accelerating evolutionary drama." His essay endorses "the skepticism of the bioconservatives as a necessary antidote to the technoscientific optimism of the transhumanists," while calling on all of us to be more humble in our predictions and more attentive to the bigger unfolding story at hand, the evolutionary story.

To conclude, transhumanism matters not because its predications are true or innovative but because it compels us to reflect about the cultural situation in which we find ourselves given the scientific and technological advances of the past half century. To appreciate the complexity of the current situation, we must go beyond the discourse of bioethics to engage in interdisciplinary inquiry that bridges the humanities, the social sciences, the natural sciences, engineering, law, and medicine. The choice of whether one wishes to be a posthuman, as Nick Bostrom does (2008), or whether one looks critically at the claim of transhumanism, as this volume attempts to do, cannot be settled by pure arguments; it reflects personal temperament, culture orientation, and a range of personal decisions. The goal of the volume is not to settle the debate on transhumanism but to show how new perspectives can both enlarge the scope of the debate and bring it into a sharper focus.

References

Agar, Nicholas. 2004. *Liberal Eugenics: In Defence of Human Enhancement.* Oxford: Blackwell Publishing.

–. 2007. Whereto Transhumanism?: The literature reaches a critical mass. *Hastings Center Report* 37, no. 3: 12-17.

Allenby, Braden, and Daniel Sarewitz. 2011. *The Techno-Human Condition.* Cambridge, MA: MIT Press.

Aronowitz, Stanley, ed. 1996. *Technoscience and Cyberculture.* New York and London: Routledge.

Badmington, Neil. 2003. Theorizing poshumanism. *Cultural Critique* 53: 11-27.

–. ed. 2000. *Posthumanism.* New York: Palgrave.

Bailey, Ronald. 2005. *Liberation Biology: The Scientific and Moral Case for the Biotech Revolution.* Amherst, NY: Prometheus Books.

Baily, Harold W., and Timothy K. Casey, eds. 2005. *Is Human Nature Obsolete? Genetics, Bioengineering and the Future of the Human Condition.* Cambridge, MA, and London: MIT Press.

Blank, Robert H. 1999. *Brain Policy: How the New Neuroscience Will Change Our Lives and Our Policies.* Washington, DC: Georgetown University Press.

Bostrom, Nick. 2003. Tranhumanism FAQ: A General Introduction, version 2.1, www.nickbostrom.com

–. 2005. A history of transhumanist thought. *Journal of Evolution and Technology* 14, no. 1. Available on http://jetpress.org/volume14/bostrom.html.

–. 2008. Why I want to be a posthuman when I grow up. In *Medical Enhancement and Posthumanity*, edited by Bert Gordijn and Ruth Chadwick, 107-36. The Netherlands: Springer Science and Business Media.

Buchanan Allen, Dan W. Brock, Norman Daniels, and Daniel Wikler. 2000. *From Chance to Choice.* Cambridge: Cambridge University Press.

Churchland, Patricia Smith. 1989 [1986]. *Neurophilosophy: Toward a Unified Science of the Mind/Brain.* Cambridge, MA, and London: The MIT Press.

Clark, Andy. 2003. *Natural-Born Cyborgs: Minds, Technologies, and the Future of Human Intelligence.* Oxford and New York: Oxford University Press.

De Grey, Aubrey, with Michael Rae. 2007. *Ending Aging: The Rejuvenation Breakthrough That Could Reverse Human Aging in Our Lifetime.* New York: St. Martin's Press.

Dinello, Daniel. 2002. *Technophobia! Science Fiction Vision of Posthuman Technology.* Austin: University of Texas Press.

Drexler, Eric K. 1986. *Engines of Creation.* Garden City, NY: Anchor Press/ Doubleday.

–. 1992. *Nanosystems: Molecular Machinery, Manufacturing and Computation.* New York: Wiley.

Drexler, Erik K., and Chris Peterson. 1991. *Unbounding the Future: The Nanotechnology Revolution.* New York: Morrow.

Frankford, David M. 1998. The treatment/enhancement distinction as an armament in the policy war. In *Enhancing Human Traits: Ethical and Social Implications*, edited by Eric Parens, 70–94. Washington, DC: Georgetown University Press.

Fukuyama, Francis. 2002. *Our Posthuman Future: Consequences of the Biotechnology Revolution.* New York: Profile Books.

Garreau, Joel. 2004. *Radical Evolution: The Promise and Peril of Enhancing Our Minds, Our Bodies, and What It Means to Be Humans.* New York: Doubleday.

Glannon, Walter. 2002. *The Moral Basis of Responsibility*. Aldershot, UK: Ashgate.
–. 2007. *Bioethics and the Brain*. Oxford and New York: Oxford University Press.
Gordijn, Bert, and Ruth Chadwick, eds. 2008. *Medical Enhancement and Posthumanity*. The Netherlands: Springer Science and Business Media.
Graham, Elaine L. 2002. *Representations of the Post/Human*. Manchester, UK: Manchester University Press.
Hansell, Gregory R., and William J. Grassie, eds. 2011. *H+ Transhumanism and Its Critics*. Philadelphia: Metanexus Institute.
Haraway, Donna. 1991. *Simians, Cyborgs, and Women: The Reinvention of Nature*. London: Free Association Books.
Harris, John. 1992. *Wonderwoman and Superman: The Ethics of Human Biotechnology*. Oxford: Oxford University Press.
–. 2007. *Enhancing Evolution: The Ethical Case for Making Better People*. Princeton, NJ: Princeton University Press.
Hayles, N. Katherine. 1999. *How We Became Posthuman: Cybernetics, Literature, and Informatics*. Chicago: University of Chicago Press.
Hefner, Philip. 2003. *Technology and Human Becoming*. Minneapolis, MN: Fortress.
–. 2009. The animal that aspires to be an angel: The challenge of transhumanism. *Dialog: Journal of Technology* 48, no. 2: 164-73
Hughes, James J. 2004. *Citizen Cyborg: Why Democratic Societies Must Respond to the Redesigned Human of the Future*. Cambridge, MA: Westview.
–. 2011. "The Politics of Transhumanism". http://www.changesurfer.com/Acad/TranshumPolitics.htm.
Hughes, Thomas P. 2004. *Human-Built World: How to Think about Technology and Culture*. Chicago and London: The University of Chicago Press.
Husband, Philip, Owen Holland, and Michael Wheeler, eds. 2008. *The Mechanical Mind in History*. Cambridge, MA: MIT Press.
Huxley, Julian. 1957. *New Bottles for New Wine*. London: Chatto & Windus.
Juengst, Eric T. 1998. What does enhancement mean? In *Enhancing Human Traits: Ethical and Social Implications*, edited by Erik Parens, 29-47. Washington DC: Georgetown University Press.
Kass. Leon. 2002. *Life, Liberty and the Pursuit of Dignity*. San Francisco: Encounter Books.
Kelly, Kevin. 2010. *What Technology Wants.* New York: Viking.
Kurzweil, Ray. 1990. *The Age of Intelligent Machines*. Cambridge, MA: MIT Press.

–. 1999. *The Age of Spiritual Machines: When Computers Exceed Human Intelligence.* New York: Viking
–. 2002. The evolution of mind in the twenty-first century. In *Are We Spiritual Machines? Ray Kurzweil vs. the Critics of Strong AI*, edited by Jay W. Richards, 12-55. Seattle: The Discovery Institute.
–. 2005. *The Singularity Is Near: When Humans Transcend Biology.* New York: Viking.
Maslow, A. H. 1971. *The Farther Reaches of Human Nature.* New York: Penguin.
Maher, Derek F., and Calvin Mercer, eds. 2009. *Religion and the Implications of Radical Life Extension.* New York: Palgrave Macmillan.
McKibben, Bill. 2003. *Enough: Staying Human in an Engineered Age.* New York: Henry Holt & Co.
Mehlman, Maxwell J. 2003. *Wondergenes: Genetic Enhancement and the Future of Society.* Bloomington: Indiana University Press.
–. 2009. *The Price of Perfection: Individualism and Society in the Era of Biomedical Enhancement.* Baltimore: Johns Hopkins University Press.
Miah, Andy. 2008. A critical history of posthumanism. In *Medical Enhancement and Posthumanity*, edited by Bert Gordijn and Ruth Chadwick, 71-94. The Netherlands: Springer Science and Business Media.
Mindell, David, A. 2002. *Between Human and Machine: Feedback, Control and Computing Before Cybernetics.* Baltimore, MD, and London: Johns Hopkins University Press.
Minsky, Marvin. 1986. *The Society of Mind.* New York: Simon and Schuster.
–. 2006. *The Emotion Machine: Commonsense Thinking, Artificial Intelligence, and the Future of the Human Mind.* New York: Simon & Schuster.
Mitchell, Ben C., Edmund D. Pellegrino, Jean Betke Elshtain, John F. Kilner, and Scott B. Rae. 2007. *Biotehcnology and the Human Good.* Washington, DC: Georgetown University Press.
Moravec, Hans P. 1988. *Mind Children: The Future of Robot and Human Intelligence.* Cambridge, MA: Harvard University Press.
–. 1999. *Robot: Mere Machine to Transcendent Mind.* New York: Oxford University Press.
More, Max. 2004. Extropian Principles 3.0, http://www.maxmore.com/extprn3.htm.
Noble, David F. 1997. *The Religion of Technology: The Divinity of Man and the Spirit of Invention.* New York: Penguin Books.
Parens, Erik. 2006. *Wrestling with Behavioral Genetics: Science, Ethics, and Public Conversation.* Baltimore, MD: Johns Hopkins University Press.

Parens, Erik, ed. 1998. Is better always good? The enhancement project. In *Enhancing Human Traits: Ethical and Social Implication*, edited by Erik Parens, 1-28. Washington, DC: Georgetown University Press.

Peters, Ted. 1996. *For the Love of Children: Genetic Technology and the Future of the Family*. Louisville, KY: Westminster Knox Press.

–. 1997. *Playing God? Genetic Determinism and Human Freedom.* New York: Routledge.

–. 2003. *Science, Theology and Ethics.* Aldershot, UK, and Burlington, VT: Ashgate.

Pepperell, Robert. 2003. *The Posthuman Condition: Consciousness beyond the Brain.* Bristol, UK: Intellect Books.

Pessig, David. 2008. *The Future Code: Israel's Future Test.* (In Hebrew) Tel-Aviv: Yediot Aharonot and Hemed Library.

Pickering, Andrew. 1995. *The Mangle of Practice, Time, Agency and Science.* Chicago: University of Chicago Press.

Postman, Neil. 1993 [1992]. *Technopoly: The Surrender of Culture to Technology*. New York: Vintage Books.

Roco, Mihail C., and William Sims Bainbridge, eds. 2002. *Converging Technologies for Improvement of Human Performance: Nanotechnology, Biotechnology, Information Technology and Cognitive Science.* Dordrecht and Boston: Kluwer Academic Publishers.

Sandel, Michael. 2007. *The Case against Perfection: Ethics in the Age of Genetic Engineering.* Cambridge, MA: The Belknap Press of Harvard University Press.

Savulescu, Julian, and Nick Bostrom, eds. 2009. *Human Enhancement*. Oxford: Oxford University Press.

Savulescue, Julian, R. ter Mueler, and G. Kahane, eds. 2009. *Enhancing Human Capacities*. Oxford: Wiley-Blackwell.

Silver, Lee. 2002 [1997]. *Remaking Eden: How Genetic Engineering and Cloning Will Transform the American Family*. New York: Perennial.

Soper, Kate. 1987. *Humanism and Anti-Humanism*. La Salle, IL: Open Court.

Stock, Gregory. 1993. *Metaman: The Making of Humans and Machines into a Global Superorganism.* New York: Simon and Schuster.

–. 2000. *Engineering the Human Germline: An Exploration of the Science and Ethics of Altering the Genes*. Oxford: Oxford University Press.

–. 2002. *Redesigning Humans: Our Inevitable Genetic Future*. Boston: Houghton Mifflin.

Tancredi, Laurence R. 2004. Neuroscience development and the law. In *Neuroscience and the Law: Brain, Mind, and the Scales of Justice*, edited by Brenner Garland, 71–113. New York and Washington, DC: Dana Press.

Tipler, Frank J. 1994. *The Physics of Immortality: Modern Cosmology, God and the Resurrection of the Dead.* New York: Doubleday.

–. 2007. *The Physics of Christianity.* New York: Doubleday.

Tirosh-Samuelson, Hava. 2003. *Happiness in Premodern Judaism: Virtue, Knowledge and Well-Being.* Cincinnati: Hebrew Union College Press.

–. 2010. Eine Auseinandersetzung mit dem Transhumanismus aus jüdischer Perpektive. In *Die Debatte über "Human Enhancement": historische, philosophicshe und ethische Aspekte der technologischen Verbesserung des Menschen,* edited by Christopher Coenen, Stefan Gammel, Reinhard Heil, and Andreas Woyke, 307–28. Bielefeld: Transcript Verlag.

–. 2011. Engaging transhumanism. In *H+: Transhumanism and Its Critics,* edited by Gregory R. Hansell and William J. Grassie, 15–94. Philadelphia: Metanexus Institute.

Waters, Brent. 2006. *From Human to Posthuman: Christian Theology and Technology in a Postmodern World.* Aldershot, UK, and Burlington, VT: Ashgate.

Wolfe, Cary. 2010. *What Is Transhumanism?* Minneapolis: University of Minnesota Press.

Young, Simon. 2006. *Designer Evolution: A Transhumanist Manifesto.* Amherst, NY: Prometheus Books

Part I:
Transhumanism and Religion

Science and the Betterment of Humanity: Three British Prophets of Transhumanism

Hava Tirosh-Samuelson

Transhumanism is a future-oriented movement, but its leading theorists insist that their vision has deep historical roots. Nick Bostrom (2005) traces the historical roots of transhumanist ideas to the ancient Sumerian *Epic of Gilgamesh*, but it is really the Renaissance of the sixteenth century, the scientific revolution of the seventeenth century, and the Enlightenment of the eighteenth century that function as historical roots of transhumanism. Thus, the foundational texts of the transhumanism are Giovanni Pico della Mirandola's *De hominis dignitate* (*Oration on the Dignity of Man*, 1486) and Francis Bacon's *Novum Organum* (1620) even though transhumanists do not engage them in depth. Yet Bostrom and other transhumanists are correct to view transhumanism as an extension of the so-called Enlightenment Project and its ideal of progress (Dear 1997). Indeed, transhumanism is best understood as *ideology of extreme progress* (Coenen 2009).

The immediate sources of inspiration for the transhumanist movement arc three British scientists and public intellectuals: Julian Huxley (1887-1975), John Burdon Sanderson Haldane (1892-1964), and John Desmond Bernal (1901-1971).[1] These accomplished scientists were close personal friends whose private lives were as rich and complex as their public careers. Two of the three – Haldane and Bernal – adopted communism as their chosen worldview and were members in the Communist Party of Greater Britain (CPGB). They influenced Huxley, who was a moderate Progressive, to endorse leftist positions that thrived in British academe during the 1930s, especially among young scientists in Cambridge. During the 1920s, these three scientists articulated a secularist vision of the future of the human species.

The future orientation of these authors and their commitment to use science for the betterment of humanity influenced the transhumanist movement more than their actual scientific works. It is important to note that the "prophets" of transhumanism advocated eugenics as the path for the betterment of the human condition, although Haldane would criticize the eugenics movement after he became a communist. As public intellectuals who popularized science, they believed that science *must* play a social role to improve the human condition. Not coincidentally, all three not only served as heads of scientific organizations or as consultants to governments but also played instrumental roles in international

1 For another treatment of these precursors of transhumanism, consult Heil 2010.

organizations committed to the betterment of humanity (e.g., UNESCO, the World Peace Council, and World Federation of Scientific Workers). As products of England's elite educational institutions – Eton, Oxford, and Cambridge – these influential writers were true heirs of the Renaissance ideal of *homo universalis*, integrating science, literature, and the arts and bridging theory and praxis. Finally, although all three repudiated theistic Christianity, they were profound idealists who secularized a shared religious impulse: to make the world a better place.

This chapter explores the views of Huxley, Haldane, and Bernal by highlighting their belief in progressive evolution, their notion that the human species verges on a new evolutionary phase, their commitment to improve humanity by means of science and technology, and their futuristic dream of transcending human biology. Moreover, our current debates about genetic engineering and directed evolution (which will be discussed in detail in the following chapters of this volume) repeat many of the issues raised during the debates on eugenics during the 1920s and 1930s (Coenen 2009, 109-14). Viewed from this historical perspective, contemporary transhumanism appears less novel, original, or outlandish.

Nonetheless, it is also important to acknowledge the differences between contemporary transhumanists and their sources of inspiration in England. Whereas the early visionaries received classical training in literature, history, and the arts, which in turn made them superb communicators of ideas, their contemporary heirs lack training in the humanities and the arts, and their vision of humanity is driven by technology; whereas the earlier thinkers endorsed socialism and/or communism, contemporary transhumanists are aligned with capitalism and enlist wealthy, private donors rather than governments to fund their projects; whereas the earlier generation believed in collectivist, planned solutions for human miseries, current proponents of the transhumanism insist on personal choice and freedom for unlimited self-expression; and whereas the early twentieth-century eugenicists recommended compulsory methods in the struggle to better the human condition, contemporary transhumanists are liberal democrats who reject any form of coercion and appeal to human self-interest as the motivating force for self-improvement. Understanding what contemporary transhumanists owe their British predecessors and where these differ will enable us to appreciate transhumanism as an ideology that tries to give coherence to our technological age.

Julian Huxley: Evolutionary Humanism and the Task of Humanity

Julian Huxley can be considered the "prophet" of transhumanism not so much because he coined the term in 1957 but because his philosophy of evolutionary humanism articulated the intellectual framework for thinking about the possibility of a posthuman age (Huxley 1992 [1954]). Huxley considered "transhumanism" as a "key concept" that "stands at the top of the organization of thought [and] imposes a pattern on it and pulls other less dominant ideals into place, modifying them in relation to the whole pattern" (Huxley 1957 [1927], 255). Huxley saw himself as a "midwife" who would deliver into the world "a new ideology" or a "new system of ideas appropriate to man's new situation." He insisted that "the truth of the transhumanist approach and its central conception is larger and more universal than any previous truth, and is bound in the long run to supersede lesser, more partial, or more distorted truths, such as Marxism, Christian Theology, or liberal individualism, or at any rate to assimilate those of their elements which are relevant to itself" (ibid., 260). Huxley considered evolutionary humanism primarily as an "attitude of mind" (1931, vi) that would address the crisis of humanity by bridging science and the arts and by using science to build a better world.

Like most English intellectuals at the end of the Victorian age, let alone the grandson of Thomas Henry Huxley, Julian Huxley could not fail to see all biological phenomena in the context of evolutionary theory. It is important to note, however, that, at the end of the nineteenth and beginning of the twentieth century, the "theory of evolution" meant at least three claims: (1) that life on earth changed over time; (2) that different species share a common ancestry and have developed over time to take their varied current forms; and (3) that "changes over time of living things from common ancestors into multiple later forms occurred through a process driven by natural selection of random inborn variants" (Larson 2004, 288). Charles Darwin, of course, came to personify the idea of organic evolution by natural selection, and all evolutionists acknowledged Darwin as their master, even though not all evolutionary theorists accepted the theory of natural selection. During the 1860s and 1870s, as scientists raised increasing doubts about the sufficiency of selection theory, Darwin revised the *Origin of Species* and added a larger dose of the Lamarckian notion that acquired characteristics also evolve. Thus, Darwin himself was distinguished from the "neo-Darwinians" who clung to the belief that a natural selection of inborn variations could sustain the evolutionary process. This view became accepted academic orthodoxy due to Thomas Henry Huxley and a few like-minded friends (known as the X-Club) who "managed to assume leadership roles in many of Britain's leading scientific societies, place supporters in prominent university and museum positions, and influence the editorial policies of scientific journals" (Lightman 1987, 94). In 1869, they founded the journal *Nature* as the mouthpiece of scientific naturalism and promoted Darwinism on its pages.

In his early childhood, Julian Huxley was very close to his paternal grandfather; there is no doubt that Julian's love of nature reflected the time he spent at T. H.'s countryside home. The elder Huxley, who coined the term *agnosticism*, clearly rejected traditional Christian tenets; but as Bernard Lightman explains, he was a deeply religious man who believed that "religion belonged to the realm of feeling, while science was part of the realm of intellect" (1987, 131). Science and religion, the elder Huxley believed, were "twin sisters" that were interdependent; the conflict was not between science and religion but between science and questionable theology.

Unlike his grandfather, Julian Huxley would actually seek to establish the relationship between science (namely, evolutionary theory) and ethics, but his desire to present a unified picture of the human being's place in nature might have something to do with the pantheistic proclivities of his mother, Julia, the niece of Matthew Arnold. Julia was a deeply spiritual person who tried to reconcile the religious tension between her own parents: her mother was an ardent Protestant, while her father vacillated between Catholicism and Anglicanism, constantly struggling to reconcile his own Catholic beliefs with the Protestantism of his wife (Huxley 1970-73, 1:16-17). Julia read chapters of the Bible to Julian and his siblings and developed her own brand of pantheistic faith to resolve the religious tensions between her parents. Her pantheism contributed to Julian's view of nature as a cosmic unity.

Julian Huxley agreed that evolution was a "series of blind alleys," but not in the case of human evolution. He saw progressive evolution as a magnificent process "that takes place in a series of steps or grades, each grade occupied by a successful group of animals or plants, each group sprung from a pre-existing one and characterized by a new and improved patters and organization" (Huxley 1992 [1954], 74). William Provine has shown that, from the beginning of his scientific career, Huxley "always and unwaveringly believed that evolution was progressive and offered hope and meaning to human existence" (1992, 166). The hope lay in raising the performance level of the human brain, in taking control of the evolutionary process itself through eugenics, and in envisioning the process of coalescence of minds into superminds. At the end of this progress, the human would be "consciously controlling his own destiny and the destiny of life upon this planet" (Divall 1992, 37). As "organ" or "agent" of the evolutionary progress, the human occupies a "cosmic office" that obligates the species to realize its highest possible spiritual experience. Despite his repudiation of religious theism, Huxley's understanding of human destiny was a secular variant of traditional Christian beliefs that assigned to humanity the task of managing God's created world (De Witt 1994).

Huxley's interpretation of evolution was rooted in solid scientific work as a zoologist, although his formal academic career was rather short. He spent a few years in Oxford (1910-12; 1919-25), Rice Institute in Texas (1912-16), and King's College, London (1925-26), but he preferred science education to the rough and tumble of academe, perhaps because he was prone to nervous breakdowns (he had a total of seven throughout his life). In the 1920s, he lectured at the Royal Institution, London (1927) and collaborated with H. G. Wells and his son in writing *The Science of Life* (1926). In the 1930s, he served as secretary of the Zoological Society of London (1935-42) and was busy writing, publishing, broadcasting for the BBC, and lecturing; out of these activities came his most important work, *Evolution, the Modern Synthesis* (1942) in which he attempted to integrate developments in ecology, genetics, paleontology, geographical distribution, embryology, systematics, and comparative anatomy. Huxley clearly saw himself as the real architect of the "new synthesis," but some biologists (e.g., Ernst Mayr, Sewall Wright, and Ronald Fisher) felt excluded by Huxley; and others, mostly younger biologists (e.g., Niles Eldredge, Stephen Jay Gould, Motoo Kimura, G. L. Stebbins, and Francisco Ayala) would debate the scientific merit of the new synthesis (Provine 1992, 171), although this debate need not concern us here.

Huxley viewed the universe as fundamentally a unity governed by the process of progress (Baker 1978, 5-56). His first published work, *The Individual in the Animal Kingdom* (1912), was an exercise in philosophical biology written under the influence of Henri Bergson's *Creative Evolution* (1907) that "argued that life was distinguished from the mechanical workings of matter because it was informed by the élan vital. One could not predict the development of life on the basis of even a complete knowledge of the workings of the material universe" (Divall 1992, 42). Prior to World War I, Bergson's theory was juxtaposed with the mechanistic materialism that underlay Herbert Spencer's Social Darwinism, but in the 1920s, there were attempts to reconcile these two opposing views by articulating the theory of "emergent evolution." Huxley accepted the doctrine of emergent evolution, which sees the emergence of the human mind as a distinctive phase in the evolutionary process, moving from biology to culture.

In *Evolutionary Humanism*, Huxley explains the uniqueness of the human:

> Man's evolution is not biological but psychosocial: it operates by the mechanism of cultural tradition which involves the cumulative self-reproduction and self variation of mental activities and their products. Accordingly, major steps in the human phase of evolution are achieved by breakthroughs to new dominant patterns of mental organization of knowledge, ideas and belief – ideological instead of physiological or biological organization. (1992 [1954], 79)

For Huxley, the emergence of mind or sentiency is "an extremely rare event in the vast meaninglessness of the insentient universe, and man's particular brand of sentiency may well be unique." Because humans alone possess mind, Huxley believed, only in humans "the transaction of the real business of evolution has been shifted from the domain of matter to that of thought. This gives a new dimension and a new flexibility to evolution and makes possible much quicker and fuller adaptation" (ibid., 253). And since evolution is one-directional and irreversible, the emergence of mind places humanity in a unique situation (ibid., 246). The destiny of humanity is to understand human nature and to actualize the possibilities of development inherent in it. Highlighting human evolving nature, Huxley urges his readers to "utilize all available knowledge in giving guidance and encouragement for the *continuing adventure of human development*" (ibid., 287). This is the core belief of the transhumanist program.

Huxley's evolutionary humanism was clearly a naturalist vision, but it was not reductionistically materialistic. It was, in fact, a statement of a *secularist faith* for a world that had to come to terms with the facts of evolution and was decidedly articulated in ethical and aesthetic terms. While Huxley opposed supernatural explanations, he deeply appreciated the mystery of existence and had no qualms using ethical and religious concepts such as "destiny" and "the sacred" to articulate his vision of and for humanity. Indeed, in his early work *Religion without Revelation* (1927), he presented his new worldview as "a developed religion" or "religious humanism" but over time changed that term into "scientific humanism," later to "evolutionary humanism," and finally to "transhumanism." The term "scientific" was intended to highlight the degree to which humankind is part of nature, and therefore subject to the same laws, and the subsequent term "humanist" was meant to highlight the centrality of the human mind in giving direction to the evolutionary process. The human mind inspires the march of progress in nature, and "the source of all truth, beauty, morality and purpose is to be found in human nature" (Huxley 1934, 7). His unified cosmic vision that privileges the human mind is remarkably similar to that of Pierre Teilhard de Chardin, the Jesuit paleontologist for whom progressive evolution led to the "noösphere" (namely, a sphere of mind as opposed to, or rather superimposed on, the biosphere or sphere of life) and later to the collective consciousness of the Omega Point (Steinhart 2008). Huxley developed his ideas sixteen years before he met Teilhard; indeed, Huxley's work exercised an important influence on the Jesuit priest. Unlike other biologists who shunned Teilhard because he blended Christianity and science, Huxley wrote an enthusiastic introduction to the English translation of Teilhard's *The Phenomenon of Man* published in 1952 (republished in Huxley 1992 [1954], 202-17).

Huxley maintained that, if the task of humanity is to actualize the immense potential of the human mind and take control of the evolutionary process itself, the human will succeed in the task "only if he faces it consciously and if he uses all his mental resources – knowledge and reason, imagination and sensitivity, capacities for wonder and love, for comprehension and compassion, for spiritual aspiration and moral effort" (Huxley 1992 [1954], 78). Here lies the connection between Huxley's evolutionary theory and his ardent support of the eugenics movement, long after eugenics was a discredited. During the 1930s and 1940s, he wrote prolifically about eugenic topics, and from 1959 to 1964, he served as the president of the Eugenics Society. A brief discussion of the eugenics movement is in order if we are to appreciate the legacy of Julian Huxley to the transhumanist movement.

The term *eugenics* (literally meaning "well born") was coined in 1883 in *Inquiries into Human Faculty and Its Development* (1919) by Francis Galton, a cousin of Charles Darwin. Galton founded anthropometric research and devised instruments for exact measurements of human physical traits, including the methods for fingerprinting. From his interest in statistics, Galton founded the Biometric Laboratory at University College in London (1884) and established the journal *Biometrics* in 1901 that published statistical research. In 1904, he founded the Eugenics Records Office, which soon became known as the Galton Laboratory at University College, London, to further scientific study of eugenics. He was named honorary president of the newly formed Eugenics Education Society (from 1908 until his death in 1911) and of the German Society for Race Hygiene. A somewhat eccentric genius with independent means, Galton traveled extensively in Africa and the Middle East during the 1850s and experienced Darwin's *Origin of Species* as an epiphany of sorts that liberated him from Christian mores. On the basis of a purportedly Darwinian process of selective human reproduction (i.e., eugenics), he turned his energy to improving humanity.

Galton held that the principles of eugenics "ought to become one of the dominant motives in a civilized nation, much as if they were one of its religious tenets" (Larson 2004, 181). He advocated *positive eugenics* – keeping superior families from falling back toward the norm – rather than negative eugenics – discouraging reproduction by the unfit – but it was *negative eugenics* that became the hallmark of the eugenics movement during the 1920s and 1930s.

In addition to England, the eugenics movement thrived in the United States and in Europe. The leading American eugenics organization, the Eugenics Record Office at the Carnegie Institution Cold Spring Harbor Genetics Laboratory, was the primary scientific institution for the promotion of research and related social policies. The eugenicists identified those who should not reproduce; their main target was hereditary forms of mental defect and deficiency. Influenced by the work of Cesare Lombroso in Italy, some eugenicists also targeted repeat criminals, prostitutes, and others who regularly manifested supposedly hereditary undesirable social behavior (Larson 2004, 192). Physical conditions such as epilepsy, hereditary blindness, and assorted gross deformities were singled out as grounds for restriction. In the U.S., the Eugenics Record Office proposed a comprehensive state program designed to sterilize one-tenth of the population every generation. Although no such mass program took place in America, the U.S. Supreme Court upheld the constitutionality of the model eugenics statute drafted by the Eugenics Record Office and enacted in Virginia in 1927. Writing for the Supreme Court, Justice Oliver Wendell Holmes wryly concluded that "three generations of imbeciles are enough."

The worst compulsory programs were enacted in Germany with the 1933 Law for the Prevention of Genetically Diseased Progeny that mandated the sterilization of persons determined by genetic health courts to suffer from congenital feeblemindedness, schizophrenia, manic depression, severe physical deformity, hereditary epilepsy, Huntington's chorea, hereditary blindness or deafness, or severe alcoholism. Some three hundred thousand persons were sterilized under this law between 1933 and 1939 when it was replaced by a euthanasia program designed to rid the Fatherland of its mentally handicapped "children." However, these compulsory programs were not limited to Germany: every Nordic nation adopted eugenic-sterilization legislation. The eugenics community focused on marriage restriction, sexual segregation, sterilization, and in the United States, especially on immigration restriction (Kevels 1995 [1985], 98).

Huxley was a vocal proponent of eugenics. As Garland Allen explains, Huxley saw eugenics less in terms of selecting individuals within family lines and more in terms of the shift of statistical means within large populations. Huxley predicted that eugenics would "inevitably become part of the religion of the future, or whatever complex of sentiments may in the future take the place of organized religion" (Allen 1992, 201). He believed that eugenicists must ask the same kinds of questions that evolutionists ask when they attempt to understand how selection operates to prevent or eliminate certain traits. Huxley held that "the future evolution of the human species depended on a two pronged eugenics approach: (1) elimination of unwanted genetic variability (genetic diseases, mental defects and so on) through negative eugenical measures coupled with selection for desirable variation through positive eugenics, and (2) encouraging the maintenance of non-deleterious genetic diversity throughout the population as the basis for future evolutionary advance" (ibid., 203). For Huxley, equalizing the environment through eugenic planning had its own social and moral rationale.

In theory, Huxley's brand of "reformist eugenics" was supposed to be different from the "old eugenics" of Francis Galton; but, in practice, there was little difference. He advocated reduction of the rate of reproduction of the lower classes or poorer ethnic groups and increase in the rate of reproduction of the upper classes or wealthier groups. He was a staunch advocate of birth control and wanted to see the dissociation of sex and love from procreation: decisions about procreation would be based on genetics and health of the off-spring (Allen 1992, 212). He anticipated opposition to his ideas, believing that 5 to 10 percent of the British population would be unable to absorb new ideas because of their innate worthlessness. Since these "unteachables" contributed the greatest percentage of hereditary defectives to the next generation because of their refusal to use voluntary birth control, Huxley *recommended compulsory sterilization.* At the beginning of the Great Depression, he proposed that unemployment relief be made contingent on the male recipient's agreeing to father no more children (Kevels 1995 [1985], 123). Throughout the 1930s and 1940s, he actively campaigned for contraception, worked to legalize voluntary eugenical sterilization in England, and lavished praise on American eugenicists for "pioneering" the passage of eugenical sterilization laws. Huxley spoke of eugenics in terms of planning and controlling human evolution. He was actively involved in various social-planning groups in the 1920s and 1930s, and he admired the Soviet Union's commitment to planning and using trained experts or technocrats in industry and agriculture. This admiration and his visit to the Soviet Union in 1931 were due to his friendship with J.B.S. Haldane and J. D. Bernal, two "converts" to communism, who led Huxley to draw the political implications of his eugenical beliefs.

The horrors of the Nazi sterilization program, their experimentation on human subjects, especially Jews, and their plan to exterminate the totality of the Jewish people discredited the eugenics movement in the postwar years. Yet Huxley remained committed to eugenics, and his association with the movement did not diminish his international reputation. In fact, immediately after World War II, he was appointed the first secretary general of UNESCO, a position he held for only two years (1946-48) due to opposition from the Americans and his own deficiencies as a manager. His continued support for eugenics and his efforts on behalf of worldwide population control received accolades in 1959 when he received an award from the Lasker Foundation in the category of "Planned Parenthood – World Population." As president of the British Eugenics Society during the early 1960s, he continued to urge people to know more about human heredity in order to think intelligently about human biological improvement. In 1965, the term *genetic engineering* was coined and rapidly came to denote "a cluster of micromanipulations of the reproductive or hereditary process, some of which, like cloning had little to do with genetics" (Kevels 1995 [1985], 265). The debates about genetic engineering, assisted reproductive technologies, and stem-cell research during the past few decades are but an extension of the controversies surrounding eugenics in early decades of the twentieth century (Holland, Lebacqz, and Zoloth 2001; Green 2001; McGee 1998).

Were Huxley alive today, it is reasonable to assume that he would be very pleased with the accelerated pace of technology and the human involvement in directed evolution. It is also reasonable to assume that he would be delighted to learn about the advances in the neurosciences and the degree to which humans are now able to control their mental life by means of biochemical substances. Similarly, the advances in artificial intelligence and the development of the World Wide Web would be to his liking since he speculated on the emergence of a supermind that would exceed ordinary human cognition. But it is also important to notice some important differences between the British visionary and the movement to which he gave a name. First, Huxley was a humanist in the original Renaissance sense of the term, namely, a person committed to the *studia humanitatis* – rhetoric, grammar, history, poetry, and moral philosophy – which today we call "the humanities." Huxley wanted to bridge the gap between the sciences and the arts, analyzed so well by his friend C. P. Snow (Snow 1964 [1959]), and he would have been dismayed to see the eclipse of the humanities and the triumph of the natural sciences. Second, Huxley was a naturalist, and his writings have strong ecological awareness, both in terms of bringing people to appreciate human kinship with nature and in terms of human responsibility to preserve nature. This ecological awareness is utterly missing in the transhumanist movement. Finally, Huxley was a humanitarian with spiritual proclivities who was devoted to the betterment of human life understood in nonutilitarian terms. He had a strong aesthetic sense and reminded his readers that "the important ends of man's life include the creation and enjoyment of beauty, both natural and man-made". Huxley cherished "all sources of pure wonder and delight, like fine scenery, wild animals in freedom, or unspoiled nature" and encouraged his fellow beings to embrace "the cosmic project of evolution." In the final analysis, Huxley's transhumanism was indeed "religion without revelation." In the grand evolutionary schema, Julian Huxley discerned "the lineaments of a *new religion* that we can be sure will arise to serve the needs of the coming era" (Huxley 1992 [1954], 76). This new religion would believe in knowledge and "will take advantage of the vast amount of new knowledge produced by the knowledge-explosion of the last few centuries." Transhumanists do not present their beliefs as "religion," but perhaps they should (Goldberg 2009) if transhumanism is to receive the attention and the criticism it deserves.

J.B.S. Haldane: Counterculture, Technological Utopianism, and Politics

The second major source of inspiration for the transhumanist movement is J.B.S. Haldane, Huxley's close friend at Eton. The son of the Oxford physiologist and philosopher of science John Scott Haldane and Louisa Kathleen Trotter, J.B.S. Haldane came from a long line of Scottish military men and leisured country gentlemen. Haldane's uncle and namesake was John Burdon Sanderson who was also a professor of physiology in Oxford, and another uncle, Richard Burdon, was a distinguished Liberal and later Labor cabinet minister. Unlike his mother who was an uncompromised Tory and fervent supporter of Joseph Chamberlain's brand of social imperialism, Haldane's father was a Liberal and a humanitarian who cared about alleviating suffering of ordinary men and women. The father investigated mining diseases and colliery explosions and imparted to his son the commitment to bettering human lives through the use of science and technology.

Haldane was clearly a child prodigy: he read English at three years of age and German at five. His intellectual talent was channeled into science by his father who treated him like a fellow scientist even before he went to Eton. Haldane took part in his father's scientific experiments (often done on themselves), and father and son published a scientific paper together when J.B.S. was but 12 years old. Haldane's closest confidants at Eton and Oxford were Julian Huxley and his younger brother Aldous.[2] Gradually, Haldane shed the conservative outlook of his mother and, to her chagrin, increasingly aligned with the Liberal side of the Haldane family. As an undergraduate at Oxford, he joined not only the University Liberal Club but also the local Cooperative Society and over the years dissociated himself from the aristocratic world of his birth. In fact, Haldane was a self-made "scientific Socialist," although it would take him a few good years to figure out what socialism means. Gradually, he shifted from being an inactive supporter of the Labour Party to being a member of the Union of Scientific Workers and eventually (under the influence of his first wife, Charlotte Burghes) to becoming a member of the CPGB.

When World War I broke out, Haldane gladly volunteered for the Scottish Black Watch Regiment and served with distinction in the Middle East. Although he was wounded twice, he cherished the wartime experience and even discovered that he liked the battlefield experience, including killing people. In the war, Haldane encountered chemical weapons and began to reflect systematically on the role of science in warfare. He came to the conclusion that chemical warfare was more humane than conventional weapons and urged the British government to accelerate its research and development in that area. He also recommended some novel ancillary projects such as training special units of black men from the colonies for chemical combat. One presumes that Haldane's scientific research found that Asians and Africans suffered less than Europeans from exposure to various gases. This view reflects his involvement with the eugenics movement, which began when he was an undergraduate at New College, Oxford. The Great War, however,

2 Aldous Huxley used Haldane as the model for the fictional character of Shearwater in the novel *Antic Hay* (1923) and Haldane's futuristic speculations about ectogenesis (i.e., birth outside the womb) played an important role in Huxley's famous dystopia *Brave New World* (1932).

was the major factor of Haldane's disillusion with his own class and with traditional liberalism. He was attentive to rapid changes in the life of working people during the postwar years and believed that their needs could be addressed only through science. The Liberals were incapable of taking appropriate action, and Haldane condemned their "gross mismanagement of the war, and more generally, the pride Britain's governors took in their ignorance of science" (Werskey 1978, 60). For Haldane, science was the answer to human social ills.

After the Great War, Haldane returned to Oxford in 1919, but in 1922, he accepted a position in biochemistry at Trinity College, Cambridge, where he taught until 1932. In Cambridge during the 1920s, he became a true cultural hero. As Isaiah Berlin attested, Haldane (along with Aldous Huxley) was seen as "one of the major intellectual emancipators" (Werskey 1978, 86). By the mid-1920s, he was a famous public figure that attracted many undergraduates and academic nonconformists because he was a larger-than-life figure. Physically, he was an imposing man with a ferocious, mercurial temper; scientifically, he was a virtuoso who covered physiology and biochemistry, as well as biometry and genetics; intellectually, he had unusual breadth mastering not only several natural sciences but also the classics, history, and political theory; and socially, he was very witty and clever, although his behavior was often mercilessly tactless.

In particular, Haldane's views on sexuality made him a celebrity in the counterculture of Cambridge during the 1920s. Both Haldane and Julian Huxley "made a point of declaring that sexual compatibility was essential to the happy marriage, that women deserved sexual satisfaction as much as men, and that there was nothing wrong or degrading about sexual pleasure dissociated from procreation. Of course, they endorsed divorce and birth control" (Kevels 1995 [1985], 125). Haldane certainly mocked many social conventions, and some people found his behavior to be simply disgraceful, but it is not clear whether his behavior was a matter of class rebelliousness or social ineptness. Haldane's affair with a journalist of the *Daily Worker*, Charlotte Burghes, who was married at the time and a mother of a child, became a much publicized scandal. In order for her to secure a legal divorce from her husband, they had to stage the adulterous affair that led the Ethics Committee at Cambridge University to dismiss Haldane from his readership in biochemistry for his "gross immorality." With the help of National Union of Scientific Workers,[3] of which Haldane was a member, he fought

3 The National Union of Scientific Workers (NUSW) hoped to represent the economic interest of a large and growing body of applied scientists. It was determined to secure for its members higher salaries, greater security of tenure, and more control over their jobs. The organization eschewed the strike as a weapon, but it was nonetheless quite militant; several pioneering negotiations with state agencies and other employers were achieved in the 1920s, although the organization collapsed in the world economic crisis after 1929.

back and won a major case against the university, protecting the rights of workers from institutional interference in their private life (Kevels 1995 [1985], 84). All these made him into an object of admiration, even if he remained rather aloof and had relatively few close friends.

In the 1920s, Haldane was not yet politicized. He did not want to leave his lab and had no desire to be involved in party politics. At that time, he felt that biologists did not have the data that would allow them to advise the government on controlling human behavior (Kevels 1995 [1985], 94). While denying that he was or ought to be politically engaged, Haldane did concede that he had a duty to preach to his audience about the *necessity of introducing the scientific attitude into politics*. He averred that the "nation's material basis is scientific, but its intellectual framework is pre-scientific." Although he acknowledged that it was impossible to predict how exactly "scientific knowledge is going to revolutionize human life," in 1924 he already had professed his belief that science "will continue to do so, and even more profoundly than I have suggested" (Haldane 1924, 80).

Haldane's main area of scientific research was population genetics. Along with Ronald Fisher and Sewell Wright, he developed the mathematical theory of natural selection that showed the direction and rates of changes of genes frequencies. Haldane was able to calculate the rate and effectiveness of selection for a character trait. While eugenics continued to fascinate him and others because of the dream of human biological improvement, Haldane's growing socialist leanings would lead him to warn against the misapplication of the science of heredity "to support the political opinions of the extreme right thereby rendering eugenics abhorrent to many democrats" (Werskey 1978, 97). As much as he disapproved of the misapplication of science, he also scolded those writers on eugenics who were not sufficiently versed in the science of heredity or who selectively manipulated scientific evidence to advance their social agenda. Haldane maintained that "in view of the demands for intellectual and manual skill in modern civilization it was an evil that the unskilled workers are breeding faster than the skilled classes, but the eugenicists were wrong to think that the best way of eradicating this evil was to prevent by force the less able part of the population for reproducing itself" (Kevels, 1995 [1985], 94). Haldane discouraged the marriage of first cousins and calculated that stopping such marriages would reduce all sorts of genetic defects, (ibid., 184), but he also believed that free and equal education and the abolition of hereditary wealth would create conditions for the betterment of the lower classes. He pushed for the removal of educational inequality and looked forward to the creation of a classless society where "far reaching eugenic measures could be enforced by the state with little injustice. Today this would not be possible" (Werskey 1978, 97). Haldane had much to say about eugenics in the ideal future society in his celebrated book *Daedalus, or*

Science and the Future (1924) where he couched the utopian vision of eugenics in scientific terms.

Daedalus is a remarkable futuristic essay that accurately predicts many of the developments of the late twentieth century. Instead of focusing on Prometheus, "the physical inventor" of Greek mythology, Haldane chose to focus on Daedalus, the first "biological inventor" – or, in our current parlance, the first genetic engineer – who oversaw the procreation of the Minotaur by arranging the coupling of Pasiphaë and the Cretan bull. Haldane reminds the reader that, whereas Prometheus was punished by the gods, Daedalus "was not punished in this world or in the next" but he was "exposed to the universal and age-long reprobation of a humanity to whom biological inventions are abhorrent" (1924, 49). Humans look at biological invention (i.e., engineering) as "indecent and unnatural," but Haldane observes that "biological invention then tends to being as a perversion and ends as a ritual supported by unquestioned beliefs and prejudiced" (ibid.). Contrasting himself to Huxley, "who could believe that while science might indeed remould traditional mythology, traditional morals are impregnable and sacrosanct to it," Haldane insisted that "we must learn not to take traditional morals too seriously," going even further to claim that "there can be no truce between science and religion" (ibid.). More removed from the values of Victorian England than was Huxley, Haldane adopted a thorough-going secularism and later made communism his secular religion, although in the 1950s, he would renounce socialism and, after settling in India, would be deeply interested in Hinduism.

Haldane's speculations on the scientific developments of the twentieth century are quite remarkable in their accuracy. His futuristic projects consist of the "gradual conquest of space and time" (Haldane 1924, 27) and include the invention of a "durable storage battery … that will enable us to transform the intermittent energy of the wind into continuous electric power" (ibid., 24). Chemistry would also transform human life, as Haldane predicts the creation of synthetic foods and the use of chemical substances for performance enhancement (ibid., 35). Human reproduction, too, will see profound changes as ectogenesis and planned breeding become universal. He reasons that "if reproduction is once completely separated from sexual love, mankind will be free in an altogether new way" (ibid., 68), echoing his own struggle for sexual emancipation.[4] He admits that "this will involve an operation which is somewhat unpleasant," but it will be "an honour" to the "ectogenetic mother" because in planned breeding only the best should reproduce. Advances in biology, Haldane went on to speculate, will bring

4 The fact that Haldane was childless in both his marriages sheds an interesting light about his speculations on the production of "test-tube babies" and his qualified support for eugenics.

about “progress in medicine” that will focus human attention not on “good death” (as Christianity has done for centuries) but “more and more on a good life” (ibid., 54). Future science will bring about “the abolition of disease,” which, in turn, “will make death a physiological event like sleep” (ibid., 73). His reflection on the relationship between science and arts is most interesting. On the one hand, he was “absolutely convinced that science is vastly more stimulating to the imagination than the classics,” but on the other hand, he observed that “the products of this stimulus do not normally see the light because scientific men as a class are devoid of any perception of literary form” (Haldane 1924, 29). He lamented the “defective education of the artists” and recommended that we “educate our poets and artists in science” and “educate our masters, labour and capital, in art” (ibid., 30).

The publication of *Daedalus* made Haldane a famous man; it sold over 15,000 copies. However, with his maturation over the years, his exuberant irreverence changed. In the 1930s, when Haldane became more involved with socialist and communist circles, he began to express dissatisfaction with unchecked eugenics. In “Possibility of Human Evolution,” while he stressed the importance of implementing eugenics policies if human beings are to overcome nature by becoming masters of their own evolution, he also argued that eugenics should not be taken too far. He averred that “the effort to eliminate all sorts of ‘Unfit’ human types is [a] very much more dubious proposition” because “many of the ‘unfit’ are unfit for society as it is today, but that is often society’s fault. The attempt to prevent them from breeding really involves the appalling assumption that society as at present constituted is perfect, and that our only task is to fit men to it.” As he moved leftward politically, he came to endorse social engineering, through education as opposed to planned breeding.

Haldane’s “conversion” to communism came gradually. In the 1920s, he had high hopes for the Labour movement, but by the end of the decade, he reversed his judgment and did not see how the ruling class would ever be able to understand enough about technology to make nationalized industries work. Conversely, he did not believe that socialist politicians, once in power, could command the loyalties of his scientific colleagues. In the 1930s, Haldane moved further to the Left. If in 1932, when he turned 40, he saw himself merely as progressive, in 1938 he declared himself a Marxist, although not yet a member of the Communist Party, which he joined in 1940. The Spanish Civil War in 1936 clearly was a contributing factor: his stepson fought with the anti-Franco forces and died in combat. Haldane’s political transformation was beginning to take shape: he decided that Marxism was true and that the prospects of achieving socialism in Britain without recourse to violent revolution were growing slimmer every year. He came to see communism as the antithesis rather than apotheosis of bourgeois liberalism and considered communism alone as the proper response to the menace of Nazism. In 1940, he joined the Communist Party and began to write his influential science column in the *Daily Worker*, teaching millions of readers how science could improve the human condition. In time, Haldane became one of the editors of the *Daily Worker* but resigned in 1954 when his infatuation with communism finally came to an end. The Lysenko affair in 1947 and Trofim Lysenko's persecution of Russian geneticist Sergei Vavilov in the early 1950s eventually led Haldane to dissociate himself from the Communist Party, even though he was reluctant to criticize Lysenko in public and believed that some of Lysenko's views on inheritance of acquired traits could be proven scientifically (i.e., through mathematical calculations of population genetics) (Clark 1968, 190-91).

Disillusioned with communism as well as with the British government's conduct in the Suez Canal Crisis of 1956, Haldane and his second wife, Helen Spurway – a physicist whose career Haldane worked hard to advance – settled in India where his socialist dreams were welcomed by the Nehru government. He headed the biometry unit at the Indian Statistical Institute and was deeply engaged in his research on human genetics and quantitative study of biology. Seeking inner peace, he became keenly interested in Hinduism, adopted vegetarianism, and became involved in an organization for the protection of animals. Haldane died in 1964 after having published several hundreds of popular essays about science, twenty-four books, and more than four hundred scientific papers. He wrote with passion about a number of social and scientific problems and often took ethics and philosophy, literature and art into consideration. Like Julian Huxley, a solid classical education at Oxford made him a humanist, but he was much more opposed to traditional religion than was Huxley. As a communist, he endorsed dialectical materialism, and some people see a connection between endorsement of materialism and his scientific work on the material basis of all life. His communist convictions made him deeply interested in bettering human life by employing science and technology, and he believed that human progress moves the species to transcend biological limitations. While Huxley was the "prophet" of transhumanism, Haldane's rebellion against traditional mores, his faith in biological engineering, and his speculations about human-brain interface capture the irreverent style of the transhumanist movement, although few transhumanists possess the literary breadth of Haldane or his depth of coverage of many branches of science – physiology, biochemistry, biometry, cosmology, statistical methodology, and all aspects of genetics (e.g., see Haldane 1964).

J. D. Bernal: Communism, Science, and the Betterment of Humanity

If Haldane speculated about the role of science in the future engineering of humanity, the person who contributed most to the professionalization of science and its cultural centrality was John Desmond Bernal. Bernal was a "fascinating, memorable and extraordinarily impressive" man; if not a genius, he was at least a uniquely gifted man (Hobsbawm 1999, ix.). Although Bernal did not receive the Nobel Prize in crystallography, he inspired several Nobel laureates (e.g., Dorothy Crowfoot Hodgkin, Max Perutz, and Maurice Wilkins), and two other Nobel laureates (Francis Crick and Aaron Klug) went out of their way to work at his lab. Despite his unusually creative mind and outstanding scientific breadth, he did not attain the highest distinction in science, partly because he spread himself too thin and partly because he devoted too much energy to local, national, and international politics. Like Haldane, who, as mentioned, served as the model for the character in Aldous Huxley's *Antic Hills*, Bernal inspired the lead character in C. P. Snow's novel *The Search* (1934). Bernal's personal charm, enthusiasm, piercing intelligence, inexhaustible energy, and unconventional approach to sexuality made him an irresistible figure, very much like Haldane, but he was more controversial than Haldane because of his refusal to distance himself from the USSR, even after the atrocities of the Stalinist regime were exposed, and because of his totally unconventional sex life. Although he was legally married, Bernal believed in sexual freedom and had children with other women, with whom he lived for extended periods without divorcing his legal wife.

Bernal was born in Ireland to Samuel Bernal, Catholic father of a Sephardic, converso descent and Elizabeth (Bessie) Miller, an American Protestant mother, one of the first females to enter Stanford University in 1891, although she did not graduate with a degree. His parents met in 1898 in Belgium where Bessie was traveling by bicycle for six months with her brother Jonathan (Brown 2005, 2). The Catholic Bernal family was quite an anomaly among the Anglo-Irish Protestant landowners of Tipperary, but it was the mother's social charm and intellect that made their life socially manageable. John Desmond (who was called Desmond by those close to him) grew up a devout Catholic and, from a very young age, was attracted to the physical world of nature. Desmond and his brother Kevin were sent to English boarding schools; the first two schools were unhappy experiences for the Bernal boys, but the Bedford School in the English Midlands (which Bernal entered in October 1914) proved a good place. He began to exhibit a deep passion for science at the expense of the conventional study of the classics and graduated from the school with a scholarship to Emmanuel College in Cambridge, which he entered in 1919 and graduated from in 1923 with work on minerals that used X-ray techniques to understand the arrangement of atoms in molecules.

During his undergraduate years at Cambridge, Bernal was politicized and gradually substituted his devotion to Catholicism with a passionate commitment to communism. At Cambridge, he also fell in love with Eileen Sprague, who introduced him to communist circles, and married her to the dismay of his mother. During the 1920s, "the Bernals seemed intent on proving that the sex life of a scientist could be as variegated and piquant as that of any painter of novelist" (Brown 2005, 56). They had a sort of open marriage and in addition to the two children with Eileen, Bernal would sire a son with another woman, Margaret Gardiner – Martin Bernal (who would later become an important historian of the ancient world) – and a daughter with yet another lover, Margot Heinemann. Along with the legal wife and the two mistresses, there was a long list of female attachments, many of whom were much younger than Bernal and often research assistants who worked in his lab. Although Bernal believed in equality between the sexes and treated the women in his lab much better than was the norm at the time (Hobsbawm 1999, 235-54), his practice of "sexual varietism," as he called it, would be considered exploitative and unacceptable by current feminist standards.

Like Haldane, Bernal was a social rebel, but unlike Haldane, Bernal's commitment to communism came earlier and lasted throughout his life. Bernal and Eileen joined the CPGB in 1923, shortly after they moved from Cambridge to London. Because the Communist Party in those days had no specific role for intellectuals in its rank, Bernal was much more active in the Holborn Labour Party, which had a particularly active, left-wing constituency, albeit divided by internal disputes and factionalism (Brown 2005, 22-24). In 1927, the Bernals moved back to Cambridge, and although Bernal's membership in the party had lapsed, a personal friend, Magda Phillips, recruited him back to the Communist Party in 1933. He remained attached to the party for the rest of his life, even though he did not carry a card (which was decided by the party). For Bernal, science and communism would emerge as two sides of the same coin: science was communism, and communism was science.

During the 1930s, Bernal played a central role in the political radicalization and mobilization of British scientists, as Marxism began to have significant impact on the natural sciences. He was the most prominent and long-lasting convert to communism among the significant scientists in Britain, many of whom were associated with the Cavendish Laboratory of Cambridge and the Cambridge Scientists Anti-War Group established in 1934, a major group of political militants among the young scientists of Cambridge (Rose and Rose 1999). These scientists were part of a reformist movement current in science who pressed for greater recognition of the social implications of science, greater scientific planning, and a greater role for science in political decision making. The antiwar scientists of the 1930s warned against the danger of aerial, chemical, and biological warfare, which they correctly predicted would be directed against noncombatants. Bernal deeply believed in trade unions and joined the NUSW in 1924 as part of his campaign to improve the wages and social conditions of scientific researchers. He helped organize the Cambridge Branch of the Association of Scientific Workers, which the NUSW had become. Due to his efforts, the organization would grow to from 1,000 to 17,000 members, and Bernal would become its president in 1949.

Political radicalization in the interwar years did not necessarily mean acceptance of Marxist ideology of scientific socialism as worthy of serious consideration. Bertrand Russell, for example, dismissed scientific socialism as philosophical quackery. Yet like J.B.S. Haldane and Joseph Needham, Bernal was most attracted to Friedrich Engels's *Dialectics of Nature*, which was published for the first time in 1927 and appeared in an English translation only in 1940, with an introduction by Haldane. Other works by Engels were available in English, leading Bernal in 1937 to publish his essay "Dialectical Materialism and Modern Science" in the Marxist journal *Science and Society*. Engels anticipated and welcomed the rupture in the framework of classical physics, recognized that the discovery of a single basic unit of life made possible the analysis of living organisms and systems of increasing complexity, and understood that diachronicity – that is, history – inevitably entered the sciences with the theory of evolution (Hobsbawm 1999, xvi). Engels's dialectical materialism not only offered a historical perspective on the processes of change and transformation, but it also justified the efforts of biologists such as Haldane and Needham to apply experiments and suitable mathematical modeling to the analysis of complex and essentially nonmechanical organisms and systems. Dialectical materialism appeared to offer a philosophical vision of the totality of the phenomena in nature that allow for both unity and limitless diversity, a theory of everything that was not mechanically reductionist. Like his friends Haldane, Huxley, and Needham, Bernal adopted an interdisciplinary or transdisciplinary outlook: he integrated science and the arts, as did Needham; Haldane combined science with philosophy, history, and political science; and Huxley mixed science, philosophy, and literature.

Following in Haldane's footsteps, Bernal also fantasized about the future where science would transform all aspects of social life and would replace religion as the dominant social force. Even more radical than Haldane's *Daedalus*, Bernal's *The World, The Flesh and the Devil: An Enquiry into the Future of the Three Enemies of the Rational Soul* expressed total commitment to science, a faith in science that can be described as secularized religious devotion. Indeed, for Bernal, "now that religion gives place to science, the paradisical future of the soul fades before the Utopian future of the species, and still the future rules." And the future concerns not only "man and his desires" but "blindly and inexorably ... the whole universe of space and time" (Bernal 1969 [1929], 3). The subtitle of the work reveals Bernal's secularized outlook: only through science (the new secularized religion) can humanity overcome the three enemies of the rational soul: "the obstacle of the physical environment, the limitations of our cellular fabric, and the darker aspects of our characters" (Brown 2005, 70). Bernal's futuristic essay argued that the three disciplines that would enable humanity to unravel the complexities of the future are history ("a storehouse of illustrative facts"), the physical sciences (a way of comprehending the whole universe of space and time), and psychology (the science of human cognition and desires).

Going beyond the short-term problem of scarcity and poverty, which were the paramount concerns of leftist circles, Bernal concerned himself with the long-term perspective for the human species. The discoveries of the nineteenth century brought about "a macro-mechanical age of power and metal, enabling humans to control the forces of nature and eventually substitute steam and electrical power in place of muscle energy" (Bernal, 1969 [1929], 11). The new discoveries in "the micro-mechanics of the Quantum Theory which touch on the nature of matter itself, are far more fundamental and must in time produce far more important results" (ibid., 12). Bernal's prediction was based on the rapid advances in quantum mechanics during the 1920s, and his ideas expressed not only deep faith in the ability of science to change the human environment but also the yearning of human beings to transcend biological and physical limitations.

In *The World, the Flesh, and the Devil*, Bernal identified "the need to acquire sufficient acceleration to escape the earth's gravitational field as the major barrier to extra-planetary travel" (Brown 2005, 71) and surmised that "the most effective method is based on the principle of the rocket" (Bernal 1969 [1929], 15). He contemplated space travel and colonization (including manned travel to the moon), considered using an airplane as an alternative to rocket power to escape the earth's gravitational pull, and even mused about "building a permanent home for men in space" (ibid., 18), admitting that a "gravitationless way of living is very difficult for us to imagine, but there is no reason to suppose that we would not ultimately adjust to it" (ibid., 22). In other words, Bernal contemplated the future transformation of the human form and believed that, in the future, "man himself must actively interfere in his own making and interfere in a highly unnatural manner" (ibid., 30). For this reason, he supported the eugenics movement; indeed "the eugenists and apostles of healthy life, may, in a very considerable course of time, realize the full potentialities of the species" (ibid.).

The central organ in the future transformation of humanity is the brain. In Bernal's schema, the brain would no longer be housed in a skull but in a rigid, lightweight cylinder, under optimal conditions. If new sense organs could be wired into the brain's circuitry, then a direct connection could be made with the brain of another "person," setting up neural networks that would permit the perfect transference of thought. Humans would acquire new "increased faculties" as their brains and their bodies would function in "television apparatus, tele-acoustic and tele-chemical organs and tele-sensory organs of the nature of touch for determining all forms of texture bodies" (Bernal 1969 [1929], 41). Although he admits that "the new man must appear to those who have not contemplated him before as a strange, monstrous, and inhuman creature" (ibid.), he considers the "mechanical man" to be the end of "normal man" who has reached "an evolutionary dead-end." The mechanical man only appears to be "a break in organic evolution" but "is actually more in the true tradition of a further evolution" (ibid., 42). Like Huxley, Bernal saw the "new man" as the logical outcome of the immense, still largely unrealized possibilities of the human brain. In the future, Bernal predicted, "connections between two or more minds would tend to become a more and more permanent condition until they functioned as dual or multiple organisms" (ibid.). Bernal made clear his own preference for a society of interlinked disembodied minds devoted to the pursuit of research and control of the universe, although he also envisioned division of labor between "the different individuals of a compound mind [who] would not all have similar functions or even be of the same rank of importance. … Thus would grow up a hierarchy of minds that would be more truly a complex than a compound mind" (ibid., 44). His youthful scientific fantasy predicted many of the technological developments of the second half of the twentieth century, and he would have been very pleased with the advances in space travel accomplished in the late twentieth century and also with the role of computers, information technology, and artificial intelligence, all of which have realized the dream of a new humanity and a new, manufactured, artificial life.

Like Haldane, Bernal foresaw the development in synthetic materials and industrial technology, but his prophetic technological forecasting is bolder and more accurate. More than any other scientist of his generation, he was aware of the new implications of scientific discoveries in relation to biology as well as to physics, and his approach drastically contrasted with that of Sigmund Freud. Bernal pondered the future of feeling and speculated that feelings would be produced and controlled by physical substances. He also forecasted that "feeling would truly communicate itself, memories would be held in common and yet in all this, identity and continuity of individual development would not be lost" (Bernal 1969 [1929], 54). He took seriously the possibility that future humanity would be divided between "one section which colonizes space and pursues the scientific enterprise to the ultimate, and the other – 'the old mankind' which would be left in undisputed possession of the earth, to be regarded by the habitants of the celestial spheres with a curious reverence" (ibid., 73). For Bernal, this prospect would satisfy scientists with their unending quest for knowledge and experience, including observation of the "human zoo" on earth, which would be "so well-managed that the inhabitants would not even be aware of it" (ibid.).

Bernal's "ode to science," so to speak, was no mere musing of a young scientist but the outline of his life-long championing of the role science must play in the betterment of humanity. In 1938, he accepted an invitation to head the Physics Department at Birkbeck College of the University of London, and remained there until the end of his academic career in 1968. A year after he arrived at Birkbeck and a decade after he published his futuristic essay, Bernal published his highly influential work *The Social Function of Science* (1939).[5] The book is divided into two parts: Part I ("What Science Does") describes the place of science in a capitalist society and demonstrates the inadequacies and shortcomings of the organization and management of science in such a world. This was the first analysis of research and development in economic terms. His critical analysis of the use and misuse of science and technology in Britain and in other countries provided the basis for what would become known as "science policy" and "technology policy," which did not yet exist in the 1930s (Freeman 1999, 119). Science policy came into its own only during World War II, and Bernal was instrumental in the efforts to harness science, technology, and large-scale planning to win the war against Germany.

In Part II of the book ("What Science Could Do"), Bernal offers prescriptive reflections about the importance of the social implications and applications of any branch of knowledge. His major concern was to define how to use science more effectively for human welfare, and his prescriptions were shaped by his communist commitment. He believed that the Soviets led the world in measurement of economic activities and their government used scientific analysis in its social policies. Here he argued for a massive increase in the scale of commitment of resources to research and other scientific activities. For Bernal, only socialist planning could rectify the gross underinvestment in science and technology, serious misallocation of resources, and inefficiency of the system. He did not simply contrast "private" and "public" science or argue that public operation and responsibility were somehow better; rather, he contrasted an idealized model of social planning with the private and public decision making of a capitalist and mixed economy. Because he identified the idealist mode of socialist planning with the actual working of the science-technology system in the USSR, his analysis is seriously flawed, especially in retrospect.

During the war, Bernal placed his scientific expertise in the service of the state, but his pro-Soviet stance made him a very controversial figure. In the postwar years, back at Birkbeck, Bernal was deeply concerned with building prefabricated homes with the use of novel materials and continued to champion the role of science in the betterment of human life worldwide. It was due to Bernal that "Scientific" was added to the title UNESCO. After the war, Bernal increasingly

---

5 An excellent summary of this book's main theme is offered in Chris Freeman's essay (1999).

devoted his energy to international peace efforts, mostly in Soviet-sponsored organizations, which earned him the nickname "The Sage." In 1946, the Association of Scientific Workers organized a conference on "Science and the Welfare of Mankind," and British scientists, including Bernal, expounded their views about the social and ethical responsibilities of science. The conference voted to establish the World Federation of Scientific Workers, with Bernal as its vice president.

Bernal continued to play on the international scene through the 1950s, especially within the framework of the Soviet-sponsored World Peace Council, but his intellectual reputation was tarnished greatly during the Lysenko affair, where he clashed with Julian Huxley, who had denounced Lysenko's theories. Bernal believed that Lysenko's theories and achievements were rooted in practical agriculture and refused to recognize the injustices that Lysenko's theories inflicted on the scientific community in the USSR. He continued to hail Stalin as a great scientist, even in his eulogy for the dictator (Bernal 1958). Bernal was a frequent visitor to the USSR in the years after the war, and after Stalin's death, he was closely associated with Nikita Khrushchev, as well as with the leaders of Communist China, Mao Zedong and Jhou Enlai (Brown 2005, 383-411). As a scientific envoy, Bernal tried to bridge the growing gap between Russia and China and was mainly concerned with scientific collaboration as a means to create a peaceful world. He summarized his vision in *World without War* (1958). Deeply committed to the principle of nuclear disarmament, Bernal always harped on his favorite theme: "the obstacles a new arms race would present to humanity's chance to benefit from scientific cooperation" (Montague 1999, 218).

Bernal's legacy for transhumanism is unmistakable. As Eric Hobsbawm succinctly put it, Bernal "was the most influential prophet of the unlimited potential of science for progress and therefore of the transformation of science and scientists into a recognized, publicly structured and funded force of production" (1999, xi). Bernal's insistence on the social function of science goes to the heart of the transhumanist outlook. For him, science is the most important activity of human beings, both short term and long term; science is its own justification, a specialized activity of a social group – the scientific community – which has a dual function: "to keep the world going as an efficient food and comfort machine, and to worry out the secrets of nature for themselves." Today, the world may be run by scientific experts even more than in Bernal's day. He believed that, as the world would become more rational and the use of brute force would diminish, real sovereignty would shift from nations to advisory bodies composed of scientists. Due to science, the immediate problems of the world (e.g., hunger, poverty, and disease) would be solved relatively quickly, freeing humanity to pursue other goals. Scarcely anything would ultimately be beyond the powers of organized scientific intelligence; even "the motions of the stars and living things could be directed." For the communist Bernal, God might not exist, but science had become God.

Transhumanists share Bernal's deep faith in science and laud his ability to forecast successfully many of the developments of the late twentieth century, even though they do not share his belief in "Communism as an inevitable consequence of the scientific and technological revolution" (Rose and Rose 1999, 137). To the extent that transhumanism is politically oriented, its leading thinkers (e.g., James Hughes and Nick Bostrom) endorse liberal democracy and leave decisions about genetic engineering in the hands of rational individuals. They maintain that the democratic process itself is the best context within which to sort out the debate about the enhancement of humanity.

Conclusion: Why Transhumanism Matters

Transhumanist ideology has generated organizations, literary documents, conferences, and even aesthetics.[6] Although the number of people formally associated with the World Transhumanist Organization is very small (only several thousand), it is a mistake to dismiss transhumanism as intellectually inconsequential. Transhumanism captures profound trends in contemporary society and culture as a result of acceleration of scientific knowledge and concomitant technological advances. By highlighting the indebtedness of transhumaism to the legacy of Julian Huxley, J.B.S. Haldane, and J. D. Bernal this essay does not wish to dismiss transhumanism as unoriginal or lacking in novelty but rather to offer some depth for the key themes of contemporary transhumanism: the notion that humanity is at the early phase of its evolutionary process, a notion that comes mainly from Huxley; the emphasis on the human capacity to engineer its material environment and itself; the belief that the salvation of humanity can come only from science and technology; and the fascination with the emergence of collective intelligence that will actualize the immense and yet largely untapped potential of the human mind.

Given recent developments in genomic, robotics, artificial intelligence, and nanotechnology, these ideas are no longer mere fantasies or musings that belong to the genre of science fiction (Hayles 1999). Rather, they have become a reality. To a great extent, we already live in a transhumanist world because we use science and technology to enhance human mental and physical abilities and aptitudes, and we

6 Natasha Vita-More has attempted to articulate a transhumanist aesthetics in her various public talks and exhibits, but she is yet to produce her vision in a full-length book. Nevertheless, her claim that Second Life, the virtual social network, expresses the distinct aesthetics of transhumanism is convincing.

try to ameliorate undesirable aspects of the human condition, especially the pain and suffering associated with aging and death. In other words, in the contemporary world of the early twentieth-first century, the human has become a design project, a piece of machinery to be tinkered with and fixed technologically. The question is not whether we want to be transhuman but rather what kind of society we wish to have given the centrality of science and technology that call on us to transcend our biological limitations and give rise to new type of a human being, the enhanced human. In the current, ambiguous state of affairs, we must engage transhumanism in a deep discussion about the feasibility as well as the desirability of our actions, or else we will abandon our responsibility, our moral duty to ourselves and to future generations.

If the prophets of transhumanism were alive today, they would be very pleased with the scientific, technological, and biomedical developments of the last four decades. However, it is also reasonable to assume that these three intellectuals would have been able to conduct the public debate about transhumanism with depth and dignity, which are sometimes missing in the current public discourse. Unlike their contemporary heirs, the three British scientists had deep respect for the humanities as expressions of the human personality. To address the transhumanist vision of and for humanity requires us to consider all aspects of being human, including values such as empathy, care, compassion, and love, which transhumanists tend to forget because they place so much faith in technology, artificial intelligence, or rational utilitarian calculus. Whether we engage transhumanism critically or approvingly, whether we think that transhumanism is the "most dangerous idea" or the best hope for humanity, we need to conduct our discourse with erudition, sensitivity, and deep concern for the well-being of human beings as they exist today: fallible, vulnerable, and mortal.

References

Allen, Garland E. 1992. Julian Huxley and the eugenical view of human evolution. In Waters and Van Helden, eds., *Julian Huxley*, 193-221.

Baker, J. R. 1978. *Julian Huxley: Scientist and Word Citizen 1887 to 1975*. Paris: UNESCO.

Beatty, John. 1992. Julian Huxley and the evolutionary synthesis. In Waters and Van Helden, eds., *Julian Huxley*, 181-92.

Bergson, Henri. 1984 [1911]. *Creative Evolution.* Translated by Arthur Mitchell. Lanham, MD: University Press of America.

Bernal, John Desmond. 1958. Stalin as scientist. *Modern Quarterly* 8: 133-42.

–. 1967 [1939]. *The Social Function of Science.* Cambridge, MA: MIT Press.

–. 1969 [1929]. *The World, The Flesh and the Devil: An Enquiry into the Future of the Three Enemies of the Rational Soul*. Bloomington: Indiana University Press.

Bostrom, Nick. 2005. A history of transhumanist thought. *Journal of Evolution and Technology* 14 (1): 1-25.

Brown, Andrew. 2005. *J. D. Bernal: The Sage of Science*. Oxford: Oxford University Press.

Calder, Ritchie. 1999. Bernal at war. In Swann and Aprahamian, eds. *J. D. Bernal*, 160-90.

Clark, Ronald William. 1968. *J.B.S.: The Life and Work of J.B.S. Haldane*. New York: Coward McCann, Inc.

Coenen, Christopher, et. al. 2009. *Human Enhancement: Study*. European Parliament (IPOL/A/STOA/2007-13; PE 417.483): http://www.itas.fzk.de/eng/etag/document/2009/coua09a.pdf; accessed July 7, 2011.

Dear, Peter, ed. 1997. *The Scientific Enterprise in Early Modern Europe: Readings from Isis*. Chicago: University of Chicago Press.

De Witt, Calvin. 1994. *Earth-wise: A Biblical Response to Environmental Issues*. Grand Rapids, MI: CRS.

Divall, Collin. 1992. From a Victorian to a modern: Julian Huxley and the English intellectual climate. In Waters and Van Helden, eds., *Julian Huxley*, 31-44.

Freeman, Chris. 1999. The social function of science. In Swann and Aprahamian, eds. *J.D. Bernal*, 101-31.

Galton, Francis. 1919. *Inquiries into Human Faculty and Its Development.* London: J.M. Dent & Co.; New York: E.P. Dutton & Co.

Goldberg, Steven. 2009. Does the wall stand? The implications of transhumanism for the separation of church and state. Paper delivered at Arizona State University, April 25, in a workshop on Transhumanism and Democracy: http://www.asu.edu/transhumanism.

Green, Ronald M. 2001. *The Human Embryo Research Debates: Bioethics in the Vortex of Controversy*. Oxford: Oxford University Press.

–. 2009. Bioethics and human betterment: Have we lost our ability to dream? In *Biotechnology: Our Future as Human Beings and Citizens*, edited by S.D. Sutton, 49-66. Albany: SUNY Press.

Haldane, J.B.S. 1924. *Daedalus: or Science and the Future*. New York: E.P. Dutton & Co.

–. 1964. *Science and Life: Essays of a Rationalist*. London: Pemberton Publishing.

Harris, John. 2007. *Enhancing Evolution: The Ethical Case for Making Better People*. Princeton, NJ: Princeton University Press.

Hayles, N. Katherine 1999. *How We Became Posthuman: Virtual Bodies in Cybernetics, Literature, and Informatics*. Chicago: University of Chicago Press.

Heil, Reinhard. 2010. Human Enhancement – Eine Motivsuche bei J.D. Bernal, J.B.S. Haldane und J.S. Huxley. In *Die Debatte über "Human Enchancement": Historische, philosophische und ethische Aspekte der technologischen Verbesserung des Menschen*, edited by Christopher Coenen, Stefan Gammel, Reinhard Heil, Andreas Wyke, 41-62. Bielfeld: Transcript Verlag.

Hobsbawm, Eric. 1999. Preface and Bernal at Birbeck. In Swann and Aprahamian, eds. J. D. Bernal, ix–xx and 235-54.

Holland, Suzanne, Karen Lebacqz, and Laurie Zoloth. 2001. *The Human Embryonic Stem Cell Debate: Science, Ethics, and Public Policy*. Cambridge, MA: MIT Press.

Huxley, Julian S. 1912. *The Individual in the Animal Kingdom.* Cambridge: G.P. Putnam's Sons.

–. 1931. *What Dare I Think?* London: Chatto & Windus.

–. 1934. *If I Were a Dictator*. London: Methuen.

–. 1942. *Evolution, the Modern Synthesis.* London: Allen and Unwin; 2d ed. New York: Harper, 1962.

–. 1957 [1927]. *Religion without Revelation*. London: Watts.

–. 1970-73. *Memories*. 2 vols. New York: Harper & Row.

–. 1971. *New Bottles for New Wine*. London: Chatto & Windus.

–. 1992 [1954]. *Evolutionary Humanism*, with Introduction by H. James Birx. Buffalo, NY: Prometheus Books.

Kass, Leon, and James Q. Wilson. 1998. *The Ethics of Human Cloning*. Washington, DC: AEI.

Kevels, Daniel. 1995 [1985]. *In the Name of Eugenics: Genetics and the Uses of Human Hereditary*. Cambridge, MA: Harvard University Press.

Krishna, Dronamraju R. 1993. *If I Am to Be Remembered: The Life and Work of Julian Huxley with Selected Correspondence*. Hackensack, NJ: World Scientific Publishing.

Larson, Edward J. 2004. *Evolution: The Remarkable History of a Scientific Theory*. New York: The Modern Library.

Lightman, Bernard. 1987. *The Origins of Agnostics: Victorian Unbelief and the Limits of Knowledge*. Baltimore, MD: The Johns Hopkins University Press.

McGee, Glenn. 1998. *The Human Cloning Debate*. Berkeley, CA: Berkeley Hills Books.

Mehlman, Maxwell J. 2003. *Wondergenes: Genetics Enhancement and the Future of Society*. Bloomington: Indiana University Press.

–. 2009. *The Price of Perfection: Individualism and Society in the Era of Biomedical Enhancement*. Baltimore, MD: Johns Hopkins University Press.

Montague, Igor. 1999. The Peacemonger. In Swann and Aprahamian, eds., *J.D. Bernal*, 212-25.

Provine, William. 1992. Progress in evolution and meaning in life. In Waterss and Van Helden, eds., *Julian Huxley.*

Rose, Hilary, and Steven Rose. 1999. Red scientists: Two strands from a life in three colours. In Swann and Aprahamian, eds., *J. D. Bernal*, 132-59.

Snow, C. P. 1964 [1959]. *The Two Cultures and a Second Look.* 2d ed. Cambridge: Cambridge University Press.

Steinhart, Eric. 2008. Teilhard de Chardin and transhumanism. *Journal of Evolution and Technology* 20 (1): 1-22.

Swann, Brenda, and Francis Aprahamian, eds. 1999. *J. D. Bernal: A Life in Science and Politics*. London and New York: Verso.

Tirosh-Samuelson, Hava, and Christian Wiese, eds. 2008. *The Legacy of Hans Jonas: Judaism and the Phenomenon of Life*. Boston and Leiden: Brill Academic Publishers.

Waters, C. Kenneth, and Albert Van Helden, eds. 1992. *Julian Huxley: Biologist and Statesman of Science*. Houston, TX: Rice University Press.

–. 1992. Introduction: Revising our picture of Julian Huxley. In Waters and Van Helden, eds., *Julian Huxley.*

Werskey, Gary. 1978. *The Visible College: The Collective Biography of British Scientific Socialists in the 1930s*. New York: Holt, Rinehart and Winston.

Wolin, Richard. 2008. Ethics after Auschwitz: Hans Jonas's notion of responsibility in a technological age. In Tirosh-Samuelson and Wiese, eds., *The Legacy of Hans Jonas: Judaism and the Phenomenon of Life*, 1-37.

Religion and the Technowonderland of Transhumanism

Linell E. Cady

Transhumanism is a slippery term. It was originally coined in the mid-twentieth century by Julian Huxley to capture the evolutionary possibilities of the human (Tirosh-Samuelson; see chapter 1 of this volume). Today it refers to the accelerating use of new sciences and technologies to engineer the human or, as some envision it, the posthuman, as enhancement technologies gain speed. It designates an ideology and movement pushing this project forward – symbolized in the uploading of the human into a computer. The lack of any clear line between therapy and enhancement and the need to redraw this boundary continually compound the interpretive and normative challenges of this accelerating trajectory. Impossible to ignore, should we celebrate, oppose, or simply resign ourselves to its advance?

Getting a handle on the perils and possibilities of transhumanism is made even more difficult by its positioning within the religion/secular framework that now deeply structures our imaginative and social worlds. Transhumanism epitomizes the power and potential of modern science and technology with its seductive promise of immortality or radical life extension achieved in and through human efforts rather than a transcendent divine being. In representing the apotheosis of science and technology and the irrelevance of a transcendent God, transhumanism positions itself as a secularist project that displaces religion.[1]

Its oppositional, often confrontational, relationship to religion is compounded by the politics of religion in American life in recent decades. A highly conservative variant of religion has dominated, trumping other more liberal interpretations of religious traditions in American public life. Not only opposed to transhumanism, the conservative religious camp typically denounces stem-cell research, cloning, and even the evolutionary premises that underlie the modern biological sciences (De Gette 2008).[2] These dynamics reinforce a picture of a deep cleavage between the religious and secular domains, lending further support to the secularist presumption and conservative religious anxiety that scientific progress is inversely correlated with religious faith.

1 The belief that religion and transhumanism are antithetical is pervasive, though some advocate a more dialogic approach: Campbell and Walker 2005; Maher and Mercer 2009; Hefner 2003; Hopkins 2005.

2 A 2006 survey released by the Pew Research Center found 42 percent of respondents "directly rejected evolution, choosing the option that humans and other living things have existed in their present form since the creation." See Keeter, Masci, and Smith (2007).

The problems with this picture are many. The cultural work of the religion/secular binary lends transhumanism the mantle of the modern, the rational, and the progressive, positioning religion as its antiquated, superstitious, and regressive opponent. Through the work of this oppositional construction, transhumanism too readily secures the legitimating credentials of an empirically grounded objective science. What is so thoroughly obscured in and through this framing is any sense of the religiosity of the transhumanist project itself or, as David Noble (1997) succinctly puts it, "the religion of technology." The modern tendency to imagine religion and secular science as fully separate or antithetical blinds us to their fusions in the Western tradition. For the past millennia, as Noble compellingly argues, technology has been "increasingly invested with spiritual significance and a transcendent meaning" (1997, 6). It has come to function as a secularized eschatology, driven by a quest for salvation. But the oppositional mapping of the religion/secular landscape has hidden this collusion of religion and technology and given unrestrained technological development a free pass.

The dominant picture of the religion/secular landscape and the politics of religion that it has spawned contribute to the perception among many that religious traditions lack the resources for negotiating the expanding transhumanist terrain. They appear to offer up blanket condemnations, employing theological visions that themselves seem to founder on the shoals of modern science and its transhumanist trajectories. The classic idea of a creator God, far from providing a compass, loses traction in this new terrain as the line between divine and human creativity blurs. Given the challenges of transhumanism to the Western theological vision, challenges that parallel those raised by Darwinian evolution over a century earlier, it is not always clear what resources, beyond denunciation, it offers to the dawning "age of enhancement" (Edmonds 2009).

In short, the cultural and intellectual work of the reigning religion/secular framework seriously compounds the interpretive and normative challenges of engaging transhumanism. It fosters an oppositional model in which transhumanism lays claim to the scientific secular, with the loudest religious voices, like the Lilliputians, shouting it down. This model conceals the religious dimensions that fuel the transhumanist project as it contributes to the presumption among many that the Western theological tradition stands fully indicted by this project, lacking any resources to navigate its currents.

This chapter seeks to illuminate the operation of the conventional model of the religion/secular framework in relationship to transhumanism and to move past its imaginative constraints. To capture the dynamics of the oppositional rendering of the religion/secular dyad within transhumanism, I will explore the writings of two of its prominent advocates: Nick Bostrom and William Sims Bainbridge. Academics who have written extensively on transhumanism, both are deeply involved in the institutional embodiment and advancement of this project. Their rhetorical positioning of transhumanism in relationship to the religion/secular classification is representative of the movement as a whole. Their bifurcated and supercessionary take on this conceptual pair is commonly taken as a universal template that maps seamlessly onto the world. In so doing, it not only fosters an essentialized and static reading of the terms, but it blocks from view alternative alignments between the religious and the secular. Prominent antisecularist religious voices offer up similarly bifurcated models, a mirror image that simply reinforces rather than undermines the dominant model. For both interpretive and normative purposes, it is essential to develop a more expansive take on the religious and secular divide and to recognize that the reigning model is one among many variations, one that has lost its emancipatory edge.

To open up space to think differently about this classification, I propose to read it through the lens of the contrast between the immanent and the transcendent, a distinction with which it is intertwined though not identical. This interpretive angle, as the works of Mark C. Taylor (2007) and Charles Taylor (2007) make clear, offers a fresh perspective on the now deeply entrenched religion/secular divide. It provides a vantage point on the Western theological tradition that discloses a broader spectrum of perspectives. In so doing, it provides a more illuminating framework for getting a handle on the challenges of transhumanism. My interest in this essay, then, is not in delving into the moral complexities of a single technological enhancement under the transhumanist umbrella but in reflecting on the broader narrative frameworks within which this ideology and movement are located.[3]

We are living at a time when the boundaries between religion and science are fraught and conflicted – clearly on display in the debates swirling around transhumanism.[4] The politics of the day push us toward exclusionary alternatives, as if we must side with transhumanism against religion or with religious faith against an antireligious science and technology. In this essay, I resist both alternatives, seeking a more nuanced position that neither simply denounces nor

3 In so doing, I am pursing the second of the two directions that Julian Savulescu and Nick Bostrom advocate in their introduction to *Human Enhancement*: zooming in on particular enhancements and zooming out to consider it in broader "big-picture" ways. They rightly argue that both approaches are essential and represent "coexisting intellectual frontiers" (Savulescu and Bostrom 2009, 19-20).

4 The public perception of perennial conflict between religion and science is widespread and pushed by the writings of popular writers such Richard Dawkins (2006) and Sam Harris (2004). Scholars typically identify a range of relations of religion and science, tracing the conflict model to developments in the nineteenth century. See Barbour (1997), Brooke and Cantor (1998), Brooke (2005).

celebrates the transhumanist project. There are resources in the Western theological tradition for the interpretive and normative engagement with transhumanism, though the encounter, as we shall see, is critically transformative for both.

Transhumanism as Ideology and Movement

The imaginings and longings of transhumanism to transcend the limitations and mortality of the body can be traced back through millennia. But these musings and desires expressed in philosophical, religious, and literary writings did not coalesce into transhumanism until scientific and technological advances brought them within tantalizing reach of being realized – at least in the eyes of some. In the past fifty years, developments in nanotechnology, biotechnology, information technology, and cognitive science, and their increasing convergence, have unleashed utopian expectations that humanity might be on the cusp of curing disease, radically extending the life cycle, perhaps even achieving immorality. Transhumanism, as one of its champions proclaims, is the "passionate belief in the transcendence of human limitations – not through religion or politics, but through *science* – product of the rational mind in the technowonderland of the modern world" (Young 2006, 6).

Only in the past two decades has this broadly diffused vision become, with the help of the Internet, a self-conscious global movement, with increasing publications, organizing, and efforts at institutionalization. These include the 1988 founding of the Extropy Institute, followed a decade later by the formation of the World Transhumanist Association (WTA) and the Italian Transhumanist Association. Each has issued a declaration or manifesto setting out its basic philosophy and principles. The movement's momentum is further evident in the recent media blitz surrounding the release of the documentary by the brilliant inventor and crusading transhumanist Raymond Kurzweil. Titled *Transcendent Man*, the film captures his inspiring life story and vision of the coming "singularity," the impending culmination of the exponential advance in technology and computing issuing in the transition to the posthuman age. In Kurzweil's futuristic vision "we will transcend all of the limitations of our biology" (Vance 2010).

Nick Bostrom and William Sims Bainbridge, key players in the institutionalization of this movement, provide an illuminating entry into its vision and values. Bostrom, an Oxford philosopher, cofounded the WTA, "the moderate and influential center" (Bainbridge 2007a) of this movement, which now boasts over five thousand members in more than one hundred countries (Hughes 2009). Recently, this organization renamed itself Humanity+, a strategic communications move foregrounding cognitive enhancement and human longevity, rather than engineering the posthuman (ibid.). Seeking to sustain the radical edge of the transhumanist movement, a breakaway group, including Bainbridge, regrouped under the rubric "Order of Cosmic Engineers" generating a new manifesto titled "Yes! To Transhumanism" (Blackford 2010). Exploring the positioning of transhumanism in relation to the religion/secular boundary in these two figures sheds light on the rhetorical framing through which this movement is commonly advanced.

Bostrom positions this movement within the Western humanist tradition as it took shape in Renaissance and Enlightenment thinking. The decisive shifts were a move away from "medieval otherworldliness" and the rise of "science and critical reasoning – rather than revelation and religious authority" as the keys to understanding nature and human life (Bostrom 2003). Transhumanism is akin to religion in offering a sense of direction and purpose, but for Bostrom, its differences are momentous: "transhumanists seek to make their dreams come true in *this* world, by relying not on supernatural powers or divine intervention but on rational thinking and empiricism, through continued scientific, technological, economic, and human development" (ibid.). The utopian dimensions of religion – whether captured through visions of immortality, heaven, or eschatology – are brought down to earth and under human control. What used to be the "exclusive thunder of the religious institutions, such as very long lifespan, unfading bliss, and godlike intelligence" are now within our grasp (ibid., 46).

Recognizing the critical need to evangelize on behalf of this movement if it is to take wing, Bostrom pens a "Letter from Utopia," designed to awaken desires to achieve the transhumanist vision (Bostrom 2008). His rhetorical strategy, borrowing from a religious playbook, is to cultivate memories of peak experiences or "bliss" that stand out from the mundane dimensions of living. These moments of "epiphany" never last, but they can, Bostrom promises, if we can summon the desire and will to take advantage of the utopian potential of modern science and technology. In such moments, we experience the "potential for a higher life," and he beseeches the reader to nurture this feeling, a feeling that is only a pale analogue of the transhumanist future that is "Beyond dreams. Beyond imagination." Bostrom also borrows standard religious tropes as points of contrast for the transhumanist trajectory: "At no point will you encounter a wall of blinding light. At no point will you have to jettison yourself over an end-of-the-world precipice" (ibid.). Echoes of the dominant narrative of modernity that envisions the secular, especially science, displacing magic and religion reverberate in the litany of practices that Bostrom invokes to track the transhumanist trajectory (Asad 2003; C. Taylor 2007): "You will not achieve this through any magic trick or hokum, nor by the power of wishful thinking, nor by semantic acrobatics, meditation, affirmation, or incantation" (Bostrom 2008). Humans have the power to *achieve* the fantastic visions of heaven that the religious imagination can only dream. Without discounting the difficulties and dangers along the way, Bostrom remains deeply optimistic: "To prevail will take your best science, your best technology, and your best politics" (ibid.).

A very similar discursive strategy characterizes Bainbridge's primary positioning of transhumanism in relationship to religion:

> Humanity is crossing an abyss on a tightrope. Behind us is the old world of religious faith that compensated wretched but fertile people for the misery in their lives. On the other side, if we can only reach it, is a new land where we no longer need to live by illusions. (Bainbridge 2007a, 247)

The rapidly emerging technologies hold out the promise that "humans could become like gods and in so doing may put conventional religion out of business" (ibid., 202). Working with a variant of the secularization narrative of modern progress, Bainbridge claims that "magic and religion arose in human culture as pseudosolutions to the problem of providing help when people were obligated but unable to offer real solutions" (Bainbridge 2005, 92). Science and technology, in his August Comte-like vision, replace magic and religion, accounting for the pervasive antagonism among the religiously affiliated to the "transhumanist heresy." In a deft though circular move to preserve the oppositional rendering of religion and technoscience and sustain his supercessionary narrative of their relationship, he paints religious orientations that embrace technology as "secularized forms of religion" (ibid.).

Both Bostrom and Bainbridge position transhumanism as a secular alternative to religion, an alternative that can actually deliver on its eschatological fantasies. They invoke a series of contrasts that work to create a bright line between secularism and religion and that consign the latter to a premodern past: reason replaces superstition; science replaces magic; reality replaces illusions. The human replaces God, with science and technology the vehicles for realizing heaven on earth. Transhumanism is the next chapter in the story of modern progress. Although displaced, religion is not absent. In claiming that transhumanism is superior to religion in its ability to achieve the ends of which religions only dream, they invoke its form and imagined aspirations to legitimate the transhumanist project. They assume, without arguing, that the traditional ends for which Western religions yearn, symbolized in God's kingdom or heaven, are equivalent to the transhumanist goals, including defeating illness, aging, and death and vastly expanding mental powers. In so doing, they exhibit the widespread belief that "'religion' and 'transcendence' can be equated" (Graham 2002, 76). Their case for transhumanism mines this very equation, at the same time that it proclaims transhumanism as a secular and successful alternative to religion, able to produce a realized eschatology rather than an endlessly deferred one.

The rhetorical strategies that both Bostrom and Bainbridge deploy to champion transhumanism draw primarily on the modern secularization narrative that envisions the differentiation of the various spheres of the market, science, and politics and the privatization if not demise of religion (Casanova 1994; Smith 2003). It is a story that envisions solid borders between these domains and effectively blocks from view the alliances and fusions that have marked their intersections on the ground. It has helped to ensure science's reputation as a pristine and thoroughly objective endeavor, hiding the ways in which scientific pursuits are "energized by emotions, motives, beliefs, and interests that transcend science. Such impulses can range from the petty and disreputable to the noble, quixotic, messianic, or marginally sane" (Slabbert 2010). The writings of transhumanists belong to a large and growing body of literature that Marilynne Robinson calls "parascience," a genre in which "some allusion to the science of the moment is used as the foundation for extrapolations and conclusions that fall far outside the broadest definitions of science" (Robinson 2010, 43). In so doing, this genre draws legitimacy from the separate-spheres model at the very same moment that it transgresses its boundaries, effectively demonstrating how to have your cake and eat it too.

Although the religious roots and inflections of technoscience are most commonly obscured by its positioning within secularism's polemic against religion, a revealing exception is evident in a secondary strand in Bainbridge's writing where he makes a case for a radical new religion of transhumanism. In his calls for a "galactic religion," Bainbridge the theologian shines a spotlight on the values that align with and fuel the transhumanist project. By daring to drop the parascientific facade that purports to be dealing with technoscience as such and to articulate the broader values and vision that animate the transhumanist project, Bainbridge makes explicit what is more commonly a subterranean current. His radical religion, which he dubs "the Cosmic Order," seeks to drive "traditional religions and retrograde cults from the field" (Bainbridge 2009). It furnishes the "transcendent motivations and perspectives" that Bainbridge believes are now needed to replenish the energy and resolve to actualize the transhumanist utopia. He fashions an updated iteration of the "religion of technology," one that is more explicitly post-Christian and committed to a posthuman future.

Bainbridge's theological aspirations are driven by his fear of the growing power of "retrograde religion" in influencing society and governments to ban the technological developments that are critical to the transhumanist project. For him, it is more than simply a worrisome trend. Although total war on traditional religion and conservative social forces is not yet mandated, Bainbridge is chillingly clear where his loyalties lie if, or perhaps better when, the time comes:

> A civilization that is not viable has no moral claim against efforts to create another. Any government that seeks to prevent technological transcendence thereby renders itself illegitimate. Clearly, many readers will not want to go very far along the line of this argument, but for sake of clarity I should state the conclusion: Well-intentioned people seeking to develop the means for transcendence of the current human condition have the right to defend themselves against any government or institution that seeks to prevent them. (Bainbridge 2007a, 224)

This passage strikingly captures the absolute value that Bainbridge places on technological transcendence. Noting that those who want "to develop banned technologies face a dilemma," he asks rhetorically, "Should they invest considerable efforts into a rational and respectable campaign to present their views, in hopes that open-minded policy leaders will refrain from instituting bans? Or should they sharpen their bayonets in preparation for total conflict against religion?" (ibid.). Bainbridge is no Rawlsian democrat.

Simultaneously playful and serious, Bainbridge's sketch of a galactic religion seeks to capture the vision and values that a singular commitment to the "transcendence of the current human condition" entails.[5] Notably, it dissolves the grounds and motivations for a shared identity of a universal humanity and its attendant moral constraints and obligations. It elevates in its stead the transhumanist vanguard. To evangelize to this elite cohort, to help them "keep faith," he contends that all those who contribute to the transhumanist future, but die before its realization, deserve immortality too. Future generations, the beneficiaries of the imagination and dedication of the early transhumanists, will owe them gratitude and more. He insists there is a "moral contract that obligates future generations to preserve and reanimate the personalities of the individuals who contributed to the development of the technologies and social institutions" leading to this transhumanist future (Bainbridge 2007b). Whether it is even feasible to upload human personalities as bits of information into computers, Bainbridge's new iteration of the religion of transcendence exposes the orienting vision that animates the more radical wing of the transhumanist project.

The freedom of the individual to pursue this new social order, to participate in its actualization, trumps and indeed provides the moral grounds to resist religious groups and governments who seek to block it. Bainbridge claims the moral high ground insofar as he insists that freedom is a universal right. As he puts it, "Transhumanism asserts that each individual has the right to become whatever

5 In 1992, Bainbridge joined the National Science Foundation (NSF) where he has held a variety of positions, including running the Artificial Intelligence and Human-Computer Interaction Program (Bainbridge 2007a). His influential positions and the significant funding that runs through the NSF preclude taking his reflections as merely the eccentric musings of an isolated thinker.

he or she wishes, so long as this does not compromise the equal rights of other people to become what they wish" (Bainbridge 2007a, 223). The utter ordinariness, indeed commonplace, appeal to the individual's right to self-determination in modern liberal societies makes it especially unsettling, and revealing, when embedded within the transhumanist project. Some, such as James Hughes (2004), seek to reign in the libertarian impulses that drive much of the transhumanist movement, with calls for democratic and more egalitarian policies. Although beyond the scope of this paper to explore, it is clearly a concern whether such brakes would actually work in a world where access to enhancements is as differentially available as is access to opportunities today. Far more likely, and ever more frightening, is the gradual shift to a new moral sensibility of precisely the sort that Bainbridge expresses, one in which the kinship and moral solidarity of the enhanced become ever more pronounced. With this turn, the danger is that the more egalitarian democratic sensibilities of a Hughes will appear increasingly quixotic, even utopian, in the neoliberal and technologically accelerating context of the twenty-first century. Bainbridge in his eccentric fashion captures the moral and political ramifications of a singular commitment to technological transcendence and serves as a cautionary tale for its overdetermined embrace.

In their articulation and defense of transhumanism, Bostrom and Bainbridge rely, primarily if not exclusively, on a dichotomous and supersessionary model of the religioous/secular classification that taps into the continuing power of the dominant secularization narrative. It is, as we have seen, a celebratory story that secularism tells of its own trajectory, from a superstitious and authoritarian religious past to a bright new world of reason, peace, and scientific progress. The transhumanists are providing another chapter to this story drawing from the same rhetorical well for their well-worn tropes and imagery but adding their own utopian twist to its ending. The oppositional model of religion and secular science fosters the conceit that these domains can be neatly separated; with that move, the politics and piety that inevitably shape scientific and technological endeavors are effaced. This polemical oppositional model is of a relatively recent vintage and, as we have seen, fails to capture any sense of the mutual aspirations fueling the religious and scientific imaginations in the Western tradition.

Bainbridge, although heavily invested in the conflict model of religion and science in his writings, recognizes the historical limitations of this picture, even more importantly its diminishing power to sustain and reinvigorate the transhumanist project. Insisting that "only a transcendent, impractical, radical religion can take us to the stars," he ventures into articulating its sacred core (Bainbridge 2009). It is a new sacred canopy for transcendent technological pursuits. Nor is Bainbridge its only practitioner. Jaron Lanier, who holds impeccable credentials within the world of technoscience, claims "what we are seeing is a new religion, expressed through an engineering culture" (Lanier 2010). Its animating vision consists of "ideas with tremendous currency in Silicon Valley; these are guiding principles, not just amusements, for many of the most influential technologists" (ibid.). It would be a mistake to dismiss these ideas as merely those of an isolated visionary or marginal fringe.

Beyond the Religion/Secular Divide

The lingering power of the modern secularization narrative with its model of religion and the secular as structural opposites continues to haunt our thinking. It is actively invoked in the rhetorical strategies of transhumanists, as well as in their religious critics who despair of humans "playing God" (Coady 2009). We often seem trapped by the dynamics of these alternatives that suggest a winner-take-all battle between distinct and contrasting pursuits. The relationship of religion and technoscience in the Western tradition, however, does not easily fit a simple conflict model, despite its evident rhetorical appeal within the transhumanist movement. Given the contentious politics at the border of religion and the secular, and the dichotomous and essentialized thinking that it spawns, it is critical to gain some leverage on these interpretive frames. To this end, I want to draw on the work of Mark C. Taylor (2007) who offers in his book *After God* a reading of the Western religious tradition through the polarity of immanence and transcendence.[6] His heuristic, elaborating on Paul Tillich's identification of the two dominant forms of philosophy of religion in Western culture, aims to track broad patterns that cut across domains in particular times and places rather than perpetuating the compartmentalized logic and isolated – and often polarized – discourses of separate spheres so evident in current ways of envisioning religion, science, and secularism.[7] Considering transhumanism in light of this polarity provides a fresh perspective on the movement and some helpful interpretive and normative tools for its engagement.

A typology of religion based on the interplay of the immanent and the transcendent in the Western Christian tradition offers a distinctively different perspec-

6 Taylor develops his typology primarily in light of the Western Christian tradition, though he suggests it has broader application, even beyond the parameters of the Western tradition. In this essay, I limit its use to developments within Western Christian traditions and cultures. For consideration of this issue in relationship to Charles Taylor's *A Secular Age* (2007) that explores the secular and secularization in the West through the distinction between the immanent and the transcendent, see Warner, Vanantwerpen, and Calhoun (2010).

7 Tillich (1964) identifies two dominant traditions, one Platonic and Augustinian and the other Aristotelian and Thomist.

tive on the modern discourses of religion and secularism. Rather than take their opposition at face value, this typology radically recasts their relations. It makes it possible to trace the religious genealogy of the distinction between religion and the secular to developments within Western religious traditions, primarily Christianity. It also makes it possible to recognize religion and the secular as a dyad constituting a distinctive formation, with its components working together. Making the case for the religious roots and inflections of secularism, Taylor argues that "modernity is a theological invention" that Martin Luther, influenced deeply by medieval nominalism, put into motion (M. Taylor 2007, 43; Milbank 1990). The signature feature of Luther's theology was a radical dualism between a transcendent and omnipotent God and a fallen world, with a primary accent on the individual standing alone before God. Luther's influence was clearly not limited to the religious domain; on the contrary, it helped to effect "a social, political, and economic revolution that continues to transform the world today" (M. Taylor 2007). Modern discourses on religion and secularism obscure this genealogy by reading secularism simplistically and polemically as simply not religion, a perspective facilitated by the deeply misleading assumption that religion can be confined to the private sphere or to its institutional forms of church, synagogue, or mosque. Effectively blocked is a recognition of the ways in which religious visions and values travel far beyond their primary institutional carriers giving shape to *varieties* of secular formations.

To escape from the politics and polemics of the religion/secular divide, Taylor identifies two dominant patterns, or schemata, in the Western Christian tradition that pivot on the polarity between immanence and transcendence. Although clothed in a variety of styles, the underlying patterns tend toward forms of monism or dualism that reflect different takes on the location of the sacred or the real, however symbolized. At one pole are "monisms in which the real is immanent, that is, in some way *present* here and now"; at the other pole are "dualisms in which the real is transcendent, that is *absent* or, more precisely, present elsewhere" (M. Taylor 2007, 297). The two models give rise to different takes on a set of related issues, including the nature of time and history, the relationship between the one and the many, identity and difference, and the form and paths to salvation. In Taylor's words,

> [t]he foundational principle of immanence entails a monistic scheme in which God, self and world are different manifestations or expressions of the same underlying reality. Transcendence shatters monism by introducing a radical Other, which forms the foundation of the principle of oppositional difference constitutive of every dualism. (M. Taylor 2007, 133)

Taylor reads the Western Christian tradition and its broader cultural contexts in terms of the dynamic alterations between these orientations or forms of religiosity. Rather than see them as static alternatives, as simply opposites, he underscores their dynamic relations, tensions, and at times reversals. When pushed to its far limit, "religiosity finally becomes indistinguishable from secularism, transcendence collapses into immanence, and dualism dissolves in monism" (ibid., 297). Recognizing these shifts allows us to see that secularization does not necessarily mean the decline of religion, as it has conventionally been understood, but its reconfiguration in new forms and places.[8]

There is something deeply inadequate about these formations, particularly in their purer iterations whether found in religion as such or beyond it in the domains of art, economics, or technology. As Mark Taylor puts it, they are "in different ways nihilistic. Dualism presupposes an otherworldliness that tends to devalue life in this world, and monism – however it is disguised – is so committed to the world as it is that every possibility of critical reflection and transformative practice disappears" (2007, 298). If the apocalyptic religious imagination that longs for the destruction of this world to usher in God's kingdom epitomizes one extreme, then the idea of life as an endless cycle of an eternal return represents the other. The normative challenge is to sustain their dynamic counterpoises, without devolving into one polarity or the other. From the early centuries of the Christian tradition, this challenge generated ideas and symbols to mediate between a transcendent God and the created order, evident, for example, in the ideas of the Incarnation and the Trinity. Although not stable or even fully coherent as worked out across the centuries, these related ideas hinted at what Taylor suggests is a third schemata only now coming into visibility.

Mark Taylor finds the resources to articulate the contours of a third schemata in the idea of complex adaptive systems that has emerged in recent decades within the biological sciences. This interpretive model rejects ontological dualisms, such as that between mind and body, spirit and matter, nature and culture, as it also rejects reductionisms that reduce wholes to their component parts. It articulates a thoroughly integrated vision of self-organizing, interactive systems. Each system or network is dynamically related to others, codependent and coemergent. Complex adaptive networks are, as Taylor puts it, "fractal – they display the same structure at every organizational level and in every operational phase,"

8 Recent genealogies of Western secularism capture its complex roots in and continuing relations with Christianity, precluding the simplistic view of the secular as simply not religion (Asad 2003; C. Taylor 2007). Charles Taylor locates secularizing developments within medieval religious reform movements. The secular continues to intersect in complex ways with Christian formations, but its emergence has also created space for more explicitly humanist and post-Christian options to flourish. Taylor compellingly argues that this variety, and the cross-pressures they exert, characterizes our secular age. For a comparative study of the varieties of secularism as they interface with diverse religious traditions in France, India, Turkey, and the United States, and more globally, see Cady and Hurd (2010).

undermining the sharp separations between biology, culture, and society (M. Taylor 2007, 21-22). In this picture humans are fundamentally embodied and embedded within interacting, contingent, and emergent processes at multiple levels. It is far removed from the modernist map that pictures the differentiated domains of nature, society, culture, and religion as neatly separated. The continued power of this modernist picture, in the face of developments in the sciences and technology, is perhaps the surprise. As Bruno Latour notes, "[T]he smallest AIDS virus takes you from sex to the unconscious, then to Africa, tissue cultures, DNA and San Francisco but the analysts, thinkers, journalists and decision-makers will slice the delicate network traced by the virus for you into tidy compartments where you will find only science, only economy, only social phenomena, only local news, only sentiment, only sex" (1993, 2). The challenge is to recognize that "all of culture and all of nature get churned up again every day" (ibid.), pointing to a network model that is integrated, dynamic, and open.

The third schemata of complex networks anchors the extreme tension between the immanent and the transcendent, countering the historical alterations that move toward forms of monism or dualism in the Western tradition. Neither monistic nor dualistic, this complex network scheme exposes the limitations of them both. In this model, the real or sacred is neither fully present nor absent. As Taylor puts it, "instead of present or deferred, the end is always emerging by forever withdrawing" (M. Taylor 2007, 41). Transcendence in this model is reconfigured, grounded in immanence that remains open to creative, transformative possibilities, an "imminent transcendence." The older conceptual vocabulary of immanence and transcendence loses traction within a model of integrated, dynamic processes that refuse reduction to either pole.

What light do these highly abstract patterns shed on the interpretive and normative challenges of transhumanism? The more expansive take on religion that informs Taylor's heuristic demolishes the rhetorical strategy through which transhumanists position and legitimate their movement as not-religion, thereby allowing them to invoke the objectivity of secularism in general and to trade on the cultural authority of science in particular. Through the prism of his typology, transhumanism presents as a form of religiosity that sacralizes the pursuit of transcendence. Pursuing this interpretive angle, Elaine Graham describes an "ideology of transcendence" that infuses technoscience, evident in a "will for transcendence of the flesh as an innate and universal trait, a drive to overcome physical and material reality and strive towards omnipotence, omniscience and immortality" (2002, 69). It is a dualistic vision blending Platonic and Christian themes that, as we have seen, invests humans with the power through technological advances to become like God, envisioned as a disembodied omnipotent, eternal spirit. What is important to underscore is that it is a particular take on transcendence, one that has been unmoored from its immanent grounding. As Graham writes, "[I]n its aspirations towards the logic of immortality, invulnerability and omniscience, transhumanism exposes its vestigial craving for a perfect transcendent world 'Apart, Beyond, Outside, Above' the messy contingencies of this one" (ibid., 174).[9] A recent article on mixed marriages between cryonic transhumanists – usually male – and their spouses captures well the existential feel of this spirituality to a nonbeliever. Commenting on her husband's desire to be preserved and stored upon death, one wife ruefully remarks, "To plan to be rocketed into the future – a future your family either has no interest in seeing, or believes we'll never see anyway – is to begin to plot a life in which your current relationships have little meaning. Those who seek immortality are plotting an act of leaving, an act of betrayal and abandonment" (Howley 2010, 51). It is the pursuit of transcendence envisioned as an escape from an embodied finite life as it is relationally constituted in a particular place and time and embedded within a thoroughly integrated world.

Far from being an entirely new phenomenon, this "religion of technology" has deep roots within the Western Christian tradition. David Nobel (1997) traces it to developments in Western Christendom during the Middle Ages when technological advances were increasingly identified with the transcendent pursuit of the divine likeness. With the rise of a millennial view of history and its unleashing of intensive reform movements, the mix of technology, transcendence, and salvation becomes the impetus for a world-changing "immanent historical project." Modern secularized language, combined with the antireligious polemic of secular ideology, has conspired to veil this merging of religiosity and science and technology, but it remains a powerful current in scientific and technological pursuits (Midgley 1992; Noble 1997; Brooke 2005; Lanier 2010).

Recognizing the comingling of Christian themes and technology in the Western tradition captures an important dynamic that escapes and undermines the secularist model, but it threatens to substitute its own ideological blinders by essentializing religion. Although it is critical to expose the religious orientation and inflections in transhumanism, it is equally important to recognize that it is one variety, albeit a powerful one, among many others. As Mark Taylor's typology makes clear, forms of religiosity vary not just across traditions but also within them. Noble's genealogy of technoscience within strands of Christian eschatology and perfectionism, for example, captures well their shared ideology of transcendence. But they are components of a particular historical formation. There are other currents within, in this case, Christianity that counter the extreme focus on a transcendence cut loose from the created world. Note that relational values have no pur-

9 Graham references Brian D. Ingraffia (1995, 92).

chase in the utopian transhumanist fantasy to be like God in terms of omniscience, omnipotence, and immortality. Love is nowhere to be found, even though it has often been cited as central to authentic Christian life. The affirmation that God is love runs through biblical, theological, and devotional Christian writings. The moral imperatives of responsibility to the stranger, to the community, living and future, and to the wider created order drop out of the transhumanist religious vision. The varied spiritual disciplines found across all religious traditions that aim to transform the self, to enhance its better nature, are not part of the picture. Spiritual practices – whether through fasting, meditation, or rituals – that seek to transform an egocentered being into a human whose identity and sensibilities locate it within a wider community are present in transhumanist writings as symbols of religion's illusory quest. Transhumanism is championed as the vehicle that can create heaven on earth, but the morally redemptive strains that are commonly pictured as integral to salvation in Christianity and other Western traditions are strikingly absent. Transhumanism is no more essentially religious or essentially Christian than it is essentially secular. The interpretive and normative challenges that it poses are not between the religious and the secular, as the transhumanists' rhetoric and their religious critics often intimate, but challenges that cross the boundaries of these formations as they are configured, contested, and reconfigured in diverse times and places.

Garret Keizer's 2010 meditation on contemporary cultural trends illuminates this fundamental point. Underscoring the imperative to address the "questions that define one's times," he cautions that they are not neatly confined to either a religious or secular box. Central to our age, he claims, is the question posed by the transhumanist project: "Do we want to be angels, or do we want to be human beings?"

> The delusion of our society is not so much its materialism as its faux spiritualism, its desire to make a heaven on earth, not as a place free of needless suffering and full of what Barbara Ehrenreich calls "collective joy", but as one in which the elect live everlastingly and communicate telepathically while flying in disembodied splendor above the heads of the Mexicans mowing the lawn. (Keizer 2010)

Rather than envision a religion and secular divide that separates distinct and discrete alternatives, we would do better to imagine a kaleidoscope (Cady 2008). In certain periods, the picture is quite settled with broad agreements on the boundaries between the explicitly religious and the explicitly secular. At other times, times like ours, the kaleidoscope is in motion, and there is little that is settled. But recognition of the tensions and conflicts that are so visible now should not blind us to their alignments, fusions, and mixes that also mark their relations over time. The influences work in both directions, as religious motivations and ends transform social and political life and as secular laws and institutions help to make and remake religion. As political scientist Elizabeth Shakman Hurd puts it, the separation of religion and the secular is not "fixed but rather socially and historically constructed" (2008, 1). It represents a particular settlement of how the ontological, the political, the sacred, and the secular should be aligned (ibid., 12). We can extend this point to include technology as well. Its dizzying pace of change has made it especially destabilizing and contentious. Perhaps more than anything else today, "technology is rearranging our world, rearranging our views of human nature, rearranging the religious question" (Hefner 2003, 12). Among the greatest challenges of our time is to work toward a new settlement, one that can negotiate the challenges, possibilities, and perils of technoscience.

Toward a New Settlement

The contours of any new settlement must move past the oppositional picture of religion and science that has fueled fundamentalist impulses on both sides. The proclivities of parascience to make grandiose claims about life and human nature that extend far beyond the grounds of science as such must be curbed. But religious fundamentalisms that resist new scientific developments and practical applications out of misplaced faith in older theological formulations or static interpretations of human nature are equally misguided. Mark Taylor's typology recasts the issue in a helpful way by breaking out of the box of the modern politics of religion and the secular to highlight the broader patterns that cross the boundaries of religion, culture, politics, science, and technology. What turns of the kaleidoscope are now called for in the face of rapidly accelerating technoscientific advances?

Especially critical is the nurturing of a form of religiosity that more adequately integrates the gyrations between varieties of transcendence and immanence. Debates today are largely shaped, as Charles Taylor notes, by the two most visible extremes, "transcendent religion on the one hand, and its frontal denial, on the other" (C. Taylor 2007, 20). As we have seen, however, its frontal denial across much of technoscience remains very much within the same magnetic field. In the transhumanist project, the transcendent God of Western theism, though rejected, persists in and through the desires and role of the human. It is, as Bruno Latour (1993) puts it, the "crossed-out God" of modernity, with divine power, agency, and control transferred to humans.

Although the roots of this shift extend back centuries, evolutionary thinking, combined with the stunning pace of technological advances, have powerfully reinforced this picture of the human. Transhumanists are intoxicated with the power to transform human life radically, to take a more directive role in the evolutionary process that had once belonged squarely to nature and nature's God. A deep moral impetus drives much of this movement, as scientific and technological pursuits hold out the promise of ending pain, curing disease, and extending life beyond its current limitations. Rather than simply learning to endure the conditions that have afflicted humans, we have the capacity, potentially, to transform them and, in so doing greatly, enhance human flourishing. Transhumanists celebrate the intensification of this capacity to intervene in the evolutionary process, to reconfigure nature through cultural aims. It is not, strictly speaking, a new capacity. As noted in the Italian Transhumanist Manifesto, "if we reason in evolutionary rather than static terms, transhumanism cannot be considered as 'unnatural'. We are rather trying to establish a new harmony between culture and nature" (Campa 2008). Although this capacity to recalibrate the line between nature and culture is not new, its elevation into a defining feature of the human is. It is also a move that collides with traditional understandings of the God-world-human interface.

Coming to terms with the human role in the creative evolutionary process and its implications for what it means to be human remains a hurdle for much religious thought.[10] We can get a glimpse of how extensive the revisioning must be from the following observations of a distinguished cosmologist and astrophysicist:

> Most educated people are aware that we are the outcome of nearly 4 billion years of Darwinian selection, but many tend to think that humans are somehow the culmination. Our sun, however, is less than halfway through its lifespan. It will not be humans who watch the sun's demise, 6 billion years from now. Any creatures that then exist will be as different from us as we are from bacteria or amoebae. (Martin Rees, quoted in Hitchens 2010)

Failing to negotiate the evolutionary turn or continuing to make humans the center of the cosmic drama or insisting on a static human nature will doom religious positions to increasing irrelevance. The question is not *if* you draw and redraw the boundary between culture and nature, but *where* and *how*. Hence, the charge that humans are "playing God" when seeking to establish a new alignment between nature and culture is neither fully coherent nor a satisfactory normative response.

That said, there is something deeply troubling about the transhumanist celebration of a dramatically enhanced interventionist role in the evolutionary process. As we have seen, ambitions extend from therapeutic technologies that cure disease to enhancement technologies that improve cognition and feelings of well-being to those that radically extend the lifespan, perhaps even secure im-

10 Although most evident among conservatives, Wesley Wildman argues (2011) that even liberal Christian thinkers have failed to come to terms with the radical implications of evolutionary thinking for understanding the nature of the human and God.

mortal life. The outsized ambitions invite images of Icaros whose heroic daring ended in tragedy. From a theological perspective, human usurption of God's role, as in the transhumanist vision, epitomizes the reversal that marks transcendence when pushed to its extreme. The religion of transcendence at its far edge collapses into an immanence that denies the transcendent principle and the relativizing features that flow from it. These include recognition of the epistemic limits of all human knowing, a sense of fallibility and humility, when contrasted to divine knowing. Substituting the human for the crossed-out God sets the stage for an exalted self-confidence in our ability to know and to act in the world. As Keizer (2010) succinctly puts it, "[T]he posthuman is merely the subhuman that results whenever people aspire to the superhuman." Evidence of such hubris and the dangers that it harbors are all around us, from foreign-policy adventures to environmental disasters. The interpretation of the human that remains after the transcendent God is bracketed carries forward some of the displaced God's characteristics, but far more dangerously insofar as the critical and prophetic dimensions of the transcendent as interpreted in the Western theological tradition are abandoned. In this sense, fear of humans "playing God," having a bloated sense of their powers to know, to intervene, and to control life processes, is very much on target.

Transhumanism rightly calls attention to the increasing powers of the human to participate in the creative process, to our role and indeed responsibility to recalibrate the boundary between nature and culture through our technological inventions and imaginative visions. In this respect, this movement poses a challenge and highlights the limitations of religious positions that embrace a static human nature or reserve creativity to a transcendent God. In aggressively promoting these enhanced capacities, transhumanism opens up and onto fundamental questions concerning the nature of the human and the world. Bracketing these questions, under the ruse that transhumanism is a secular scientific successor to religious imaginings, makes it harder to engage the interpretive and normative challenges of the technosciences.

Transhumanism extends in a secularized idiom a form of transcendent religiosity that has deep roots within the Western Christian tradition. Although illuminating to trace these roots and continuities, this tradition includes other currents, sometimes called sacramental or incarnational, that have pulled in different directions. Although the historical record clearly captures the failures to achieve it, the Western theological tradition, interpreted broadly, has sought to sustain the dynamic tensions of, as classically expressed, the God-world relationship. This conceptualization has increasingly foundered on the shoals of a collapsing natural/supernatural distinction and an evolutionary vision that undermines the sharp divide between divine and human creativity. The challenge today is in nurturing a form of religiosity that more adequately sustains the dialectical tensions between transcendence and immanence. In this regard, the model of complex adaptive systems shows promise. Interpreting the human and life processes in terms of complex adaptive systems provides an integrated model that makes room for a transcendence that remains bound to life as it is embodied and embedded in particular times and places. It is a vision that acknowledges the accelerated mixing of nature and culture; but, insofar as all life forms are networked, codependent, and coevolving, it precludes the apotheosis of the human, the imaginative product of a crossed-out, otherworldly, disembodied God. It offers resources to rethink transcendence in a way that ties it to bodily, material existence. It is a way that is more life affirming and, we may hope, more life sustaining.

Within this interpretive horizon, transhumanism can be faulted, but not because it advocates taking on the role, responsibility, and risks of recalibrating the line between culture and nature. Rather, it far too aggressively embraces this role, with a zeal for enhancements and intervening control of the evolutionary process that is blind to the complex, relational webs within which life unfolds and tone deaf to the chords of love and responsibility that reverberate through any life worth living. It embraces an interpretation of the human that is far too spiritually truncated and isolated to serve as a model of human flourishing, let alone perfection. Religious traditions are rich repositories of robust and extended reflection on the nature and ends of human life. Rather than allow the burgeoning genre of parascience to consign these perspectives to our premodern past, it has become ever-more critical to introduce them into the mix as we debate the contours of a new settlement.

References

Asad, Talal. 2003. *Formations of the Secular: Christianity, Islam, Modernity.* Stanford, CA: Stanford University Press.

Bainbridge, William Sims. 2005. The transhuman heresy. *Journal of Evolution and Technology* 14 (2): 91-100: http://jetpress.org/volume14/bainbridge.html.

–. 2007a. *Across the Secular Abyss.* Lanham, MD: Lexington Books.

–. 2007b. Trajectories to the heavens. *The Journal of Personal Cyberconsciousness* 2 (3): http://www.terasemjournals.org/PCJournal/PC0203/wb1.html, accessed July 10, 2011.

–. 2009. Religion for a galactic civilization 2.0. http://ieet.org/index.php/IEET/more/bainbridge20090820/, accessed July 10, 2011. This is a revised version of an essay that was originally published in Eugene Emme, ed., *Science Fiction and Space Futures* (San Diego, CA: American Astronautical Society, 1982).

Barbour, Ian G. 1997. *Religion and Science: Historical and Contemporary Issues*. Rev. ed.). San Francisco: HarperSanFrancisco.

Blackford, Russell. 2010. On the yes! Statement by the order of cosmic engineers. *Institute for Ethics and Emerging Technologies*, April 4. http://ieet.org/index.php/IEET/more/blackford20090123, accessed July 10, 2011.

Bostrom, Nick. 2003. The transhumanist FAQ: A general introduction. Version 2.1: http://www.transhumanism.org/resources/FAQv21.pdf, accessed July 10, 2011.

–. 2008. Letter from Utopia. *Studies in Ethics, Law, and Technology* 2 (1): 1-7: http://www.nickbostrom.com/utopia.html, accessed July 10, 2011.

Brooke, John Hedley. 2005. Visions of perfectibility. *Journal of Evolution and Technology* 14 (2): http://jetpress.org/volume14/brooke.html, accessed July 10, 2011.

Brooke, John Hedley, and Geoffrey Cantor. 1998. *Reconstructing Nature: The Engagement of Science and Religion*. Edinburgh: T&T Clark.

Cady, Linell E. 2008. Royce, Dewey, and the religion/secular classification: Toward a kaleidoscopic model. *American Journal of Theology and Philosophy* 29 (3): 231-52.

Cady, Linell E., and Elizabeth Shakman Hurd, eds. 2010. *Comparative Secularisms in a Global Age*. New York: Palgrave Macmillan.

Campa, Ricardo. 2008. *Italian Transhumanist Manifesto*. July 29: http://ieet.org/index.php/IEET/more/campa20080722/, accessed July 10, 2011.

Campbell, Heidi, and Mark Walker. 2005. Religion and transhumanism: Introducing a conversation. *Journal of Evolution and Technology* 14 (2): http://jetpress.org/volume14/specialissueintro.html, accessed July 10, 2011.

Casanova, Jose. 1994. *Public Religions in the Modern World.* Chicago: University of Chicago Press.

Coady, C.A.J. 2009. Playing God. In Savulescu and Bostrom, eds., *Human Enhancement*.

Dawkins, Richard. 2006. *The God Delusion*. Boston: Houghton Mifflin.

De Gette, Diana. 2008. *Sex, Science and Stem Cells: Inside the Right-Wing Assault on Reason.* Guilford, CT: Lyons Press.

Edmonds, David. 2009. The age of enhancement. *Prospect Magazine*. September 3. http://www.prospectmagazine.co.uk/2009/09/the-age-of-enhancement/, accessed July 10, 2011.

Graham, Elaine L. 2002. *Representations of the Post/Human: Monsters, Aliens and Others in Popular Culture*. Manchester, UK: Manchester University Press.

Harris, Sam. 2004. *The End of Faith: Religion, Terror, and the Future of Reason.* New York: Norton.

Hefner, Philip. 2003. *Technology and Human Becoming*. Minneapolis, MN: Fortress Press.
Hitchens, Christopher. 2010. The catastrophist. *The Atlantic*: http://www.theatlantic.com/magazine/archive/2010/01/the-catastrophist/7820/, accessed July 10, 2011.
Hopkins, Patrick D. 2005. Transcending the animal: How transhumanism and religion are and are not alike. *Journal of Evolution and Technology* 14 (2): 11-26: http://jetpress.org/volume14/hopkins.html, accessed July 10, 2011.
Howley, Kerry. 2010. Until cryonics do us part, *New York Times Magazine*, July 7: http://www.nytimes.com/2010/07/11/magazine/11cryonics-t.html, accessed July 10, 2011.
Hughes, James. 2004. *Citizen Cyborg*. Cambridge, MA: Westview Press.
–. 2009. A progressive interpretation of transhumanist politics (interview with Michel Bauwens), posted February 13: http://blog.p2pfoundation.net/a-progressive-interpretation-of-transhumanist-politics/2009/02/13, accessed July 11, 2011.
Hurd, Elizabeth Shakman. 2008. *The Politics of Secularism in International Relations*. Princeton, NJ: Princeton University Press.
Ingraffia, Brian D. 1995. *Postmodern Theory and Biblical Theology: Vanquishing God's Shadow*. Cambridge: Cambridge University Press.
Keeter, Scott, David Masci, and Gregory Smith. 2007. Science in America: Religious belief and public attitudes: http://pewforum.org/Science-and-Bioethics/Science-in-America-Religious-Belief-and-Public-Attitudes.aspx, accessed July 11, 2011.
Keizer, Garret. 2010. Why dogs go after mail carriers. *Harper's Magazine*, September, 6-9.
Lanier, Jaron. 2010. The first church of robotics. *The New York Times*. August 9. http://www.nytimes.com/2010/08/09/opinion/09lanier.html, accessed July 11, 2011.
Latour, Bruno. 1993. *We Have Never Been Modern.* Trans. Catherine Porter. Cambridge, MA: Harvard University Press.
Maher, Derek F., and Calvin Mercer, eds. 2009. *Religion and the Implications of Radical Life Extension*. New York: Palgrave Macmillan.
Midgley, Mary. 1992. *Science as Salvation*. New York: Routledge.
Milbank, John. 1990. *Theology and Social Theory*. Oxford: Blackwell.
Noble, David. 1997. *The Religion of Technology*. New York: Knopf.
Robinson, Marilynne. 2010. *Absence of Mind*. New Haven, CT: Yale University Press.
Savulescu, Julian, and Nick Bostrom, eds. 2009. *Human Enhancement*. Oxford and New York: Oxford University Press.

Slabbert, N. J. 2010. Promoting the universe. *The Chronicle of Higher Education.* June 10: http://chronicle.com/article/Promoting-the-Universe/65959/, accessed July 11, 2011.

Smith, Christian, ed. 2003. *The Secular Revolution.* Berkeley: University of California Press.

Taylor, Charles. 2007. *A Secular Age.* Cambridge, MA: Harvard University Press.

Taylor, Mark. 2007. *After God.* Chicago: University of Chicago Press.

Tillich, Paul. 1964. Two types of philosophy of religion. In *Theology of Culture,* ed. Robert Kimball. New York: Oxford University Press.

Vance, Ashlee. 2010. Merely human? That's so yesterday. *The New York Times.* June 11: http://www.nytimes.com/2010/06/13/business/13sing.html?pagewanted=all, accessed July 11, 2011.

Warner, Michael, Jonathan Vanantwerpen, and Craig Calhoun. 2010. *Varieties of Secularism in a Secular Age.* Cambridge, MA: Harvard University Press.

Wildman, Wesley J. 2011. The ambiguous heritage and perpetual promise of liberal theology. *American Journal of Theology and Philosophy* 32 (1): 43-61.

Young, Simon. 2006. *Designer Evolution: A Transhumanist Manifesto.* New York: Prometheus Books.

Jewish Perspectives on Transhumanism

Norbert Samuelson and Hava Tirosh-Samuelson

This chapter compares and contrasts some transhumanist utopian visions of the ultimate end of humanity with a variety of conceptions in Judaism of the messianic age and the End of Days. There are at least two reasons for expecting such an engagement to be intellectually interesting and conceptually fruitful. First, Judaism as a modern religious tradition uniquely defines membership at least in part in biological terms. Although birth is not the only way to become Jewish, anyone whose natural mother is considered by the Jewish community to be Jewish has indeed been regarded as a Jew, at least until the present day.[1] Thus, by defining group membership in relation to genetics, Jewish communal interests can easily be related to a philosophy such as transhumanism that focuses on the biological improvement of a human collective, be it a nation state or an ethnic group. Second, the Jewish community, relatively speaking, is remarkably open to biotechnology, although the degree of openness is subject to debate, varying between different Jewish subgroups. In part, the debate is caused by how we interpret statements of openness by Jewish religious leaders (Shatz 2009, 93-117, 139-76). Still, even the most conservative religious spokespeople are more positive about the value of at least technology than are their most conservative counterparts in other religious traditions.

Comparisons

Transhumanism

Transhumanism envisions the augmentation of human capabilities and health by means of science and technology. We are asked to believe that a new phase of human evolution will come about as a result of the confluence of recent developments in the life sciences (e.g., stem-cell therapies, genetic enhancement, and artificial genes), bioengineering (e.g., robotics and biomaterials), materials science (e.g., nanotechnology), and the neurosciences (e.g., neuropharmacology and artificial intelligence). Although it is evident that these innovations are making important strides toward eliminating devastating diseases such as cancer,

1 Rabbinic Judaism decreed that Jewishness is transmitted through the mother, but, in 1985, Reform rabbis decided that Jewishness can also be transmitted through the father. As a result, there is no consensus today about the Jewishness of individuals.

diabetes, and AIDS, we are also told that future technologies will produce human beings with enhanced capabilities who will not only be able to live longer but also will be able to create and modify new forms of life. In the transhuman age, so the promoters claim, the successors of humanity will become their own makers, transforming their environment and themselves.

James Hughes, a leading transhumanist, summarizes the transhumanist vision most succinctly when he predicts that, in the present century, human beings will achieve

> things previously imagined only in science fiction. Life spans will extend well beyond a century. Our senses and cognition will be enhanced. We will gain control over our emotions and memory. We will merge with machines, and machines will become more like humans. These technologies will allow us to evolve into varieties of "post humans" and usher us into a "transhuman" era and society. (2004, xii)

In effect, Hughes sees the disappearance of humanity as a distinct species, as all forms of living things (both plants and animals) will merge with inorganic beings to form a single kind of universal being. Hughes and fellow transhumanists are enthusiastically optimistic about this future scenario; this is indeed an eschatological vision, a scenario for the ultimate end of the human species.

Judaism

From a historical perspective, Jewish literature is foundational for all of Western culture, from the biblical period through medieval Christian and Muslim civilizations to modern secular post-Christian culture. The premodern Jewish world and life views all reality as a directed flow of events from a prehistorical origin (called "creation") to a posthistorical conclusion (called "redemption"). Both the origin and the end come in sophisticated religious and scientific premodern thought to be understood as asymptotes that do not so much describe events in time as set yardsticks for understanding the past conceptually and establishing moral criteria by which to evaluate future acts – the past conceptually because all events are seen as consequences of the act of creation and the future morally because all events are critically evaluated in terms of their contribution to bringing about the hoped-for (or prayed-for or even anticipated) cosmic final vision.

1. Racial Theories about the Jewish People. For centuries, the embodiment of the Jews – especially the symbol of Jewish embodiment, the circumcision of Jewish males – has been a bone of contention between Judaism and Christianity. In antiquity, Christians used circumcision to denigrate the carnal nature of Jews, which presumably prevents them from seeing the spiritual truth of Christianity

(Gager 1985; Hirshman 1996). The intense polemics between Judaism and Christianity during the Middle Ages and the early modern period (Stow 1992; Cohen 1994; Chazan 1997) created a negative image of Jews designed to explain and justify their spiritual inferiority. Nonetheless, in the premodern world, Jews could opt out of being Jewish through conversion to Christianity, and many took the path of conversion. In the modern period, by contrast, when the secularization of European culture diminished the effectiveness of religious polemics against the Jews, the Jewish body became the differentiating mark between Jews and non-Jews (Gillman 1985, 1987). In the nineteenth century, as Mitchell Hart succinctly put it, "medicine and race coalesced around nationalism to produce a coherent anti-Semitic ideology that cast the Jew as essentially different from and dangerous to civilization and culture. … Judaism and the Jews were often represented as pathological and pathogenic, as diseased and as the cause of disease" (2007, 7). Thus, racial ideas made it impossible for Jews to *improve* their social status through conversion or even to fight social exclusion and marginalization. Ironically, in the secularized modern period, Jewishness could never be erased or transcended; it marked a person for life or worse, as in the Nazi ideology and policies, for extermination.

Race theory, interestingly enough, was advanced not only by anti-Semitic non-Jews but also by philo-Semitic Jews. A good number of Jewish biologists, anthropologists, and physicians in Europe, England, and the U.S. participated in and contributed to this academic discourse, and they had no qualms defining the Jews as a "race" in order to defend the uniqueness and distinctiveness of the Jews (Efron 1994; Hart 1999, 2000; Weidling 2006). Not unlike the transhumanists of today, these Jews believed that science, especially the (pseudo-) science of eugenics, would improve Jews individually and collectively, eliminating specific diseases, unhealthy mental proclivities, or undesirable social tendencies.

The debate about the meaning of being Jewish at the turn of the twentieth century bears some resemblance to the debate about the meaning of being human raised by the transhumanist discourse. In both cases, at stake is the relationship between the embodied and nonembodied aspects of the human in the pursuit of perfection. This chapter maintains that just as to be Jewish involves more than a fact of birth and embodied existence, so to be human cannot be reduced to the genetic makeup of the human body or to its biochemical functions.

The complex relationship between embodied and nonembodied aspects of being Jewish is exemplified most acutely in the case of Zionism, the modern movement of Jewish nationalism that responded to modern racial anti-Semitism by seeking to gather all Jews to the ancestral home in the Land of Israel (Shimoni 1995; Almog et al. 1998). A utopian movement, Zionism believed in the perfectibility of humanity, especially with regard to the Jews. Desiring to create

"Muskeljudentum," as the physician Max Nordau put it in 1892,[2] Zionism envisioned a new breed of Jews free from the negative physical and mental traits of Diaspora Jews. Zionist ideologues and technocrats had no qualms resorting to eugenics to ensure the elimination of undesirable dispositions exhibited prominently in Jewish populations.

We will discuss below the Zionist endorsement of eugenics for the physical improvement of the Jews in light of the transhumanist program for improvement of human nature by means of genetic engineering. We will argue that, to the extent transhumanism and Zionism equate being human with having a particular kind of body and physical traits, these programs are conceptually and morally problematic. Having a body is necessary for being human and for being Jewish, but neither being human nor being a Jew can be reduced to embodied existence.

Judaism, Science, and Technology

Whereas believing Christians, especially Roman Catholics, have felt deep anxiety about the current biotechnology revolution (Song 2002; Cole-Turner et al 1996; Dean-Drummond 2001), Jews by and large have welcomed biotechnological advances and have taken an activist stance toward it (Wahrman 2002). In the heated debates about biotechnology – namely, about stem-cell research (Ruse and Pynes 2006; Gruen et al 2007), reproductive technologies (Chapman 1989), and human cloning (McGee and Caplan 2004; McKinnon 2000) – several Jews have been quite prominent, but there is no consensus about the Jewish position on biotechnology. Among the most thoughtful critics of biotechnology is Leon R. Kass, the past chairman of the President's Council on Bioethics under President George W. Bush, who has cautioned us about biotechnology:

> [W]e now clearly recognize new uses for biotechnical power that soar beyond the traditional medical goals of healing disease and relieving suffering. Human nature itself lies on the operating table, ready for alteration, for eugenic and neuropsychic "enhancement," for wholesale redesign. In leading laboratories, academic and industrial, new creators are confidently amassing their powers and quietly honing their skills, while on the street their evangelists are zealously prophesying a posthuman future. For anyone who cares about preserving our humanity, the time has come to pay attention. (2003, 10)

Kass's caution is not universally accepted in the Jewish community, neither in North America nor in Israel. Jewish legal thinkers, bioethicists, and theologians

2 Nordau was the author of *Degeneration* (1892) in which he tried to account for the problems of modernity as symptoms. His call for the creation of "muscular Judaism" is a Jewish variant of and a response to the ideal of "muscular Christianity" advocated by Evangelicals who "translated the belief in a robust body and mind into a battle cry against all sinfulness" (Mosse 1996, 49).

across the spectrum of modern Judaism are rather supportive of assisted reproductive technologies, stem-cell research for medical purposes, genetic screening, testing, and even engineering. Unlike Kass, who argues for restraint based on the "virtues of mortality," Reform, Conservative, and Orthodox rabbis and ethicists tend to be strongly in favor of "more life, longer life, new life," as Kass derogatorily put it (2003, 258). The probiotechnology stance of the major Jewish denominations – Reform, Conservative Judaism, and Modern Orthodoxy – makes Judaism a religious tradition particularly suitable for reflection on transhumanism.

All forms of modern Judaism are responses to the emancipation of the Jews and the need to respond to the challenge of modernity. *Reform Judaism* advocated the emancipation of the Jews and their integration in Western society and culture by modernizing Jewish religious rituals and highlighting the rationalist core of the Jewish religion. Reform Judaism defined itself in rationalist terms as a belief in the God-Idea (i.e., ethical monotheism) and denied that there can be tension between Judaism and science. The rationalist spirit of Reform Judaism intended to strip Judaism from the morass of ossifying, legalistic minutiae and bring to the fore the timeless, universal truths of the religion. During the nineteenth century, the rationalist temper of Reform Judaism did not necessarily mean endorsing the most challenging scientific theory of the nineteenth century – Darwinism – but in the twentieth century, Reform Judaism has generally accepted the authority of science as the arbiter of truth.

Reform Judaism views healing as a righteous obligation rather than merely as a profession. In the case of controversial stem-cell research, Reform Judaism considers it a *moral imperative* to pursue scientific research into stem-cell regeneration because it holds the promise of finding new and effective treatment for many diseases. In 2003, the General Assembly of the Union for Reform Judaism adopted a resolution that supports research using both adult and embryonic stem cells, not limited to the existing lines currently approved for funding by the U.S. government. The movement has also supported research and funding of somatic gene therapy, in contrast to germ-line gene therapy, which poses serious medical and moral concerns. However, in accordance with its commitment to moral autonomy, the Reform movement places the responsibility for the employment of stem-cell research on each individual who wishes to use it, rather than on the scientific community. While the movement supports therapeutic cloning, it opposes reproductive cloning.

Conservative Judaism also endorses accommodation to modernity and integration to Western society and culture, but it seeks to preserve traditional rituals and the collective identity of the Jews expressed in the Hebrew language, Jewish law (*halakha*) and Jewish folkways. Conservative Judaism regards Jewish law as binding on modern Jews but acknowledges that the legal tradition has changed over time in response to historical circumstances and through human interpretation and action. Conservative Judaism regards science – especially its application in technology – and scientific research as both possible and potentially fruitful and contemporary interpretations of *halakha* must be informed by the advances in science and technology (Dorff 2003 [1998]; Mackler 2000; Sherwin 2000, 110-26; 2004). Yet scientific activity cannot be undertaken for its own sake alone because scientific means and ends have to be evaluated in terms of religious values and those values in principle transcend any modern scientific methodology.

The leading Conservative jurist and bioethicist, Rabbi Elliot Dorff, has asserted that "Jews have the duty to try to prevent illness if at all possible and to cure it when they can, and that duty applies to diseases caused by genes as much as it does to disease engendered by bacterial viruses, or some other environmental factors" (Dorff 2003, 157). On the controversial issue of stem-cell research, Rabbi Dorff has stated that

> the Jewish tradition would certainly not object to such research; it should actually push us to do as much as we can to learn about these lineages so that hopefully one day soon we can help people avoid cancer, or, failing that, cure it. This attitude follows from the fundamental Jewish approach to medicine, namely that human medical research and practice are not violation of God's prerogatives but, on the contrary, constitute some of the way in which we *fulfill our obligation to be God's partners in the ongoing act of creation.* [emphasis added] (ibid.)

As for the cloning to produce children, Dorff recognizes arguments against the technology, but he concludes that "human cloning should be regulated, not banned" (ibid., 322). He allows cloning "only for medical research or therapy," and his view is derived from the requirement to help other people escape sickness, injury, and death. Medical research serves the religious commandment to heal and to imitate God's healing power by extending cure to the sick.

The third main movement in contemporary Judaism, *Modern Orthodoxy*, also emerged in nineteenth-century Germany. In its response to the challenges of modernity, Modern Orthodoxy reaffirms the divinely revealed status of Jewish law and regards the principles of Judaism to be timeless and true. The law does not change, but it must be constantly and creatively reinterpreted to discover how its eternal principles apply to the changing world. In the modern period, these changes include science. According to Orthodox jurists, scientific and technological advances can help resolve many practical details of religious practice, especially in matters that concern the human body. Therefore, medical ethics is a primary area in which a fruitful interaction between science and Judaism exists. Modern Orthodox jurists evaluate each and every new technology not in terms of its impact on the society at large but in terms of its permissibility within the principles and reasoning procedures of Jewish law.

Orthodox theologians see the human being as God's "partner in the work of creation." The idea is derived from Talmudic sources that teach that "three partners (God, man and woman) are required for the creation of a human being" (Babylonian Talmud Niddah 31 a; Kiddushin 30b; Shabbat 10a), meaning that humans cannot accomplish procreation alone and must receive divine involvement. To be a "partner of God" is understood to mean that humans have an obligation to improve and ameliorate what God has created. Rabbi Abraham Steinberg expresses the Orthodox view when he states, "We are permitted to interfere in nature. ... [W]e are obligated to interfere, obligated to improve the world" (Wahrman 2002, 72). Therefore, science and technology can and should be used for this purpose "as long as the act of perfecting the world does not violate halakhic prohibitions or lead to results that would be halakhically prohibited" (ibid.). In terms of human cloning, Rabbi Azriel Rosenfeld (1972), for example, has concluded that cloning can be permitted because this productive method does not involve a sex act; therefore, it is not halakhically forbidden. Rabbi Fred Rosner (1979), who initially did not approve of cloning because "cloning of men negates identifiable parenthood and would thus seem objectionable to Judaism," in a later ruling concluded that it is permissible (Wahrman 2002, 71).

The Orthodox endorsement of reproductive technologies including research that will lead to cloning humans is most notable in the State of Israel, where legal reasoning and public policies are openly informed by Jewish religious values no less than by secular considerations. A recent study noted that "technologies that are controversial in other parts of the western world, such as embryonic stem cell research, prenatal genetic testing and human cloning have not caused heated public debates in Israel and generally enjoy a liberal regulatory framework" (Prainsack and Firestine 2006, 34). In Israel, biotechnology regulation is characterized by a relatively permissive approach and a low regulatory density. Because the Israeli government has viewed science and technology as matters of national priority (Penslar 1991), scientists do not have to protect themselves from intervention by "nonscientists." As for human cloning, in 1998 the Israeli parliament, the Knesset, passed a law that bans human cloning and germ-line therapy for a period of five years, but that law still permitted research on the activation of cells and production of human embryonic tissue "without actually getting to a human clone."

Regarding Jewish support of biotechnology and demographic stresses, it is not difficult to explain why Jews today are quite enthusiastic about the new genetics and its accompanying biotechnology. Beyond the religious commandment to procreate (Genesis 1:28) and the obligation to heal the sick and alleviate or prevent suffering, the Jewish endorsement of the new genetics reflects the deep anxiety about the demographic weakness of the Jewish people. The anxiety arises from a serious demographic crisis. The loss of one-third of the Jewish people in the Holocaust combined with the fact that Ashkenazi Jewry, the community that suffered most from the Nazi extermination policies, also exhibits preponderance to inherited genetic diseases (e.g., Tay-Sacks disease, cystic fibrosis, Fragile X syndrome, Gaucher's disease, and breast cancer) deepens the Jewish resolve to remedy genetic ailments by resorting to the new genetics (Goodman 1979; Goodman and Motulsky 1979; Bonné-Tamir and Adam 1992). In postindustrialized, Western democracies, the demographic threat to Jewish existence is further exacerbated by the combined effect of modernization, acculturation, assimilation, and social mobility, which have not only destabilized Jewish collective and personal identities but also contributed to the shrinking of the Jewish family. As a result of late marriage age, the choice to have fewer children, the common use of abortion among nonreligious Jews, and genetic and environmental factors that contribute to infertility, the Jewish family today is unable to replenish itself. The current situation stands in marked contrast to the Jewish religious obligation to procreate.

In the State of Israel, moreover, these demographic pressures receive a special significance given the on-going struggle between Israel and its Arab neighbors. According to the demographer Arnon Soffer (2001), the non-Jewish population in Israel plus Gaza and the West Bank is expected to have outnumbered Israel's Jewish population by 2020 (eight million non-Jewish Palestinians in contrast to 6.6 million Jews).[3] It is no wonder, therefore, that medical genetics is a recognized medical specialty in Israel where thirteen clinical genetic centers offer genetic testing, genetic screening, and infertility treatment to a population of only six million, and Orthodox and Ultra-Orthodox rabbinic authorities provide religious justifications for a wide range of reproductive technologies (Kahn 2000, 2002; Portuguese 1998).

The new genetic technologies have complicated the very question of Jewish embodied existence. What does it mean to be Jewish? Even if one agrees with the rabbinic norm that Jewishness is transmitted through the mother, the question has no simple answer. As Susan Martha Kahn has convincingly argued, "[T]his transmission becomes less straightforward: is it the mother's egg that transmits Jewishness, or is it the act of gestation and parturition that makes a child Jewish?" (2005, 10). In the modern period, the definition of *Jewishness* became ambiguous and contested matter, open to conflicting interpretations.

---

3 According to Sofer's analysis, within the pre-1967 borders, the development is similarly pessimistic for the Jewish majority: the current population of more than five million Jews and 1.2 million Arabs will change to a ratio of 6.6 million Jews to 2.1 Arabs (Muslim, Christian, and Druze) in Israel proper.

This ambiguity is most evident in the case of Zionism, the Jewish nationalist movement that emerged at the end of the nineteenth century to solve once and for all the "Jewish Question" that haunted Europe since the emancipation of the Jews. Zionism too struggled to find the balance between the somatic and nonsomatic (i.e., cultural, spiritual, or religious aspects of being Jewish) and the Zionist commitment to the improvement of the Jewish body. This struggle exemplifies the tensions already inherent within the utopian discourse of human betterment. The Zionist attitude toward the improvement of the Jews sheds a new and somewhat somber light on the transhumanist discourse of human betterment, since both programs endorsed eugenics.

Zionism and Eugenics

In the second half of the nineteenth century, Europe was preoccupied with the "Jewish racial question," "the Jewish Question," and the "Jewish problem," terms that were "used interchangeably to refer to aspects of Jewish society, or to Jews themselves, that were considered to be objectionable and in need of improvement" (Efron 1994, 3). Throughout the nineteenth century, the belief in racial difference was given intellectual respectability by race science that provided supposedly anthropological, biological, and statistical proof for human differences. Anti-Semites appropriated the scientific discourse to prove the inherent inferiority of the Jews and their innate inability to integrate into European society and culture. Indeed, race science was a major cause for the failure of political liberalism and the emancipation process. But in response to anti-Semitism, there was also a discourse about the "healthy Jew," in which an effort was made to represent Judaism and Jewry as robust and link them to the history of Western medicine and science. Some of this discourse was meant for Jewish audiences and written in Yiddish to educate the Jewish masses, but there were also many texts written by Jews and non-Jews in English, German, and French for scientifically educated and medically trained readers (Hart 2007).

The concept of race was central to this scientific and medical discourse. Jewish scientists, especially physical anthropologists and physicians, "employed the discourse and methodology of race science and ethnography in order to meet the claims of their opponents" (Efron 1994, 7). Among the Jewish race scientists, Joseph Jacobs (1854-1916), Samuel Weissenberg (1867-1928), Elias Auerbach (1882-1971), Felix Theilhaber (1884-1956), and Ignaz Zollschan (1877-1948) devoted much of their professional careers to defining the Jews in new scientific terms. To place Judaism on firm scientific foundation they asked several questions: What are the Jews? Are the Jews a race? If so, do they form a stable racial type, or are they made up of many races? What are the unique characteristics of the Jews? Are the Jews more susceptible to certain diseases? Are these dispositions hereditary or environmental? (ibid. 8).

The Jewish race discourse was supported by statistical evidence compiled by the Bureau for Jewish Statistics, and the major scholarly venue for the publication of scientific research was the *Zeitschrift für Demographie und Statistik der Juden* (Efron 1994, 167). This information was meant to effect rational and scientifically based *amelioration of the Jewish condition*, and many essays were devoted to the question of racial purity and its relationship to intermarriage. Jewish scientists concerned themselves with certain disagreeable features of Jewish behavior, for example, Jewish involvement in crime, but also with the susceptibility of Jews to certain diseases or, conversely, the high representation of Jews in professions such as medicine and law. The discourse was suffused with Social Darwinism, and evolutionary and eugenic ideas articulated by researchers such as Francis Galton and Charles Davenport were applied to understand Jewish history and Jewish survival (Hart 2007, 107).

The language of eugenics was deemed legitimate and necessary for analyzing issues of collective identity and survival (Hart 2007, 110-14). The discourse on eugenics and hygiene allowed Jewish medical writers to demonstrate that Jews and Judaism anticipated the modern state's central interest and that Jewry posed no danger to the state's and society's vision and interest in this crucial matter. Jewish scientists and physical anthropologists who supported the Zionist cause developed a contrary discourse. Recognizing the depth of European anti-Semitism and agreeing that Jewish life in the Diaspora was degenerate and diseased, Zionist race scientists rejected the desire of Jews to assimilate in Europe and predicted that Jews would have no future in Europe. Instead, they claimed that only in their national ancestral home – the Land of Israel – could the Jews achieve their full potential and express their innate creativity. Like their universalist Jewish counterparts, Zionist physical anthropologists utilized race theory and were open to eugenics. This was not surprising since, as Nicholas Gillham notes, "the opening decades of the twentieth century found the educated classes in England primed to welcome eugenics. ... This notion soon became popular not only in England, but in much of Europe and the United States as well" (Gillham 2001, 98).

Brian Gratton, in this volume, demonstrates that the victims of eugenics during the early twentieth century were by no means only Jews and that racialist discourse was inseparable from the debates about immigration and about national identity. Similarly, Diane Paul reminds us that the proponents of eugenics in

> Germany and America were able to play on racialist fears that cut across class lines; eugenics was often aimed at "outsiders." In Germany, Jews were damned; in the United States and

Canada, the foreign-born. But reflecting Britain's sharp class divisions, the target of eugenics in that country was almost exclusively the urban poor. (Paul 1995, 73)

The science of eugenics was endorsed by Zionist physicians, especially after the new science of genetics was established (Falk 2006, 148). For example, the physician Redcliffe Nathan Salaman (1874-1955) published an essay in the *Journal of Genetics* in which he documented the excellent physique of early Zionist settlers as natural selection in action. There were also Jewish physicians who wrote in Hebrew about eugenics but rejected the claims that Jews have hereditary diseases. Thus, Shneor Zalman Bychowsky (1865-1934) in his essay "Nervous Disease and the Eugenics of the Jews" rejected attempts to explain diseases by reference to hereditary or environmental causes. Instead, he saw the appalling living conditions of the Jews as responsible for Jewish nervous afflictions (ibid., 149-50).

Eugenic ideas were even more prevalent among Zionist physicians in Palestine who created the health system of the nascent Jewish polity during the 1920s and 1930s. For the physician Israel Rubin, the Zionist enterprise was a "great eugenic revolution in the life of the nation" whose essence is "the production of a New Hebrew type restored and improved" (Falk 2006, 151). For another Zionist physician, Abraham Matmon, "the task of modern hygienic is to protect humanity from the flood of inferiors and block the way for them from penetrating humanity, by denying them the possibility to inherent their delinquency to later generations" (ibid., 151-52). The eugenics discourse was not limited to theory; it also informed the practice of "choosing the human material" for the Zionist home. Thus, Arthur Ruppin (1846-1943), a contributor to the Bureau of Jewish Statistics before he became a Zionist and later the head of the Palestine office of the Zionist Federation in Jaffa (1908), had no qualms talking about "purifying the Jewish race" and stressed that "in Palestine we want to develop particularly what is Jewish" (ibid., 155). In 1904, Ruppin published *Die Jüden der Gegenwort* (The Jews of the Present) that stated that the Jewish claim to nationhood was based on biology, history, culture, and religion. In 1919, he published an article titled "Der Jude" where he argued that "it would be better if only healthy people with all their needs and their powers would come to Palestine so that new generations would arise in the country that are healthy and strong" (ibid., 159). Many Zionists accepted the notion that "the ingathering of the Diaspora" (*kibbutz galuyot*) should be directed from a eugenic perspective at creating "a new Hebrew type, restored and improved" (ibid., 160).

Precisely because the Zionist project was conceived in utopian terms (Ravitzky 1991), the settlement of Jews was accompanied by a fierce debate about control of immigration to Palestine. In historical hindsight, the Zionist willingness to exclude other Jews from immigrating to Palestine seems astonishing given the restriction on Jewish immigration in the U.S. during the 1920s and 1930s and the tragic ramifications of this restrictive policy for those who tried to flee the Nazi regime. But at the time, the commitment for the betterment of the Jews in Palestine helped forge a positive attitude toward the science of eugenics. Although one could argue that Jewish physicians were not the leading intellectuals of the Zionist movement, their publications demonstrate that Zionist physicians and technocrats had no qualms defining Jews as a race, identifying certain racial traits distinctive to Jews, or recommending eugenics to eliminate negative traits highly representative among Jews.

After the Holocaust, the discourse of scientific racism lost its validity (Barkan 1992), and concern with the physical improvement of the Jewish people shifted toward saving Jewish survivors and reconstructing the Jewish people. In the nascent State of Israel during the early 1950s, a fierce debate took place about medical selection criteria for the waves of Jewish immigrants entering the country, mostly from North Africa and the Middle East. In that decade, genetic studies based on blood-group polymorphism were carried out in different communities in Israel, and increasing scientific effort was directed to uncovering the common Jewish genetic characteristics and to trying to establish links with the more exotic communities, namely, Jews in more remote locations. After the discovery of the DNA in 1953 and the emergence of the more precise methods of molecular genetics, new studies proliferated whose goal was not only to identify the distribution of Jewish genetic material so as to reconstruct the history of the Jews and their geographic dissemination but also to identify which genetic traits are amenable to manipulation, i.e., to eugenics (Falk 2006, 159).

Since the 1950s, the discipline of molecular biology has thrived in the State of Israel, and this science is routinely applied to contemporary Israeli political life. For example, there are studies of the Y-chromosome sequences among Yemenite Jews and the Hadhramaut, as well as the Lemba Tribe of Zimbabwe and South Africa (Parfitt 2000; Parfitt and Egorova 2006; Goldstein 2008). Other studies focus on Ashkenazi Jews and indigenous Iraqi Jews who share the same mutation of blood-clotting factor XI. There are also studies about DNA sequencing that seem to show that all present-day Jews, both Ashkenazi and Sephardic, can claim a single hereditary line of evolution from the Middle East. These genetic studies have important implications for both the political and the religious life of the Jewish people and the utopian spirit of Zionism. Some of the studies concern the degree of intermarriage between Jews and non-Jews in the past two thousand years; others support the claims of the African and Middle Eastern tribes whose religious myth of origins include a reference to Jews and Judaism; and still others are used to prove the legal right of these same people to Israeli citizenship under the Law of Return. In short, molecular biology provides a scientific underpinning for attempts to establish claims about the Jewish people as well as to improve the bodies of Jews by eliminating certain diseases that are highly represented among Jews on account of past inbreeding. In sum, the formerly discredited science of eugenics has today been revived as the science of genetics and is fully supported by Israeli medical policy in its determination to eliminate Jewish genetic diseases.

The evidence above might lead one to think that the Jewish tradition is especially amenable to the transhumanist project. But the story gets much more complicated when we turn to modern Jewish religious thought and examine how three leading modern Jewish philosophers – Kaplan, Buber, and Rosenzweig – reflected on the utopian project. Their speculation presents us with a critical perspective to view the transhumanist project in the light of any ideology that closely links the end of humanity to the betterment of the individual human body.

The Ideal End: Beyond Human Embodiment

Three prominent Jewish philosophers in the twentieth century – Mordecai Kaplan (1881-1983), Martin Buber (1878-1965), and Franz Rosenzweig (1886-1929) – bolster a critical engagement with transhumanism. Kaplan and Buber were cultural Zionists, and, to at least that extent, their visions of the future of humanity have something in common with the utopian vision of the transhumanists. As Zionists, Kaplan and Buber looked forward to an improved humanity who would live within an improved human community in this world. In this sense, they share with the transhumanists a futurist vision of an idealized *embodied humanity*. However, transhumanists tend to be individualists, while Kaplan was a nationalist. Like the transhumanists and contrary to Kaplan, Buber tended to envision his ideal in individualistic rather than collectivist terms. But whereas Kaplan, like the transhumanists, tended to be humanist and modernist, and consequently physicalist, Buber intellectually came out of the romantic rebellion against modernism in the years following World War I. As a result, he understood the human ideal in profoundly spiritual rather than in physical terms. In the language of Buber's phenomenology, what we are here calling "the physical" is encompassed by his category of the "I–It," which is associated with negative moral value, while the spiritual is encompassed by Buber's category of the "I–Thou," which is almost identical with positive moral value. Hence, while Buber never negated human embodiment,[4] clearly the ideal end is associated with the nonembodied domain of the spiritual.

4 Quite to the contrary, with the sole exception of God (who is called "The Eternal Thou"), everything else in reality, including human beings, exist through both I–It and I–Thou relations. This means that God and only God can be said not to be embodied.

The most profound critique of the transhumanism comes from the German-Jewish philosopher Franz Rosenzweig who described the ultimate end of everything as a state that transcends all physical nature, including the human body. To be more precise, the ultimate end consists of the elimination of everything in realizing the absolute reign of God. Most ingeniously, however, Rosenzweig visualized this eschatological end in the shape of a human face, the very thing transhumanism seeks to erase by reducing humans to superintelligent machines.

Jewish philosophical reflections on the ideal end should be understood in their proper historical context. The discourse of Jewish philosophy (both premodern and modern) involves a dialogue between the Judaic tradition and non-Jewish culture, especially philosophy and science. Premodern Jewish philosophy arose out of the engagement between the prevailing philosophy of those periods and the accepted canon of the Hebrew scriptures (Samuelson 1994, 2002, 2003, 2009). Modern Jewish philosophy results from the dialogue between what Jews have learned from their knowledge of their inherited religious and cultural tradition of authoritative texts and what they learn from the scientific and cultural authoritative texts in their contemporary society. The difference between premodern and modern Jewish philosophy lies not so much in their respective procedures as in the tenets of science that each takes to be authoritative. In terms of an eschatological vision, modern-thinking Jews derive the sources of their scientific judgments about the End of Days from both the modern physical sciences associated with cosmology and the modern biological sciences associated with evolution. The latter make predictions about the long-term future of humanity, while the former make predictions about the long-term end of the entire universe. Since modern scientific judgments about both clusters are significantly different from anything a premodern Jewish thinker would have affirmed, contemporary Jewish philosophers must always reexamine their views on all subjects, especially in regard to the rabbinically central notion of redemption and the eschatological end. Out of this historical perspective, we will now investigate the relevant religious thought of each of these three Jewish philosophers to focus our comparison of teachings of Judaism with transhumanism's vision of an ideal end.

Mordecai Kaplan

Mordecai Kaplan was deeply aware of the radical gap between the intellectual values of traditional rabbinic Judaism and what he calls "modernity", and he shared the prognosis that Judaism cannot survive if the rupture is not healed. For Kaplan, the tension between the premodern and the modern is most evident in terms of politics, sociology, and economy. Whereas traditional Judaism favorably presupposes theocratic monarchy as the most desirable system of government, modern political philosophy affirms democratic nationalism as the ideal. Whereas traditional Judaism holds obedience to the commandments of the Torah to be the standard by which human virtue is to be judged, modern economic philosophy affirms both that human happiness consists of maximum pleasure with minimal suffering and that the use of money to acquire goods plays the critical role in its achievement. Similarly, whereas traditional Judaism sees the sensible, material world to be only one part of a greater spiritual reality, modern philosophy equates the physical with the real. This modern view can be summarized as "scientific humanism," and it is exemplified most potently in transhumanist ideology. This outlook is humanist because it holds that life should be about human beings rather than about God, and it is scientific because the physical and human sciences are the sole source of knowledge.

As a Zionist, Kaplan understood redemption in terms of an ideal Jewish global politics. His *Judaism as a Civilization* presents a secularized vision of the messianic age. This claim might startle some readers familiar with the book because the book is commonly seen more narrowly as a treatise in Jewish political philosophy, its intent being to provide political and sociological reforms to enable Jewish communal life to prosper in the twentieth century. Yet the concluding paragraph book states its intent along the lines proposed here:

> In sum, those who look to Judaism in its present state to provide them with a ready-made scheme of *salvation* in this world, or in the next, are bound to be disappointed. The Jew will have to save Judaism before Judaism will be in a position to save the Jew. The Jew is so circumstanced now that the only way he can achieve *salvation* is by replenishing the "wells of *salvation*" which have run dry. He must rediscover, reinterpret and reconstruct the civilization of his people. To do that he must be willing to live up to a program that spells nothing less than a *maximum of Jewishness*. True to his historic tradition he should throw in his lot with all movements to further social justice and universal peace, and bring to bear upon them the inspiration of his history and religion. Such a program calls for a degree of honesty that abhors all forms of self-delusion, for a temper that reaches out to new consummations, for the type of courage that is not deterred by uncharted regions. If this be the spirit in which Jews will accept from the past the mandate to keep Judaism alive, and from the present the guidance dictated by its profoundest needs, the contemporary crisis in Jewish life will prove to be the birth-throes of a new era in the civilization of the Jewish people. (Kaplan 1934, 521-22; italics added for emphasis)

Kaplan's redemption is a secularized reconstruction of the version of Jewish messianism that can be traced all the way to the Hebrew Bible, especially to the prophecies of Ezekiel. Under the influence of the American pragmatism that he absorbed from his study at City College and Columbia University, Kaplan strongly believed in the epistemic authority of what William James called "radical empiricism," the kind of democratic liberal polity that John Dewey promoted and the kind of collective worldwide Jewish identity advocated by Ahad Ha'am in his cultural Zionism (Zipperstein 1993). He believed that the Jewish people were entering into a new world, a "world-to-come" that would replace the old so-called "this world" of the past. At the center of this Jewish world would be a democratic nation-state established in the Land of Israel for the Jewish people. It would function as an intellectual or spiritual (for Kaplan, these two words were interchangeable) sun around which would orbit a world of reconstructed Jewish communities in every nation on earth. These Diaspora Jewries would function as states within states. In Kaplan's utopia, nations would be ethnically pluralistic democracies whose cultural, economic, and political life would be largely autonomous. (Only in the new State of Israel would the Jewish polity be completely autonomous.)

Kaplan's utopia is a confederation of polities where power is vested in the constituent members. The primary collective identity of each individual would be as members of a family. The families would be part of a "Bet Am," a political organization for urban neighborhoods. (Kaplan did not think about Jewish life in agrarian villages outside large urban areas.) The Bet Am would combine the features of early twentieth-century North American synagogues, Jewish community centers, and Jewish philanthropic agencies. In turn, each Bet Am would belong to a city-wide government called a "Kehillah," which regulated collective life between neighborhoods. Similarly, each Kehillah would be part of a "General Assembly" at the level of the nation itself.

The form of government of each unit was to be democratic. The families would elect leaders of the Bet Am who would represent the neighborhood in the Kehillah. Similarly, each Kehillah would elect leaders who would represent the city in a national General Assembly, and the General Assembly would elect an Executive Council both to govern the national internal affairs of the national Jewish collective and to represent the nation in global deliberations directed to preserve and prosper world Jewry. On Kaplan's model, nations would function more or less as the United Nations functions. Just as nations are autonomous members of the UN, so Kaplan thought that ethnic groups should become largely autonomous members of their host nations.

Kaplan believed that his political program was realistic. However, despite his immense influence on American Jewish intellectuals in the 1930s and 1940s, it never was adopted successfully anywhere. Its fatal flaw in terms of the this-worldly reality of North America was that he failed to take capitalism sufficiently seriously. No community structure could provide the kinds of services Kaplan envisioned as essential to a prosperous Jewish community (notably worship, education, and charity) without money, but those who could give the money would not give it to an institution (be it Jewish or not) that they could not trust to do what they thought should be done. Consequently, no Jewish communal structure could succeed (especially in a nation as firmly committed to enlightened capitalism as is the United States) that was not an oligarchy of wealth. Hence, Kaplan's vision of Jewish life survives simply as a futuristic hope for a more enlightened time that even he would call, in the spirit of his reconstruction of rabbinic language, the "messianic age."

Although Kaplan's utopian vision had nothing to do with transhumanist agenda, his political vision offers a certain indirect critique of the transhumanist approach to human life. Transhumanism is inherently individualistic, viewing human beings as bodies that can improve their performance through genetic engineering. Kaplan tells us that human beings are members of communities and that human perfection can happen only through communal interaction. By contrast, transhumanist thought is decidedly individualistic, concerned with the happiness of individuals who have no collective identity and who do not concern themselves with social welfare.

Martin Buber

Another cultural Zionist was Martin Buber, the recognized intellectual leader of German Jewry from 1933 to 1938 and the most influential Jewish thinker, whose philosophy of dialogue inspired many non-Jewish thinkers (Brenner 1996, especially chapters 4 and 7). Buber's philosophy cannot be explored here in any detail, but it is important to recognize that his hope for the future was no less Jewish and no less political than was Kaplan's. However, Buber presented a vision for the future that is rather universalist, akin to the teachings of the prophet Isaiah rather than to the nationalist and particularist vision of the prophet Ezekiel. The work of Buber's that most closely parallels Kaplan's *Judaism as a Civilization* is *Paths to Utopia* (1967).

Like Kaplan, Buber wrote in response to the severe crisis of survival facing all of Jewry in the Western culture, and both men sought to solve this problem out of a commitment to some form of socialism in the minimalist sense of the term, namely, a belief that the happiness of individuals is intimately tied to correct moral choices and sound social policy by government. However, for the American Jew, Kaplan, the political ideal envisioned for the world was a form of representational democracy, while for the German Jew, Buber, the political ideal was a form of direct democracy. Kaplan's model was developed out of his involvement in Jewish community city planning (notably in New York City and in Pittsburgh) for absorbing anticipated poor Jewish immigrants from Europe to the United States, while Buber's model for good government was his ideal of what the Kibbutz movement in Israel should strive to become as it also prepared for mass Jewish immigration from Europe. In this sense, the difference between them had more to do with their contemporary cultural identities as Jews in their new homelands, North America and Palestine, not with their backgrounds of European Jews.

In *Paths to Utopia*, Buber instantiated his general dialectic in the institution of the Kibbutz movement, which was founded on the ideal that people through personal relationship would be able to move beyond objectification and self-interest and find a shared collective way to live. However, even the *Kvutzah* (a distinctive, smaller form of agricultural collectives) needed to merge into some "higher social unit" (Buber 1967, 146). At first, the cooperatives were sufficiently small that all the members could come together and achieve a consensus. However, their success in working together led them to expand to even larger cooperatives so that they could accomplish even more, until the collective finally reached a point where consensus on every issue was no longer practical.

The need of the newly born cooperative to lead a normal life of doing things like raising food and educating children led the comrades eventually to delegate responsibility and, with delegation, arose the necessity for their society to evolve into something both more communist and federalist, both of which required the differentiation and, therefore, objectification of the fellows into different roles. People were divided by what they could do for the good of the whole; as such, the people themselves ceased to live as a whole (Buber 1967, 147-48).

The logic of Buber's dialectic suggested that, in the end, the seeming growth of the political units would fail to produce the desired solidarity and sense of mutuality because the units would have simply become too large for continued direct relationship, and, indeed, the actual history of the Kibbutz movement supports this conclusion. However, this was not the conclusion Buber drew. Rather, he adds, "but the trend towards a larger unit is far from having atrophied in the process." Buber saw the inevitable direction toward death, either into (by implication) something resembling the dreaded capitalist exploitation system of the United States or the nightmare of impersonal bureaucracy of the Soviet Union. Buber refused to accept this conclusion for the Jewish polity in Israel. In stubborn (and conscientious) opposition to all that his sharp intellect had revealed in this retrospective on his life-long commitment to socialism, Buber's final words in this book are the following:

> So long as Russia has not undergone an essential inner change – and today we have no means of knowing when and how that will come to pass – we must designate one of the two poles of Socialism between which our choice lies, by the formidable name of "Moscow". The other, I would make bold to call "Jerusalem".

As a product of early twentieth-century German socialism, Buber saw no hope for the future continuing to practice the nineteenth-century political values of individualism, democracy, and materialist utility that formally capitalist and democratic countries such as the United States continued to advocate as a global ideal after World War II. Without question, Buber believed that the future was socialist. However, socialism appeared in two forms, one dark and the other light. German Nationalist Socialism was the dark form, representing the greatest extent to which any society in history had overcome the *Ich-Du* (I–Thou) for existence in the form of *Ich-Es* (I–It). It became the society that, before World War I, Franz Kafka had predicted as the future in his surrealist fairy tales. Buber had hoped for the other side, a society of pure *Ich-Du* relationship where living beings had learned to overcome their material need to objectivize. He saw the Soviet Union becoming fascist and feared that the same could happen to the *Kvutzah*.

Buber's hope for the Jewish state over the increasingly apparent fate of the Russian state was grounded in Jewish messianism. For him, the Kibbutz imitated the ideal of "Jerusalem," and the Jerusalem that fed this hope was the messianic Jerusalem rabbinic tradition extracted out of the prophecies of Ezekiel and Isaiah.

Already thirty years before he published *Paths to Utopia*, his messianic ideal for redemption, he had deduced a logical imperative from the past into the present in *I and Thou* (1970, 168). Buber used his dialectic of subjective and objective language to analyze the development of language, history, and theology. His analysis of the history of language focused on the role of what he called the "foundational word" (*Das Grundwort*) through a human social history that culminates in (by implication) the history of religions. Corresponding to the term *word* in language is the term *revelation* (*die Offenbarung*) in religion.

Buber ends the body (there is also an "Afterthought") of this central text in his philosophy with these thoughts: "The word is present in revelation, at work in the life of the form, and becomes valid in the dominion of the dead form." This sentence introduces the conclusion of his book. Walter Kaufmann notes that the sentence in the original ("Das Wort ist in der Offenbarung wesend") is "utterly unidiomatic German." The reason is that here, as often in his (and Rosenzweig's) writing, Buber is speaking German but thinking biblical-rabbinic Hebrew. The "word" is "DIBBUR," which in this context is an allusion to "the word of God", i.e., to revelation. The German term for revelation, *Offenbarung*, literally means that state of being open to receive something. When God reveals, what he reveals is Himself, not mere (objective) content. Revelation is a relationship in which one person makes herself completely open (even naked) to another person. Hence, a word is not some thing stated, and revelation is not some thing revealed. It is a (the) form of life between persons. "Thus the path and counter-path of the eternal and eternally present word in history" (Buber 1970, 168). God uniquely is the only living subject who can never be object. Thus, in Buber's language, God and God alone is "the eternal You" (*das ewige Du*) (ibid. 160). However, humans, like all created living things, live between the subjective and the objective. Hence, religions, namely, all societies that live or try to live in relationship to God, share in the historical movement from birth as pure *Ich-Du* toward death in pure *Ich-Es*. However, each life-to-death is only a stage in an ongoing cycle, for each death is overcome by a new birth that begins the cycle all over again (ibid.).

This cycle will not last forever. There is a hope that beyond each future "Moscow" in human history, there will be a final "Jerusalem." The path is not a circle. It is the way. Doom becomes more oppressive in every new eon, and the return more explosive. And the theophany comes ever *closer* to the sphere *between beings* – comes closer to the realm that hides in our midst, in the "between." History is a mysterious approach to closeness. Every spiral of the path leads us into deeper corruption and, at the same time, into more fundamental return. But the God-side of the event whose world-side is called return is called redemption (Buber 1970).

This one concluding paragraph of *Ich und Du* lays out with astounding brevity of expression Buber's entire philosophy of redemption. Writing at the end of World War I, Buber prophesies that worse coming. We are not yet in "the days of the messiah." The cycle is, in fact, not a cycle, because in a cycle there is no progress. Each beginning is nothing more than the earlier beginning, and each end is nothing more than the previous end. Hence, there is no change. That is what "pagans" have thought, but it is not the hope affirmed here of the Jewish philosopher. In each cycle, the darkness becomes greater, which, in turn, produces a greater light. Here, the true prophet Martin Buber predicts that, after that darkness, there will be a greater light. The creation of the State of Israel is not the End of Days. Redemption still, even with the Kibbutz, lies in a future. However, it will come. At least, that is the hope of the Jew Martin Buber.

Franz Rosenzweig

Buber's closest friend and collaborator on the translation of the Bible into German was Franz Rosenzweig, perhaps the most profound Jewish thinker in the twentieth century. The socialism that informed the Jewish conceptions of redemption shared by both Kaplan and Buber (as we have seen, Kaplan more than Buber) reflects the latest stage of a political and ethical direction in Western European utopian thought that traces its origins at least to the eighteenth-century ideals of the American and French Revolutions. In its broadest outline, that model of messianism defined modernity as secularist and humanist. As such, the modern vision of the world – past, present, and future – is a radical break with the earlier rabbinic conception of the world that was spiritualist and theocentric. In this most fundamental respect, the conceptions of redemption affirmed by both Kaplan and Buber are modernist.

Rosenzweig's vision of the End was deeply indebted to all the strands of premodern Jewish thought. In fact, it was an intentional critique of any modernist reinterpretation of Jewish messianism found in either liberal religious versions of Judaism (of which Kaplan's conception is one paradigm) or Zionist versions of Jewish identity (of which Buber's conception is one ideal). Rosenzweig's analysis of redemption is presented here as a model of postmodern, contemporary reflection in Jewish philosophy that contains the most profound, albeit implied, critique of transhumanism.

Although Rosenzweig was indebted to post-Hegelian German philosophy for a politically charged, contemporary, secularist vision of what Jews and Christians call "the kingdom of God" (*malkhut shamayim*), it is crucial not to misunderstand his own eschatological vision. For Rosenzweig, the human will indeed be transformed in the eschatological end, but the "End" pertains to absolutely everything and not just to human beings. What Rosenzweig presents is not an argument, not even a prediction, but what can only be called a *prophetic vision of the end of absolutely everything.*

Rosenzweig's vision of the End is of a human face, and into that final humanity disappear both the world and the divine. In the End, the human becomes everything. Dissolved of everything physical as well as mental except for a "face," the human becomes, in Nietzsche's words, "superhuman." But Rosenzweig's *Übermensch* is not Nietzsche's; instead, Rosenzweig has in mind the homiletically conceived reconstitution of the first human (*ha-Adam ha-Rishon* in Hebrew) created by God at the origin of absolutely everything.

Rosenzweig's conclusion that redemption is to be envisioned as a face is itself homiletical. In Hebrew *countenance* (German, *das Gesicht*) is *panim*, and the obvious implicit allusion of this term is to Deut. 34:7, which says "Never again did there arise in Israel a prophet like Moses – whom the Lord singled out, face to face (*panim el panim*)." In all other cases to look on God's "face" causes the viewer's death. Yet, even here, Deut. 34:6 says, "Moses, the servant (*'eved*) of the Lord, died there in the land of Moab, at the command of the Lord (*'al-pi YHWH*)." *'Al-pi* literally means "by the mouth of," which the Midrash and subsequent traditional rabbinic commentaries take to mean that God kills Moses with a kiss (Greenberg 1996; Meir 2006).

Rosenzweig here understands Moses's death by the kiss of God to express human perfection. The Midrash identifies Moses as the ideal human being; his death is his "end," and by "end" the rabbis mean perfection. Hence, on Rosenzweig's interpretation, the death of Moses expresses the ultimate perfection of humanity, and that end is caused by a kiss from God. As Mosaic (here meaning ultimate human) revelation occurs "face to face," so the redemption of all of creation occurs "mouth to mouth," i.e., as a kiss, from the mouth of God on the mouth of Moses.

The kiss is an action of loving, and this loving is human. But the human is more than human. Kissing is an act by what the human is intended to become, and that becoming is understood on Rosenzweig's suggestion in light of Nietzsche's prediction of the transformation of the human into the superhuman. Although we cannot prove it here, Rosenzweig's conception of the End is entirely rooted in rabbinic, philosophic, and kabbalistic sources; but the relevant point for us is that his notion of human redemption (*Erlösung* in German, *Ge'ulah* in Hebrew) is comparable to (but not identical with) how transhumanists understand what they call "the Singularity" (Rosenzweig 1971, 265). Rosenzweig describes his understanding of what the Hebrew scriptures say about the End of Days as a single point of time, a moment, at the end of the line of time whose starting point, also a single moment, is creation. With respect to time, both creation and time are nothing substantial. All they are, from the perspective of the positive thinking of naturalist science or philosophy, is a point. The history of our world can be measured on a time line that is finite with respect to both its origin and its end, and that beginning/end is only a point – a moment, a (so to speak) nothing in time. As the world was created from nothing, so the world will end as nothing.

Yet the nothing posited for the End is full of meaning: it is not only the end of the world; it is also its redemption. Here redemption is not to be understood in the this-worldly political-utopian terms that the Ezekiel tradition was transmitted through both the modernist Kaplan and the romantic Buber. Rather, Rosenzweig draws a picture of a world beyond all worlds that is portrayed as a single cosmic light that overcomes all darkness. Rosenzweig in all likelihood derived this notion of the ultimate End from the conception of redemption in medieval Jewish rationalism and mysticism, even though he does not quote these sources. Instead, he bases his judgment on the Psalms, especially Ps. 139. The Psalms are chosen because, for Rosenzweig, literature, like science, is a way of knowing about something, but prayer is a form of action. In the case of prayer, the object is redemption, and the words of prayer do more than describe redemption: their communal utterance is the way that redemption is brought about.

Conclusion: Evaluations

We have presented transhumanism and Judaism in order to provide the background needed to make a comparison. In the case of Judaism our survey focused on two questions. First, what are the variety of premodern and modern positions that the intellectual leaders of Jewry have expressed and exhibited toward science and technology? Second, how, in comparison with the transhumanists, have Jewish intellectuals, both premodern and modern, envisioned the future of humanity and, beyond humanity, the End of the universe? All the issues for evaluation arise with respect to the second question.

Transhumanism presents a technological utopia that is challenging from the perspective of Jewish philosophy in three respects. First, the transhumanist vision of the End is profoundly secular; second, it is inherently materialistic; and third, it is utopian. In general, transhumanist discourse calls not only for improving the human condition by biological augmentation but for transcending humanity altogether.

The techno-optimism that characterizes the transhumanist movement has little basis in reality. The more we know the history of the human species the less plausible transhumanism becomes as a scenario about the future of humanity. Jared Diamond (1992) shows how human beings throughout the world have destroyed their environment and, by so doing, ultimately themselves. There is no reason to believe that, in the future, human beings will be able to save their inhabitable world more than they have been able to do so in the past.

In this respect in particular, the Jewish tradition offers intriguing perspectives on the transhumanist vision. On the one hand, the Jewish historical experience has made Jews particularly interested in improving the human body and made them welcome the science of eugenics. In the secular variants of Judaism – especially Zionism – eugenics has been endorsed as a means to improve the Jewish bodily condition. To this extent, Judaism shares a good deal with transhumanism. On the other hand, Jewish eschatological reflections expose the limits of transhumanism because they make clear that human existence cannot be reduced to embodiment. The ultimate End of life cannot be envisioned merely as physical betterment or even perfection: it must transcend embodiment. Furthermore, the ultimate End cannot reflect the narrow perspective of humans; instead, it must pertain to the End of the universe as seen from the perspective of God.

This Jewish perspective is better understood in contemporary physics than in biology. For example, the physical cosmologist and Nobel Laureate Steven Weinberg explains how the physical universe began and, based on its present trajectory, how it will end. *The First Three Minutes* ends with the following judgment: "the more the universe seems comprehensible, the more it seems pointless" (Weinberg 1993, 154). We know that the universe began in a singularity as a single positive, nearly infinitely small globe of nearly infinite density, at nearly infinite temperature. This singularity imploded, and the implosion produced an expansion of the initial energy into the emptiness of the surrounding space. The story of this expansion is the history of the cosmos. As time goes on, everything becomes more remote from everything else, so that everything that is becomes less dense and colder. This story can have one of two possible endings. Which ending will actually occur depends on the density of the universe. If it is sufficiently great, then the rate of acceleration of the universe will be negative, so that, with time, the expansion will slow down and will eventually reverse. On this scenario, the universe will end as it began, namely, as an infinitely small, infinitely hot, single thing. Conversely, if the density of the universe is sufficiently small, then the things within the universe will continue endlessly to expand. The universe will never end, but it will end for any practical purpose. In the end, what there is will be infinitely remote from anything else in a state of near infinite cold. However, whatever the "it" is that will be, it will not have anything to do with anything that in anyway has anything to do with being human. In the end, all will be one or nothing, but this "End" is, in Weinberg's words, something that, while "comprehensible" is utterly "pointless."

This is the major difference between the Jewish religious tradition, as interpreted most creatively by Rosenzweig, and contemporary science, or, by extension, transhumanism. Unlike contemporary science, the Judaic vision of the ultimate End is not pessimistic. The "End" is indeed universal death, as science teaches, but is has a positive and hopeful scenario. God alone, the ultimate reality, will remain; all multiplicity, diversity, and imperfection will vanish. From this religious perspective, this End is not "pointless" or depressing, as the secularist Weinberg claims, but a hopeful vision that enables us to gain the proper perspective on human life in its futile attempt to transcend human limitation and become superhuman. This attempt is misguided because it mistakenly defines the "ultimate end" in human terms and because it identifies perfection with the well-being of the human body. Rather, traditional Judaism asserts that only when human beings acknowledge God as the one and ultimate reality can they live meaningfully with a genuine eschatological hope in accord with what modern science teaches about the universe. The traditional Jewish position lacks the pessimism of Weinberg's position because it does not lead to nihilism or despair.[5]

5 The issue in this concluding paragraph has been conflicting conceptions of the cosmos and not different accounts of causation. Both sets of issues are part of the broader question of what is commonly called "Naturalism" and "Supernaturalism," and while there is some logical connection between the two sets of questions, one set does not necessarily entail judgments within the other . On the special logical complexity involved in issues of occasionalism, strong and weak naturalism, and secular and religious naturalism, see Shatz 2009, 179-208).

References

Almog, Shmuel, Jehuda Reinharz, and Anita Shapira, eds. 1998. *Zionism and Religion*. Hanover, NH: University Press of New England for Brandeis University Press.

Barkan, Elazar. 1992. *Retreat of Scientific Racism: Changing Concepts of Race in Britain and the United States between the World Wars*. Cambridge: Cambridge University Press.

Bonné-Tamir, Batsheva, and Avinoam Adam, eds. 1992. *Genetic Diversity among Jews: Diseases and Markers at the DNA Level.* New York: Oxford University Press.

Brenner, Michael. 1996. *The Renaissance of Jewish Culture in Weimar Germany.* New Haven, CT: Yale University Press.

Buber, Martin. 1967. *Paths in Utopia.* Boston: Beacon.

–. 1970. *I and Thou.* Translated by Walter Kaufmann. New York: Scribner. In German: M. Buber, *Ich und Du.* Heidelberg: Lambert Schneider, 1958.

Cantor, Geoffrey, and Marc Swetlitz, eds. 2006. *Jewish Tradition and the Challenge of Darwinism*. Chicago: University of Chicago Press.

Chapman, Audrey R. 1989. *Unprecedented Choices: Religious Ethics at the Frontiers of Genetic Science*. Minneapolis, MN: Augsburg Press.

Chazan, Robert. 1997. *Medieval Stereotypes and Modern Antisemitism*. Berkeley: University of California Press.

Cohen, Mark R. 1994. *Under Crescent and Cross: The Jews in the Middle Ages.* Princeton, NJ: Princeton University Press.

Cole-Turner, Ronald, Maureen Junker-Kenny, and Lisa Sowel Cahill, eds. 1996. *The Ethics of Genetic Engineering.* London: SCM and Maryknowll: Orbis.

Dean-Drummond, Celia. 2001. *Biology and Theology Today: Exploring Boundaries*. London: SCM Press.

Diamond, Jared. 1992. *The Third Chimpanzee: The Evolution and Future of the Human Animal*. New York: HarperCollins.

Dorff, Elliot N. 2003 [1998]. *Matters of Life and Death: A Jewish Approach to Modern Medical Ethics*. Philadelphia: Jewish Publication Society.

Efron, John. 1994. *Defenders of the Race: Jewish Doctors and Race Science in Fin-de-Siecle Europe*. New Haven, CT: Yale University Press.

Falk, Raphael. 2006. Zionism, race, and eugenics. In G. Cantor and M. Swetlitz, eds., *Jewish Tradition and the Challenge of Darwinism*, 137-62.

Gager, John. 1985. *The Origins of Anti-Semitism: Attitudes toward Judaism in Pagan and Christian Antiquity*. New York: Oxford University Press.

Gillham, Nicholas Wright. 2001. *A Life of Sir Francis Galton: From African Exploration to the Birth of Eugenics.* Oxford: Oxford University Press.

Gilman, Sander. 1985. *Difference and Pathology: Stereotypes of Sexuality, Race, and Madness*. Ithaca, NY: Cornell University Press.
–. 1987. *Jewish Self-Hatred: Anti-Semitism and the Hidden Language of the Jews*. Baltimore, MD: Johns Hopkins University Press.
Goldstein, David B. 2008. *Jacob's Legacy: A Genetic View of Jewish History*. New Haven, CT: Yale University Press.
Goodman, Richard M. 1979. *Genetic Disorders among the Jewish People*. Baltimore, MD: John Hopkins University Press.
Goodman, Richard M., and Arno G. Motulsky. 1979. *Genetic Diseases among Ashkenazi Jews*. New York: Raven Press.
Greenberg, Yudit K. 1996. *Better than Wine: Love, Poetry and Prayer in the Thought of Franz Rosenzweig*. Atlanta, GA: Scholars Press.
Gruen, Lori, Laura Grabel, and Peter Singer, eds. 2007. *Stem Cell Research: The Ethical Issues*. Malden, MA: Blackwell Publications.
Hart, Mitchell 1999. Racial science, social science, and the politics of Jewish assimilation. *Isis* 90: 268-97.
–. 2000. *Social Science and the Politics of Modern Jewish Identity*. Stanford, CA: Stanford University Press.
–. 2007. *The Healthy Jew: The Symbiosis of Judaism and Modern Medicine*. Cambridge: Cambridge University Press.
Hefner, Philip. 1993. *The Human Factor: Evolution, Culture and Religion*. Minneapolis, MD: Fortress Press.
Hirshman, Marc. 1996. *A Rivalry of Genius: Jewish and Christian Biblical Interpretation in Late Antiquity*. Albany: State University of New York Press.
Hughes, James. 2004. *Citizen Cyborg: Why Democratic Societies Must Respond to the Redesigned Human of the Future*. Boulder, CO: Westview Press.
JPS Hebrew-English TANAKH. 1999. Philadelphia: Jewish Publication Society.
Kahn, Susan. 2000. *Reproducing Jews: A Cultural Account of Assisted Conception in Israel*. Durham, NC: Duke University Press.
–. 2002. Rabbis and reproduction: The uses of new reproductive technologies among ultra-orthodox Jews in Israel. In *Infertility around the Globe: New Thinking on Childlessness, Gender and Reproductive Technologies*, edited by M. C. Inhordn and F. Van Galen. Berkeley: University of California Press.
–. 2005. Are genes Jewish? Conceptual ambiguities in the new genetic age. David W. Belin Lecture in American Jewish Affairs. Ann Arbor: Jean and Samuel Frankel Center for Judaic Studies; The University of Michigan.
Kaplan, Mordecai M. 1934. *Judaism as a Civilization*. New York: Macmillan.
Kass, Leon R. 2003. *Life, Liberty and the Defense of Dignity: The Challenge for Bioethics*. San Francisco: Encounter Books.

Mackler, Aaron L., ed. 2000. *Life and Death Responsibilities in Jewish Biomedical Ethics*. New York: Jewish Theological Seminary of America.
Manuel, Frank E., and Fritzie P. Manuel. 1979. *Utopian Thought in the Western World*. Cambridge, MA: Harvard University Press.
McGee, Glenn, and Arthur Caplan, eds. 2004. *The Human Cloning Debate*. 4th ed. Berkeley, CA: Berkeley Hills Books.
McKinnon, Barbara, ed. 2000. *Human Cloning: Science, Ethics, and Public Policy*. Urbana: University of Illinois Press.
Meir, Ephraim. 2006. *Letters of Love: Franz Rosenzweig's Spiritual Biography and Oeuvre in Light of the Grittli Letters*. New York: Peter Lang.
Mosse, George L. 1996. *The Image of Man: The Creation of Modern Masculinity*. Oxford: Oxford University Press.
Parfitt, Tudor. 2000. *Journey to the Vanished City: The Search for a Lost Tribe of Israel*. New York: Vintage Books.
Parfitt, Tudor, and Yulia Egorova. 2006. *Genetics, Mass Media, and Identity: A Case Study of Genetic Research on the Lemba*. Abingdon, UK: Routledge.
Paul, Diane B. 1995. *Controlling Human Heredity: 1865 to the Present*. Atlantic Highland, NJ: Humanities Press.
Penslar, Derek J. 1991. *Zionism and Technocracy: The Engineering of Zionist Settlement in Palestine, 1870-1918*. Bloomington: Indiana University Press.
Portuguese, Jacqueline. 1998. *Fertility Policy in Israel: The Politics of Religion, Gender and Nation*. Westport, CT: Praeger.
Prainsack, Barbara, and Ofer Firestine. 2006. Science for survival: Biotechnology regulation in Israel. *Science and Public Policy* 33 (1): 33-46.
Ravitzky, Aviezer. 1991. *Messianism, Zionism, and Jewish Religious Radicalism*. Chicago: University of Chicago Press.
Rosenzweig, Franz. 1971. *The Star of Redemption*. Translated by William Hallo. New York: Holt, Rinehart & Winston. In German: F. Rosenzweig, *Mensch und sein Werk, Der: Gesammelte Schriften. 2. Abteilung: Der Stern der Erlösung* (Haag: Martinus Nijhoff, 1976).
Rosenfeld, Azriel. 1972. Judaism and gene design. *Tradition* 13: 71-80.
Rosner, Fred. 1979. Recombinant DNA, cloning and genetic engineering in Judaism. *New York State Journal of Medicine* 79 (9): 1439-44.
Ruse, Michael, and Christopher A. Pynes, eds. 2006. *The Stem Cell Controversy: Debating the Issues*. Amherst, NY: Prometheus Books.
Samuelson, Norbert M. 1994. *Judaism and the Doctrine of Creation*. Cambridge: Cambridge University Press.
–. 1999. *A User's Guide to Franz Rosenzweig's Star of Redemption*. Richmond Surrey, UK: Curzon.

–. 2002. *Revelation and the God of Israel*. Cambridge: Cambridge University Press.
–. 2003. *Jewish Philosophy: An Historical Introduction*. London and New York: Continuum.
–. 2009. *Jewish Faith and Modern Science: On the Death and Rebirth of Jewish Philosophy*. Lanham, MD: Rowman & Littlefield.
Shatz, David. 2009. *Jewish Thought in Dialogue: Essays on Thinkers, Theologies, and Moral Theories*. Boston: Academic Studies Press.
Sherwin, Byron. L. 2000. *Jewish Ethics for the Twenty-First Century: Living in the Image of God*. Syracuse, NY: Syracuse University Press
–. 2004. *In Partnership with God*. Syracuse, NY: Syracuse University Press.
Shimoni, Gideon. 1995. *The Zionist Ideology*. Hanover NH: University Press of New England for Brandeis University Press.
Soffer, Arnon. 2001. *Israel: Demography 2000-2020: Risks and Possibilities* [in Hebrew]. Tel Aviv: University of Tel Aviv, Center for the Study of National Security.
Song, Robert. 2002. *Human Genetics: Fabricating the Future*. Cleveland, OH: The Pilgrim Press.
Stow, Kenneth R. 1992. *Alienated Minority: The Jews of Medieval Latin Europe*. Cambridge, MA: Harvard University Press.
Wahrman, Miryam Z. 2002. *Brave New Judaism: When Science and Scripture Collide*. Lebanon, NH: University Press of New England for Brandeis University Press.
Weidling, Paul. 2006. The evolution of Jewish identity: Ignaz Zollschan between Jewish and Aryan race theories, 1910-40. In G. Cantor and M. Swetlitz, eds., *Jewish Tradition and the Challenge of Darwinism*, 116-36.
Weinberg, Steven. 1993. *The First Three Minutes: A Modern View of the Origin of the Universe*. New York: Basic Books.
Zipperstein, Steven J. 1993. *Elusive Prophet: Ahad Ha'am and the Origins of Zionism*. Berkeley: University of California Press.

Ideals of Human Perfection: A Comparison of Sufism and Transhumanism

Farzad Mahootian

Sources of Islamic Religious Thought

Islam is a complex religious civilization and worldview that cannot be reduced to a single tenet or characterization. Like all religious traditions, Islam is not a monolithic entity but a product of ongoing conflict, concordance, and synthesis from the time of the Prophet Mohammad to the present. Conflicts about the "true religion" of Islam were alive during the Prophet's lifetime (572-633), and flared up immediately on his death. The major schism of Islam, between Sunni (literally "traditional") and Shi'a (literally, "sectarian"), arose around the question of the legitimate successor to Mohammad as spiritual and political authority of the faithful (Berkey 2003, 70-71). Similar to the development of Christianity (Herrin 1987), Islam also evolved out of debates about scriptural interpretation, especially in regard to the authenticity of prophecies and the authority of prophets. The act of scriptural interpretation is a religious and philosophical imperative in Islam, and its literary product is the living tradition of the *hadith*, very similar to Rabbinic Judaism, which was present in the Hijaz at the time of Mohammad.

The *hadith* provide much of the basis for interpretations and applications of Qur'anic revelation. The *hadith* consist of collections of stories and interpretations of the Prophet Mohammad's life and sayings. Functionally, the *hadith* bear strong similarities to the Jewish Midrash: their application to Islamic jurisprudence has developed into a vast body of work over the centuries to the present day.

Two schools of Islamic orthodoxy emerged from the first two centuries after the rise of Islam: the Mu'tazilite and Ash'arite. The former tended to emphasize the metaphorical and symbolic interpretation of the Qur'an's many allusions to the attributes of God, while the latter accepts them *bila kayf*, that is, without further qualification or investigation. It is generally agreed that the Ash'arite school of orthodoxy has prevailed throughout the Islamic world (Netton 1994, 4). The differences between these two schools of theology need not concern us here except to note that the Ash'arite approach represents a selective suppression of logic and inquiry in matters theological. By contrast, the Mu'tazilite applied logic, allegory, and symbolism to develop interpretations that could reconcile a variety of conflicting statements in the Qur'an about God's immaterial essence with his physical properties.

A third major source of Islamic religious thought and practice is Sufism, the mystical form of Islam. Annemarie Schimmel, a leading scholar of Sufism, defines Islamic mysticism as follows: "Mysticism can be defined as love of the Absolute – for the power that separates true mysticism from mere asceticism is love. ... This love can carry the mystic's heart to the Divine Presence 'like the falcon which carries away the prey'" (Schimmel 1975, 4). From the eighth to the fourteenth centuries, various Sufi orders and numerous individual thinkers generated deep reflections about the inner meaning of Islam. However, over time, the reluctance of Sufis to engage in politics and their commitment to esotericism prevented Sufism from dominating Islamic culture and social institutions. Furthermore, the domination of the Ash'arite orthodoxy since the fourteenth century resulted in a culture that became increasingly legalistic, autocratic, and closed; it focused on the letter of the law rather than its inner spirit, and opposed discovery and explorations in philosophy and science.

The Sufi tradition in Islam cannot be understood apart from yet a fourth intellectual strand, namely, philosophy. Islam spread in the Hellenized Middle East during the seventh and eighth centuries, but instead of destroying the cultural riches of the region, Islam preserved them. The Abbasid caliphs of Baghdad supported a massive translation project that made Greek and Hellenistic philosophy and science available in Arabic. This literature not only gave rise to the systematization of Islamic theology in the various schools of *kalam* but also to rationalist philosophy that was a hybrid of Platonic, Neoplatonic, and Aristotelian elements. This unique blend of philosophy and mysticism is vividly captured in the Illuminationist philosophy of Shahabuddin Yahya Suhrawardi (1155-1191), the focus of this chapter's discussion.

Sufism was not opposed to orthodox Islam; it employed orthodox concepts but transformed them greatly in theory as well as praxis. In general, Sufism absorbed Neoplatonic ontology that viewed the world as emanating from the mind of God. In this view, the goal of human life is the attainment of gnosis, that is, experiential knowledge of God. Such knowledge is understood as the means of "return" and "reunion" of the human soul with the Godhead. This union is attained only when the practitioner annihilates the human self in God (*fana*) after which he or she returns to the world only to serve God's will (*baqa*). Sufi spiritual practices sometimes came into conflict with the literalist tradition of orthodox Islamic theology, *kalam* (which literally means "speech" or "words"). The stifling legalistic bureaucracy that eventually grew around the *kalam* tradition ultimately ended the outward expansion of Islam as an integrative and cosmopolitan civilizing power just as Europe was beginning its period of colonial expansion. Chief among the ideas shared by Islam's orthodoxy and Sufism, by Sunni and Shi'ite alike, is the concept of the perfect human, *insan-i kamel* (literally, "complete" or "universal human"). Sufi mystical practice, religious devotion, and moral development are all guided by the notion of this concept of human possibility.

This chapter engages transhumanism from the Sufi perspective. The notion of a "perfect human nature" makes a comparison with transhumanism compelling. If in Christianity Jesus Christ embodies the human ideal, in Islam the discourse on "perfect human nature" centers around Mohammad. The Qur'an presents itself as the continuation of revelations that began in the Hebrew Bible, recounting the lineage of prophets beginning with Adam and finding its completion in Mohammad, the "seal of prophecy."

There are many other similarities between Islam, Judaism, and Christianity, too many to analyze here, but these include some themes of interest to our discussion, namely, physical assumption into heaven of certain prophets (Elijah, Jesus, and Mohammad); theologies of light; theologies of love; the creation of the human being in the image of God; divine authorship of human destiny; bodily resurrection; the Day of Judgment; and the End of Days. A closer look at the Islamic idea of "perfect human nature" will give us a vantage point from which to reflect on the transhumanist project of improving the flaws of human nature.

The Quest for the "Perfect (or Universal) Man" in Sufism

Seyyed Hossein Nasr, a leading Islamic scholar, summarizes the idea of perfect man:

> The Universal Man is then the sum of all degrees of existence, a total mirror before the Divine Presence and at the same time the supreme archetype of creation. It is the prototype of man, the reality that man carries potentially within himself and can always realize if there is aspiration, persistence, and of course divine succor. It is enough for man to realize the total possibility of his own existence, to become fully conscious of himself, to gain that treasure of true felicity and peace which he seeks outwardly here and there but never seems to find. (Nasr and Chittick 2007, 66)

In Islamic metaphysics, human nature is divine. Schimmel (1975, 188) notes that according to the Qur'an, "man was created 'by God's hands' (Sura 38:75), an idea that tradition elaborated: God kneaded Adam's clay forty days before He gave him life by breathing into him with His own breath (Sura 15:29, 38:72)." The shared breath expresses how intimately human nature shares in God's divinity. Furthermore, the human being is the "channel of grace for nature" (Nasr and Chittick 2007, 67). The Islamic concept of humanity's special place carries with it the necessary role of stewardship: "nature has been entrusted to us, as we are God's vicegerents on Earth" (Ozdemir 2003, 27).

Given this understanding of humanity in the Qur'an, the question is how human beings fulfill this function for nature. In the *hadith* of the "Hidden Treasure," God answers the question of the prophet David regarding the purpose of creation: "I was a treasure that was not known, so I loved to be known. Hence I created the creatures and I made Myself known to them, and thus they came to know Me" (Chittick 1983, 47). As the *hadith* indicates, the bidirectional reference inherent in "knowledge of God" here means both knowledge of God as the subject and object of human knowing and, reciprocally, humanity as the object and medium of divine knowing and divine self-knowledge. The renowned thirteenth-century Andalusian Sufi writer ibn al-Arabi, puts it thus, "When my Beloved appears / With what eye do I see Him / With his eye, not with my mine / For none sees Him except Himself" (quoted in Schimmel 1975, 266).

Many other Sufis (e.g., Hallaj, Suhrawardi, Rumi) have expressed the intimacy of knowing and being known by God as divine love, wherein lover and beloved merge in love. As Schimmel notes,

> The mystics have found numerous allusions in the Koran to prove man's lofty rank. One of their favorite verses in this respect is: "And we shall show you signs on the horizons and in yourselves – do you not see?" (Sura 41:53), a verse that they interpret as God's order to look into their own hearts to find the source of knowledge and, eventually, the divine beloved, who is "closer than the jugular vein." (Sura 50:16)
>
> From this feeling the *hadith* "*man arafa nafsahu faqad arafa rabbahu,*" "who knows himself knows his Lord", must have developed; it may originally have been an adaptation of the Delphic *gnothi theuton, "know thyself.*" (Schimmel 1975, 190)

Here knowledge in its ultimate form – divine knowledge – is an ideal form of self-knowledge; as the *hadith* indicates, the entire purpose of creation is for the sake of God's desire to be known in and through human self-knowledge. Plato's *Symposium* and *Phaedrus* dialogues present the human encounter with beauty on the cosmic stage, highlighting love as the divine path to self-knowledge.

According to ibn al-Arabi's reading of this *hadith*, the whole cosmos is a mirror created to reflect the glory of God, but it is an *unpolished* mirror, and the role of the human being is to polish it. The metaphor of polishing may be interpreted in terms of various human activities (i.e., of knowing, thinking, seeing, and doing), but at its most basic level, it is the conscious act of bearing witness (*shahada*) to the handiwork of the creator. In a word, it means bearing witness to *cosmic theophany*, i.e., the showing forth, or self-disclosure of God on the scale of all existence and, simultaneously and comprehensively, so on the human scale. The simultaneity of *disclosure and recognition* is the epistemological point of departure for Suhrawardi's philosophy of illumination, as we shall see in the following section.

Illuminationism and Knowledge in Sufism

Shahabuddin Yahya Suhrawardi was a Persian Sufi, martyr, and originator of the "philosophy of illumination." Some have characterized Suhrawardi as primarily a theosophist who synthesized ancient Persian wisdom with Greek philosophy, integrating Islamic revelation and his own mystical experiences (Nasr 1964; Corbin 1979; 2003). Others have presented Suhrawardi's illuminationism as an analytic system of philosophy that reforms the Aristotelian, or "peripatetic," philosophy of his day and reconciles it with visionary experience, i.e., with direct intuitive knowledge (Ziai 1990, 1996; Walbridge 2001).

Suhrawardi's philosophical system explicitly provides a framework to integrate religious experience with the intellectual requirements of logic. One perspective on this position is that it explicitly treats extraordinary (i.e., mystical) experience as a source of first premises for logical arguments, in this sense, on a par with other empirical and semiempirical sources of scientific argumentation. Whether the subject of thought is physical (astronomy) or visionary (involves encounters with prophets and angels), Suhrawardi maintains that the analysis and discussion of such observations must be subject to the same consistent standards (Ziai 1996, 450). In so doing, Suhrawardi's philosophy attempts to provide epistemological and ontological foundations for *theurgy*, i.e., the conscious self-transformation of human nature into divine nature by means of mystical practice and visionary experience, what Corbin calls "active imagination." At the center of this effort is self-knowledge. In illuminationist epistemology, an act of self-knowledge underlies the possibility of every act of knowledge. In this view, knowledge is an act that simultaneously requires illumination by, and comprehension of and by, God. There is a direct analogy of this with Suhrawardi's theory of eyesight: eyesight requires no medium, only the visible object, the healthy eye, and a source of illumination/light (whose speed he thought was infinite). The act of vision is a simultaneous coupling of eyesight, ambient light, and the visible object. So too in the case of knowledge, no medium is present (it is nonrepresentational) and no time is required (it is instantaneous): it requires only an intelligible object (ultimately, all reality, i.e., God), a healthy mind, and a source of illumination/intelligibility (ultimately, God). So, knowledge by direct mystical experience requires *no* duration: God's self-disclosure (i.e., theophany) is coincident and simultaneous with direct human intuition. So intertwined is God in every act of being, every act of human knowledge and self-knowledge, that theology becomes theurgy by necessity.

According to Suhrawardi, self-consciousness is direct presentational knowledge because "the perception of one's own self-consciousness (*idrak al-ana'iyya*) is the same as the direct perception of what a thing is in itself (*idrak ma huwa*

huwa), and not perception by means of an idea (*mithal*) of self-consciousness. This is true of all things that are self-constituted and cognizant of their own essence" (Ziai 1990, 150-51). Furthermore, for Suhrawardi, any self-conscious entity is an "abstract light," as distinguished from concrete light, i.e., the phenomena studied by physical science. As an abstract light, the self-conscious human soul plays an essential part in the continuity of the illuminationist cosmology, for, in the context of the divine luminous emanation of the Light of Lights,[1] the "perfect human" emerges through a series of acts of self-consciousness in which the soul understands (and so transcends certain of its limits) and thereby becomes closer to God. Self-perfection through self-consciousness is the role of the human in the cosmos.

This was the common aim of various flavors of Neoplatonism during Suhrawardi's time and characterizes the essence of the vast majority of Sufi poetry (Schimmel 1975, 287ff). The epistemological significance in Suhrawardi's philosophy of poetic and symbolic expression is an important consequence of overcoming the limits of discursive thought (Ziai 1996, 451), and overcoming separation in song. The sublime interplay of loss and return, desire and separation, is illustrated in this excerpt of the song of the reed from Persian poet Rumi (1207-1273):

> "Since I was cut from the reedbed, I have made this crying sound."
> Anyone apart from someone he loves understands what I say
> Anyone pulled from a source longs to go back ... (Barks and Moyne 1995, 17)

Suhrawardi's unique innovations were twofold. On the one hand, there are formal projects, including a detailed critique and reform of Aristotle's logical categories, theory of description, epistemology, and a return to Pythagorean expression of Neoplatonic emanation cosmology (Walbridge 2001, 8). On the other hand, his appeal is to the "oriental" philosophy, mysticism, and theurgy of ancient Iranian religion. The key is the tone of dynamic tension set by the inclusion of both mystical experience and logical consistency. As we shall see, the conscious effort to balance these two is absent in transhumanism. Suhrawardi explicated the co-limitation of these two modes of knowledge: in the introduction to his treatise the *Philosophy of Illumination,* he warns readers interested in observational astronomy to pursue the excellent and readily available works of Peripatetic philosophers. The philosophy of illumination is for those who seek to understand inner observation of spiritual objects, the "apocalyptical lights," that are no less real than the lights of sun, moon, and stars but that illuminate spiritual rather than physical things (Ziai 1990, 176).

In Suhrawardi's system, the cosmos emanates from the One, the Light of Lights, via a series of lights (First Light, Second Light, etc.). There are several

1 This is a reference to God as light in the famous Qur'anic Light Sura 24:35.

subsidiary lights that facilitate the emanation process. Suhrawardi scholar Hossein Ziai explains:

> On the cosmic level, every "abstract light" [such as, a human soul] "sees" the "lights" that are above it in rank, while the higher "lights" instantaneously, at the moment of vision, illuminate the lower in rank. The Light of Lights (*Nur al-anwar*) illuminates everything. … Thus every being comes to know its own degree of perfection, an act of self-knowledge which induces a desire (*shawq*) to "see" the being just above it in perfection, and this act of "seeing" triggers the process of illumination. By means of the process of illumination, "light" is propagated from its highest origin to the lowest elements. (Ziai 1990, 156)

The dynamic of desire and self-knowledge described here bears strong resemblance to the Platonic notion of desire (*eros*) as essential to knowledge of the Good (Friedlander 1969, 61). Even in its most abstract heights, Suhrawardi's philosophy follows Plato in remaining true to the simple Socratic exhortation to "know thyself." The nature of visible light, its pervasive continuity through seemingly infinite degrees of intensity, gives Suhrawardi the analogical basis to render his entire system consistent with two simple *hadith* in which Mohammad tells his followers that "Who knows himself knows his Lord" and that "No one knows God but God." Through diligent practice, human self-knowledge is cultivated to the point to receive illumination; when this occurs, knowledge is given as

> visions of the "apocalyptic lights" … Human souls who have experienced the "apocalyptic lights" are called "abstract souls" because they have torn away from the physical body. They obtain an "[image] of the light of God" (*mithal min nur Allah*), which the faculty of imagination imprints on the "tablet of the *sensus communis*". By means of this [image], they obtain control over a "creative light" which ultimately gives them power to know. (Ziai 1990, 157)[2]

The creative light, as its name indicates, bestows the active power of poesy: this is not passive experience, not a mere "spectator theory" of knowledge. All this takes place in *alam al-mithal*, the imaginal world; the attempt to describe events of *alam al-mithal* overburdens literal language, but poetry inspired by the creative light sets language free from its worldly restrictions and guides the self-conscious soul to greater depths and brighter intensities. Discovering the limits of any given level of knowledge prepares one for illumination from the level above it and results in transcendence of one's present stage of limitation, thereby reinforcing the inward trajectory toward the truth of one's own existence.

In "The Apocalypse of Islam," N. O. Brown compares the Qur'an with James Joyce's *Finnegans Wake* with regard to their devastation of human language. He quotes Nasr on this point:

---

2 I have substituted "image" for Ziai's translation of *mithal* as "idea" in this quote. I believe *image* is better suited to the Arabic *mithal*, which we have encountered in the term *alam al-mithal*, the *imaginal* world. The term *idea*, with its formal, intellectual connotations, introduces ambiguity here.

> It is neither like a highly mystical text nor a manual of Aristotelian logic, though it contains both mysticism and logic. ... The text of the Quran reveals human language crushed by the power of the Divine Word. ... The Quran displays human language with all the weakness inherent in it becoming suddenly the recipient of the Divine Word and displaying its frailty before a power which is infinitely greater than man can imagine. (Brown 1984, 168-69)

Self-knowledge about the frailty of language necessitates poetry because, in poetry, language may overcome its finitude, at least to some limited extent. The dynamic of illumination by self-knowledge is at work most clearly in the extensive and rich collections of Sufi poetry.

Approaches such as Suhrawardi's, which conceive knowledge as a union of object and subject, tend to startle the rational mind, take it by surprise for a moment. In that moment of suspension, the mind realizes the limits of its arsenal of concepts, its tools of thinking; and, in that realization, when ignorance and knowledge merge, the mind knows itself truly – but there is more than *merely itself* at play here. That is, in the context of conceptual paradox, there is an *existential* paradox that challenges the human mind to know itself and gain power in finding out its own limits. The power of self-limitation incorporates mastery over the self, as well as a bearing witness to that act, in a simultaneous act of love. The latter involves cultivation of the Sufi's inner witness, the inner guide, Socrates's *daimon*. The gift of the inner companion is self-knowledge via the disclosure and understanding of limits and surmounting these in manner resembling Platonic dialectic,[3] while highlighting the compassion that accompanies the act of knowledge.

In Sufism, the dialectical structure of the growth of knowledge and the growth of human perfection is fleshed out in visionary recitals, not unlike those of Socrates, as well as mystical elaborations of Qur'anic prophetology. In the prophetology, the idea of the completed, perfected, and universal human is systematically elaborated in a way that appealed both to the orthodox Muslim and the Sufi. In both cases, it was not seen as a merely intellectual structure but as the consummation of human experience. To summarize, every step along the Sufi path involves "polishing the heart," the organ of inner perception, of self-perception and self-recognition. In Islam, the ultimate archetypes or models of perfect humanity are present in the lineage of prophets from Adam to Mohammad. For Sufis, the prophets are exemplars of the way of life. While the prophets are considered to be perfect humans in Islam, they are not on this account identical with one another. According to the Sufi philosopher Alaoddawleh Semnani (1261-1336), the succession of states of exaltation experienced by the Sufi practitioner mirrors the succession of the prophets. In Semnani's words, by attaining the "Adam of

---

3 As demonstrated, for example, in *Republic* 507-20 (the Sun, Line, and Cave), *Symposium* 210-12, and *Phaedrus* 251-57.

one's soul" – the Noah, Moses, and Jesus of one's soul, and so on – the Sufi is enriched and enabled to continue striving for and attaining the "Mohammad of one's soul" (Corbin 1978, 124-25). Each attainment brings the adept closer to participating in the ultimate possibility for humankind: the perfect, the "complete" human (*insan-i-kamel*). The Arabic term *kamel,* which so often is translated as "perfect," actually means *complete*, as in *whole, comprehensive, total, universal.* So the dialectical succession, whether of knowledge or of prophets, is *not linear*: the last step is *not* its destination but its completion. It is important to bear this in mind as we consider transhumanist visions of endless upgrades on the path of human enhancement. We shall see in the following section that some transhumanists already anticipate a break, indeed a radical discontinuity – the *Singularity* – to occur between the human and the ideally enhanced "posthuman" of the future. Literal interpretation of prophetology misconstrues the intention of idealizing the lives of the prophets. For Sufis, the effort is primarily that of the archetypal imagination, not that of dogged replication of historical acts and events.

The pursuit of human perfection is as central to Islam as it is to Jewish and Christian faith traditions. Such a pursuit presupposes the notion of human self-transformation rooted in the assumption that "the transformative act is predicated on a transcendent vision that ontologically we are infinitely better and therefore more worthy than we actually are" (Tu Weiming, in Chittick 2007, 114). Self-transformation is a moral imperative in Islam, Judaism, and Christianity, inseparable from the eschatological hope of the faithful.

Transhumanism's Misguided Approach to Perfection

With a better sense of Islamic approaches to the pursuit of perfection as a striving for perfection within the divine, we may now examine the transhumanist project, especially its fascination with human enhancement and endless "progress." There are important differences between the transhumanist and the Sufi pursuit of perfection. For the Sufi, all knowledge is there to help answer the key question of "What does it mean to be human?" In Islam, only God knows the answer, and it is the human quest to divine that answer.

Transhumanists are also on a quest, but they disavow any teleological answer to the question and any assumption of finality. Such disavowals are aimed, consciously or not, at a *static* notion of perfection. Transhumanists reject a static, essentialist idea of human nature. A flat denial of static human nature justifies a goal of endless improvement, endless upgrades. But explicit consideration of dynamic, process-based metaphysics is absent from transhumanist literature. Transhumanist appeals to evolution are common: whether evolution is understood to be driven by differential rates of reproduction in the classical sense or by systematic genetic modification of individuals via government-sponsored technological means, e.g., germ-line manipulation (Mehlman 2003).

The key unquestioned assumption, however, is that questions of enhancement can be practically and meaningfully answered by science and technology. Significantly, this assumption is unaffected by one's position on the existence of a fixed human essence or ideal toward which humans ought to strive – consequential as these positions may be. But a commitment to science as the royal road to human improvement is problematic. Even where Nick Bostrom, a leading transhumanist thinker, voices some skepticism about the goal of endless human enhancement, he does not doubt the key role of science in striving for this goal. Bostrom discusses a number of what he calls "existential risks" that might derail the pursuit of endless improvement (Bostrom 2002, 5-6). But the gist of Bostrom's essay is that if we are sufficiently clever, creative, careful, and caring, rational thought will enable us to improve ourselves indefinitely. While he admits the limits of rationality, he still considers rationality to be self-corrective and does not fathom any other alternative. In his view, scientific rationality is without rival, and we have no real choice in the matter of how *real* knowledge about anything is best attained. Whereas Islam places ultimate faith in God, believing that the purpose of human life, the perfection of human consciousness, and the experience of bliss terminate in God (Chittick 2007, 140), transhumanists firmly and unselfconsciously believe that science and technology can and will pave the way to endless improvement and human happiness. At the very least, they believe that science and technology are by far the best bets.

A strong argument in support of the transhumanist faith in a technology-mediated process of infinite improvement, at least from the epistemological perspective, may be the self-correcting nature of scientific inquiry. The logic of self-correction was developed by the American philosopher of logic Charles Sanders Peirce (1839-1914). Most recently, Peirce's ideas on the logic of inquiry have been adopted by artificial intelligence (AI) developers (e.g., Josephson and Josephson 1994; Magnani 2000). This is especially interesting in connection with the place that AI holds in the predictions of Ray Kurzweil (2006), an influential spokesman for a transhuman vision of the future enhancement, and eventual surpassing of human intelligence via its merger with AI. Scholars of religion such as Geraci (2008) have already noted the strong apocalyptic tendencies in the works of Kurzweil, Hans Moravec, and Marvin Minsky and have appropriately dubbed their vision "Apocalyptic AI". Geraci avers:

> Apocalyptics hope that God, as arbiter of absolute justice and rectifier of a corrupt world, will radically reconstruct the world. Apocalyptics, despite their criticism of the present world, are not pessimistic in their outlook. They are "passionately concerned, even obsessed, with the possibility of goodness". As this world is so miserably sinful, apocalyptics look forward to the time when God creates a new, infinitely good world. (Geraci 2008, 143)

Apocalyptic AI identifies humanity with rational thinking and rationality with self-corrective computation. Given the acceptance of these presumptions, or ones very like them, the idea of limitless, automated, autonomous self-improvement seems plausible, even inevitable, as Ray Kurzweil argues (2003, 197). Yet, given the obviously mythical nature of such claims, their apocalyptical stature cannot escape notice: Kurzweil uses the device of dialogues with *Molly 2104*, an AI agent from the future, to present his vision of the glorious technomediated destiny that await those who "heeded the signs" and began taking the right steps in 2004 (Kurzweil 2006, 141).

The limits of rational thought were addressed very early in the history of philosophy and science. Plato, one of the most influential exponents of such limitation, was a master of suspending opposite tendencies of thought without resolving the tension. The creative tension between logical, discursive thought – *logos* – and inspired, mystical thought – *mythos* – is featured explicitly and implicitly in most of his dialogues. Suhrawardi advanced this insight with reference to logical and the mystical tendencies present in the Islamic culture of his era. Like Plato, Suhrawardi understood that it is preferable to maintain tension about some issues rather than to force their resolution and declare a victory of one side over the other.

The attraction of these primal modalities continues to draw on human aspirations. Both mythic and logical thinking permeate the content of scientific ideas, as well as the pursuit of these ideas in actual practice. Examples from the frontiers of physics and medicine abound in the literature of science and technology studies. Some of the currently predicted panaceas will turn out to be snake oil, some the elixir of life; and inevitably, many theories of everything will turn out to be theories of not much. Most often, however, it is never so clear: an idea or approach may display decades, or more, of effectiveness even though it is wrong-headed or just wrong. Ptolemaic astronomy is a paradigm case.

Though it disavows the idea of perfection as an outmoded "medieval" concept, transhumanism opts for unlimited enhancement as the best way to human well-being. Therefore, transhumanism measures progress as improvement relative to the present state of affairs and aims to remove or repair human flaws without prejudgments about what is "ideal" or perfectly human. Kurzweil echoes a basic conviction of transhumanism when he questions the "inevitability of death." The irony is that the "posthuman" state toward which transhumanists strive is here defined negatively: the *denial* of death is emblematic of its mission to eradicate a host of natural flaws and "design errors." When stated positively, the aims of transhumanism are often couched in terms of amplification of existing human qualities currently judged to be valuable. Though transhumanism is not a religion, religious ideals continue to shape the quasi-mythical nature of many its ideals.

Transhumanism's Religious Aspirations

I argue that, while transhumanism shares certain ideals traditionally found in the world's religions (e.g., transcending biological limits, overcoming death, achieving superhuman traits, and attaining a state of bliss), it understands and pursues these ideals in fundamentally flawed ways. First, transhumanists tend to literalize the ideals expressed by various religions (Hopkins 2005; Hughes 2007; Geraci 2008), thus trading meaning for a tangible material result that, at least temporarily, satisfies the simple aspiration that "we can be better than this" (Hopkins 2005, 26). Second, transhumanists reduce erstwhile religious ideals to products and processes that are more or less technologically plausible. By contrast, the Sufi perspective offers us a nonliteral, nontechnological ideal of human perfection as a vantage point from which to critique central transhumanist proposals.

In agreement with some of the other essays of this volume, I see transhumanist thought as a secularization of religious themes long present in Western religions. The "prophets" of transhumanism, Julian Huxley, J.B.S. Haldane, and J.D. Bernal (see Tirosh-Samuelson, this volume), were scientists and public intellectuals who acted on their principles with keen deliberation and articulate openness. Though the term *transhuman* was not introduced (by Huxley) until 1957, the concept was already articulated by each of the three scientists in the 1920s. Haldane's *Daedalus* (1924); Huxley's *Religion without Revelation* (1927), and Bernal's *The World, The Flesh and the Devil* (1929) explored the possibilities of a wholehearted, systematic application of science and technology to human enhancement. Even allowing for the fact that these works were addressed to the general public, it is of singular importance, I believe, that each author selected explicit religious and mythological themes in their titles. Of the three men, Huxley was most substantively aware of the religious dimension of transhumanism. He considered the transhumanist enterprise to be a replacement for, or rather an *upgrade* of, religion. When it comes to contemporary transhumanists, however, there seems to be less self-awareness or else a lack of concern about foundational questions of motivation and history, as if the idea of progress and futurity somehow trumps legacy.

Contemporary transhumanists have written about religion, though the dialogue seems more than a little one-sided. James Hughes, executive director of the Institute for Ethics and Emerging Technologies and author of *Citizen Cyborg* (2004), wrote an article on the compatibility of religious and transhumanist perspectives (Hughes 2007). In it, he presents the results of a survey of religious sentiments of members of the World Transhumanist Association (WTA): 62 percent of members are secular, atheist, or agnostic, while 24 percent identify with some form of religion or spirituality and 14 percent indicate "Other/Don't know." Throughout much of his presentation, Hughes discusses areas of overlap and agreement to show that religions are not at odds with transhumanism. While this is not the place for a thorough analysis of his article, a few points should be highlighted. To a large extent, the cases discussed by Hughes demonstrate how science can aid in bringing about much of what various religions hold dear. He translates the aims of a given religion into something that science and technology *can* address. In this, he follows Julian Huxley. This tendency becomes especially obvious in the case of apocalyptic discourse. Hughes maintains his approach of showing the literal compatibility of transhumanism and religion at the expense of the latter's symbolic and mystical dimensions. As long as religious prophecies and practices are interpreted in a materialistic, factual, and historical perspective, Hughes's brand of transhumanism agrees with *all* of them.

Hughes acknowledges and builds on Patrick Hopkins's analysis of similarities and dissimilarities between transhumanism and religion. Hopkins articulates same areas of stark incompatibility but finds that the compatibilities are based in the shared desire to transcend what he calls the "animal account" of human nature (Hopkins 2005, 24). Hughes illustrates Hopkins's claims with a variety of examples, ranging from created cocreator theologies to technologically and chemically mediated moral improvement and religious experiences. In all of Hughes's illustrations, the underlying assumption is one that Hopkins states clearly: "Technology lets us see religious ideals as *literally* realizable" (Hopkins 2005, 26).

The shape of scientific theories and the direction of technological development in any age are influenced by the way in which a civilization deals with the ever-present rational and mystical tendencies of human thought. I argue that the presence of this pair of tendencies is common to both transhumanism and Sufism, but the intersection is often unconscious and relatively undifferentiated in the former case and relatively well- differentiated in the latter. I contend that, although transhumanists are moved by the same transcendental urges, they act on them in ways that are ultimately futile at best or, at worse, self-defeating. Though he disagrees with this argument, Hopkins states it as follows: "[T]ranshumanism is pointless and distracting: material technology will never accomplish what it seeks, so the pursuit of it simply wastes time, money, and energy" (2005, 24) While I generally agree with this statement, I would not put it in these terms. The key point of difference revolves around modern culture's tendency to valorize literal, rational, and historical thinking as opposed to symbolic, metaphorical, and metahistorical thinking (Brown 1984). This point is developed further in the final section of this chapter when we consider transhumanist approaches to resurrection and immortality.

The transhumanist wish list includes many of the same divine gifts that we find in the ancient mythologies of every human culture, chief among these being eternal life and the transcendence of physical, or at least bodily, limitations: it's the end of the world as we know it. Robert Geraci's discussion of "Apocalyptic AI" neatly sums up transhumanism's apocalyptical tendencies:

> Longstanding religious dreams of purity, perfection, and immortality can be realized, say the Apocalyptic AI advocates, as long as we see them through scientific and technological lenses. … Only by eliminating the physical and embracing the virtual, say Apocalyptic AI authors, can we return to the undifferentiated wholeness of the good. (Geraci 2008, 160)

The Imaginal World of Sufism and the Transhuman Imagination

Our comparison of Sufism and transhumanism is brought into sharper relief by examining the use of the imagination in both traditions. A distinctive feature of Suhrawardi's philosophy is *alam al-mithal,* literally, the "world of images or likenesses." Henry Corbin, famed scholar of Islam, dubbed it the *mundus imaginalis* or the imaginal world:

> [B]etween the two [sense and intellect] is placed an intermediate world … '*alam al-mithal*', the world of the Image, *mundus imaginalis*: a world as ontologically real as the world of the senses and the world of the intellect, a world that requires a faculty of perception belonging to it, a faculty that is a cognitive function, a *noetic* value, as fully real as the faculties of sensory perception or intellectual intuition. This faculty is the imaginative power, the one we must avoid confusing with the imagination that modern man identifies with "fantasy." (Corbin 1976, 9)

I maintain that the ontological status of the imaginal world is consistent with the status of certain products of the scientific imagination that are constructed by blending empirical findings and theoretical models – most of the knowledge that the sciences produce falls into this category. As products of theoretical thinking, the abstract entities formulated by science and engineering enable us to interact in powerful ways with the world of the senses. Abstract entities are not strictly speaking *material*; while they are not on the same ontological level as empirical objects, nevertheless, they are of tremendous benefit in manipulating the world of empirical objects. Neither are these abstract entities what Plato would have called "pure ideas," like numbers or other purely formal concepts.

While abstract entities are, at least in my view, at home in the imaginal world, they are not the only denizens of this realm. The Sufis populate this realm with countless cities, people, landscapes, and wonders that defy description – all meant for those religious practitioners seeking to perfect themselves. There are similarities between the eschatological vision of the Sufis and those of some transhumanist who resonates with Kurzweil's view of the postsingularity world of the future. In both cases, we find familiar rewards promised by various religious traditions.

Can the imaginal world, whether Kurzweil's or Suhrawardi's, be distinguished from pure fantasy? Suhrawardi applies logical criteria equally to all three worlds: empirical, imaginal, and intellectual. If we take internal coherence and consistency as primary criteria of what belongs in the imaginal world, we would have to admit all kinds of products of scientific imagination, including biochemical formulas and the genetic code – the latter, as its metaphorical name clearly indicates, is a construct blended from empirical observations and theoretical concepts. I believe that these items – and the long wish list of real and imagined transhumanist products that promise to extend life, intelligence, and maturity – all belong in *alam al-mithal*. However, a number of scholars commenting on the work of Suhrawardi and ibn al-Arabi (e.g., Corbin 1979; Cheetham 2003) would exclude the items I have mentioned because, in their view, *alam al-mithal* has a moral and spiritual tone that is incongruent with the command-and-control approach shared by Western science and much of the transhumanist project. I acknowledge the point; but on purely ontological grounds, I cannot see how to exclude these and certain other blended products of scientific imagination from *alam al-mithal*.

Perhaps the key difference is the contrast between the nonutilitarian, classically apocalyptic understanding of human aspiration in Sufism and the largely utilitarian nature of scientific and technological development. The first commits one to a never-ending and, strictly speaking, impossible quest to mirror the infinite beauty of the divine within the finite vessel of a human life. The second commits one to a never-ending and, strictly speaking, all-too-possible and even technologically necessary quest to upgrade and surpass the previous generation of devices, from the lowest frivolous gadget to the most sophisticated medical instrument.

For the spiritually minded Sufi philosopher, the imaginal world is not a workshop for inventing an endless series of new gadgets ... or is it? Sufis are not, by and large, hermits, nor are they doctrinally against scientific knowledge. During the peak of Islamic civilization, before the *kalam*-based theocracy achieved full strength and infiltrated every facet of intellectual culture, Sufis were among the ranks of great inventors and discoverers of scientific and technological novelties. I doubt that any of them would have refused better laboratory equipment. Nevertheless, though science and technology are not in principle incompatible with Sufism, the main intention of entering the imaginal world was never utilitarian for Sufis. Rather, it is seen as the locus of the human soul between the "two blasts of the Trumpet." The first blast separates souls from their corporeal bodies at the point of bodily death; the second awakens the soul to its resurrection body and its afterlife judgment. The period "between the blasts" is spent in the inter-world of *mundus imaginalis*, a space of spiritual creativity, where the object of creativity is the spiritual body of the itinerant soul of the mystic. While *mundus imaginalis* is the dwelling place of all souls during dreams and after death, it is also the chosen habitation of mystical adepts while still awake and alive. Suhrawardi and ibn al-Arabi refer to this as the "world of prophecy," meaning that accounts of revelation and miracles witnessed or performed by prophets "took place" in *alam al-mithal*, not in the world of everyday sense-based experience (Corbin 1979). It is only here that the human soul finds transcendent meaning. The quest for the empirical referent of miracles would, in this view, be a meaningless and wrong-headed activity. Given this understanding, Kurzweil's eschatological scenarios are largely meaningless, if partially achievable, fantasies.

The status of the imagination is most relevant to the ideal of eternal life in Sufism and transhumanism. The idea that science and technology could bring about the final defeat of death by resurrecting the body has been articulated by the Nikolai Fedorovich Fedorov (see Clay, this volume). Preoccupation with resurrection of the body is also of deep concern to Sufis of the illuminationist school. However, for the Sufis, these are apocalyptic events that take place in *alam al-mithal*. The Sufi Shaikh Ahmad Ahsai and his followers (late nineteenth century to the present) focus not on the physical body but on the *subtle* body, the body of light that dwells "in the cities of *alam al-mithal*." Not only is the subtle body directly involved in the final destiny of the soul (the Day of Judgment), but also in its incremental refinement and improvement (Corbin 1979, 180-83). It is in the intermediary world of *alam-al-mithal* that each soul builds the pattern of its resurrection body, i.e., the template on which the resurrection will occur at the sounding of "the second blast of the Trumpet" at the end of the world.

Transhumanism's Enlightenment and the Limits of Reason

In "A History of Transhumanist Thought," Nick Bostrom (2005) sees transhumanism as a continuation of the eighteenth-century European Enlightenment ideals. But he fails to acknowledge the strong mythic commitments in Enlightenment thinking that undermine its claims for pure rationality. The "shadow" side of the Enlightenment contains much of what had passed for legitimate intellectual production over several centuries of premodern Europe culture. A number of interesting historical studies have traced the transition of European thought into the modern world with a focus on pivotal figures like Francis Bacon (1561-1626), Johannes Kepler (1571-1630), and Isaac Newton (1643-1727): visionaries who saw far beyond the world into which they were born (Merchant 1980; Shapin and Schaffer 1985; Dobbs 1975). These studies indicate that scientific rationality was anything but pure during the Enlightenment. The case of Newton is interesting given his iconic status in the history of science: he is the textbook case of rational thought chasing away the last vestiges of the "spook-filled" medieval world. But in actuality, it is a textbook case of revisionist history.

Thanks to extensive studies of Newton's nonscientific manuscripts that were sold at auction in 1936 (Dobbs 1975, 13), a very different picture of Newton has emerged. John Maynard Keynes, who purchased the manuscripts, noted that "Newton was not the first of the age of reason. He was the last of the magicians" (Keynes 1947, 27). It became apparent that his writings on theology, alchemy, and biblical history far outstrip the volume of his magnificent writings in physics and math. There are two morals to Newton's story. First, rational thought did not free itself from mythic thinking in the case of the most celebrated genius of "The Century of Genius." Second, if the public understanding of Newton is any indication (Gleik 2004), many academics and the general public are still in a state of ignorance or denial about certain nonrational aspects of the Enlightenment's intellectual achievements. Nearly seventy-five years have passed since the public auction of Newton's "occult" writings, and there is still widespread ignorance of his ardent devotion to theological and alchemical matters – what most people today wouldn't hesitate to call irrational thinking. This trend is well exemplified by Bostrom's nostalgia for Enlightenment rationality. Simply declaring independence from mythico-religious thinking does not make it go away. The ideal, according to some schools of Sufism, including those discussed in the present paper, is to maintain a dynamic balance between the two aspects of thinking.

Bostrom upholds "empirical science and critical reason – rather than revelation and religious authority – as ways of learning about the natural world and our place within it and of providing a grounding for morality. Transhumanism, has roots in rational humanism" (Bostrom 2005, 3).

Let me ignore the false dichotomies Bostrom posits between revelation and science, reason and religious authority, to focus on the important issue of "grounding." The moral systems that emerged from the historical period that Bostrom sets up as exemplary are largely centered on the individual as the moral subject, the ultimate unit of moral consideration. The moral perception of eighteenth-century Europe is largely refracted through the lens of scientific empiricism and critical reason. While the resulting moral philosophies are not wrong, strictly speaking, they suffer from severe blind spots that subsequent generations of moral reflection have taken centuries to correct. For example, after many decades of philosophical debates, many ethicists now hold "the environment" to be a moral subject deserving consideration and protection (Callicott and Palmer 2004). Since the civil rights and feminist movements of the 1960s, we have become more keenly aware that rational humanism had important blinds spots. Indeed, until relatively recently, the term *moral subject* implicitly referred to the "privileged, white Christian male of European descent." In the past few decades, "new" voices have started changing the shape and content of moral discourse in the academic world. Is it surprising that it should take critical reason well over two hundred years to reflect on the deficiencies of this stance as a starting point for moral reflection – and only then by social forces largely external to academia? Perhaps it should not be a surprise that "pure" reason is limited in itself and always stands in need of external stimuli. But if we delimit the applicability of pure reason – as Kant (1999 [1781]) himself attempted to do – what is left to us? What happens to empirical science and historical thinking? And can we think coherently without viewing the individual subject as the starting point and progressing linearly, logically step by step, to rational conclusions about the world?

Certainly, the *denial* of these and other weapons in our intellectual arsenal would be self-defeating. But arguing for their *limitation*, on the other hand, is tenable. That has been done by scores of thinkers in the past – and many of them did so during the Middle Ages. Nearly a century has past since Kurt Gödel and Werner Heisenberg presented mathematically rigorous statements about the limits of mathematics and physics, respectively (Gödel 1951; Heisenberg 1930). But Bostrom makes no mention of these major milestones of twentieth-century thinking. He does question the usefulness of fictional scare tactics employed by Aldous Huxley, George Orwell, and Leon Kass; and his rehearsal of George Annas's laughable *Planet of the Apes* us-vs.-them paranoia about the posthuman subjugation of (natural) humans is especially amusing (Bostrom 2005, 24-25). Heisenberg and Gödel were not making appeals to emotion but rather to sustained logical and mathematical arguments about the limits of logic, math, and observational science. Bostrom is guilty of facile stereotyping, as he begins his history by trotting out the old image of the medieval era as a period of great intellectual stagnation. A cursory survey of discoveries, explorations, and innovations in many fields of human endeavor, extending from Europe through the Middle East to China (Huff 2003), give lie to that stale image – one as old as the Enlightenment itself and as narrow-minded and selective in its choice of evidence.

Apocalyptic Islam and the Transhumanist Denial of Death

Whereas Enlightenment humanism and moral theory center on the individual, the medieval world of Islamic civilization in its prime was shaped by religious imagination and apocalyptical vision. The transhumanist enhancement of Enlightenment humanism strives to transcend human limits via a historical sequence of technoscience-mediated improvements to the human condition. By contrast, the apocalyptic religious vision presents a metahistorical reading of present history as the ever-unfolding revelation of archetypal tales that have been told and retold from prehistoric times up to the present moment. It presents a vision of human enhancement that is interpreted neither literally nor historically.

While the apocalyptic mode of religious experience is present in Judaism and Christianity, it is often subordinated to strictly historical accounts of God's interactions with the world. The key difference between the Bible and Qur'an – and, hence, the distinct religious sense of Islam – lies in the fact that the relationship between history and apocalypse is reversed. The historical sense of the Qur'an is so often submerged that many non-Muslim commentators have questioned its narrative coherence.

In his "Apocalypse of Islam," N.O. Brown (1984) recalls the comment by the eminent twentieth-century orientalist R.A. Nicholson: "Mohammed with his excitable temperament does not shine as a raconteur." And there is the less charitable assessment of the Qur'an by Thomas Carlyle, a Victorian-era defender of Mohammad:

> "I must say, it is as toilsome reading as I ever undertook. A wearisome confused jumble, crude, incondite; endless iterations, long-windedness, entanglement; most crude, incondite; – insupportable stupidity, in short!" (Brown 1984, 155)

Although the Qur'an proclaims itself as the continuation and final chapter of the prophetic tradition of Abraham, it is a mistake to think of it as an attempt to update and reconcile the stories and histories of the Bible. The Qur'an is not intended to supersede what it reveres as Holy Scripture with an account that is more palatable to the rational, historical mind of the modern reader. Quite the contrary, it routinely dissolves the facts of the latter in the dreamy waters of myth and folklore and distills new spirits from familiar tales. Rather than setting the record straight, it bends it further away from factual claims and shifts consciousness from history to meaning, from prediction to prophecy:

> Islam is committed by the Koran to project a meta-historical plane on which the eternal meaning of historical events is disclosed. It is that plane on which Moses and Elijah are seen conversing with Jesus in Matthew chapter XVII; that plane on which Dante's *Divine Comedy* unfolds; and Blake's prophetic books; and *Finnegans Wake*. History *sub specie aeternitatis*. (Brown 1984, 167)

Brown has captured some of the purpose of Suhrawardi's recurrence to symbolism and visionary recitals. The illuminationist tradition posits an ontology within which the prophetic has all the reality of sensual and historical experience but is free from its material conditions and linearity. In this way, the "mute speech" of events and things continues as a medium of communication without restricting or redirecting the mind to the single correct answer to the question "What actually happened here?" The apocalyptic vision stimulates consciousness of the separation

> between "what actually happened", events as seen by the eye of historical materialism, and "what is really going on", events *sub specie aeternitatis*, as seen by the inward, the clair-

voyant eye, the second sight ... between literal meaning and something beyond – in Islamic terminology between *zahir* and *batin*, between outer (exoteric) and inner (esoteric); between external-visible-patent and internal-invisible-latent; between materialist and spiritual meanings. (Brown 1984, 162)

Transhumanism – especially the variety that subscribes to what Geraci (2008) calls "Apocalyptic AI" – is what you get when you strive for transcendent values but refuse to separate the worldviews that Brown described. Geraci's use of the term *apocalyptic* is ironically bereft of the depth of Brown's traditional usage. Geraci wishes to lay bare the transhumanist confusion of inner and outer worlds in a triumphal reduction of religious apocalyptic goals into technologically achievable "solutions" to the human problem.

Perhaps the earliest, and certainly one of the more outlandish, version of the transhumanist project of technology-mediated eschatology is found in the work of Nikolai Fedorovich Fedorov (1829-1903). Like contemporary transhumanists, Fedorov's enemy was death, which he called the "greatest evil." His solution: abolish death ... but not just going forward; he exhorted his contemporaries to join together in the great task of resurrecting all dead ancestors! I believe this goal goes much further than any transhumanist on record, including Ray Kurzweil, who is currently pursuing the project of resurrecting his deceased father through cloning and artificial intelligence (Lyons 2009).

While Kurzweil is admittedly motivated purely by individual sentiment, Fedorov's ultimate project of "scientific resurrection" was borne out of his unique response to a central issue in Christian theology. His innovation was to use science and technology to bring about literal resurrection by means of resuscitation. He interprets the "Day of Resurrection" as a world historical project and a religious imperative that would unify all humankind in a "common task," as he called it. When examined in its religious context, it becomes clear that Fedorov was taking on an issue central to the history of Christian theology, namely, the resurrection of Christ and the thorny questions of how to reconcile Christ's humanity and mortality with His divinity and eternality (see Clay, chapter 5 in this volume). In the context of transhumanist ideals, Fedorov anticipated and, in fact, inspired the futurists who started the Russian space program and other influential figures and philosophies at the heart of transhumanism.

The great Russian philosopher of the twentieth century, Nikolai Berdyaev (1874-1948) presents Fedorov as an odd coincidence of opposites and a "monstrous duality of religio-conservative and the revolutionary-progressive ... [and] positivist-rationalist approaches towards mystical matters." In short, a very Russian mix of utopianism, realism and materialism:

> The fantastic and the utopian for Fedorov are bound up namely with his realism, with his materialism. These bold projects are directed particularly at this material and empirical world, and they are attempts to transform and manage it. He is hostile to the contemplation

> of other worlds, he demands actions in this world. He employs the word "mystical" always in a negative sense, and it means the same for him as that which is unreal, the idealistic, the fantastic, although his own fundamental idea outside of mysticism is bereft of all meaning. (Berdyaev 1915, sec. I)

Berdyaev was a philosopher of politics and religion and a proud Russian (Clarke 1950; Lowrie 1960). While expressing sympathy for Fedorov's selfless, romantic, religious fervor, Berdyaev did not shy away from exposing the latter's blindspot. Celebrating the centenary of Fedorov's birth, Berdyaev closes with the following:

> Fedorov sees in death the source of evil, and in victory over death the primary task of mankind. In this is his truth. But he underestimates the mystical meaning of the passage through death as the inner moment of life, i.e. the redemptive meaning of the Cross and of Golgotha. (Berdyaev 1950, 130)

This is as appropriate an assessment of Fedorov's project as it is of today's transhumanists. The fact that Berdyaev employs the central symbols of Christianity to critique the sense of Fedorov's oversight does not in any way diminish its applicability to transhumanists, whether they self-identify as atheists, Buddhists, Jews, Christians, or Muslims.

Conclusion

Nothing is perfect. This statement of the obvious betrays, at one and the same time, simple realism and an awareness, perhaps a desire for transcendent perfection. Reflections on human perfection have "launched a thousand ships" bearing cargo and crew of mixed origins and of negotiable, sometimes questionable value. This is our inescapable cultural legacy.

Every response to the question of human perfection is of mixed lineage. Separating the mythical and mystical from the literal and realistic is not a trivial task but keeping them balanced in a productive tension is even more difficult. All too often, transhumanist authors have decided that rational scientific and technological discourse is always the best approach to the question, so a scientific and technical answer, with reasonable allowance for moral and humanitarian ideals, will be the right one. Suhrawardi strove for a balance of the two co-limiting tendencies within the rigidly religious world of his time. Though his solutions are worthy of consideration, they do not exactly fit our world and our time. We would benefit from applying a similar sense of balance to the operation of these two tendencies of thought in the current debates about human enhancement. As it stands, the emphasis on scientific and technological arguments is excessive, and any awareness of the positive relevance of nonscientific considerations is dim or nonexistent.

What if we were to consider the value of nonliteral, nondiscursive thinking and assume for a moment that our premodern ancestors were *not* completely mad?

Can we understand that their reverence for song, poetry, and story was not idle and that their religious reflections about the meaning of human life actually got at something meaningful? How would our discussion of human enhancement appear to them, and where would it go from here?

I believe that, if Suhrawardi and ibn al-Arabi were to return magically to our time, or slightly in the future, they would stroke their beards, smile and say, "*Your brilliant imaginations have borne so many irresistible fruits, magical fruits that promise to increase your physical, mental and spiritual capacities, fruits that promise you longer life – Marvelous! But tell me: is there one that makes you wise in your choices of which fruits to eat, how much to eat, how to combine and enjoy your increased capacities? And who is making your music, your poetry these days? Do you know if these are improving, their quality increasing? Or do you have some fruit that increases your capacity to respond with bliss to any music regardless of its inherent quality?*"

References

Barks, Coleman, and John Moyne. 1995. *The Essential Rumi*. New York: Harper Collins.

Berdyaev, Nikolai A. 1915. "The religion of resusciative *[sic]* resurrection", translated by S. Janos: http://www.berdyaev.com/berdiaev/berd_lib/1915_186.html, accessed July 12, 2011.

–. 1950. N. F. Fedorov. *Russian Review* 9 (2): 124-30.

Berkey, Jonathan Porter. 2003. *The Formation of Islam: Religion and Society in the Near East, 600-1800*. New York: Cambridge University Press.

Bernal, J. D. 1970 [1929]. *The World, the Flesh and the Devil: An Enquiry into the Future of the Three Enemies of the Rational Soul*. London: Jonathan Cape.

Bostrom, Nick. 2002. Existential risks: Analyzing human extinction scenarios and related hazards. *Journal of Evolution and Technology* 9: http://www.nickbostrom.com/existential/risks.html, accessed July 12, 2011.

–. 2005. A history of transhumanist thought: http://www.nickbostrom.com/papers/history.pdf, accessed July 12, 2011.

Brown, N.O. 1984. The apocalypse of Islam. *Social Text* 8: 155-71.

Callicott, J. Baird, and Clare Palmer, eds. 2004. *Environmental Philosophy: Critical Concepts in the Environment*. New York: Routledge.

Cheetham, T. 2003. *The World Turned Inside Out: Henry Corbin and Islamic Mysticism*. Putnam, CT: Spring Publications.

Chittick, William C. 1983. *The Sufi Path of Love*. Albany, NY: SUNY Press.

–. 2007. *Science of the Cosmos, Science of the Soul: The Pertinence of Islamic Cosmology in the Modern World*. Oxford: One World Publications.

Clarke, Oliver Fielding. 1950. *Introduction to Berdyaev*. London: G. Bles.
Corbin, Henry. 1969. *Creative Imagination in the Sufism of ibn Arabi*. Princeton, NJ: Princeton University Press.
–. 1976. *Mundus imaginalis: Or, the Imaginary and the Imaginal*. Translated by Ruth Horine. Ipswich: Golgonooza Press.
–. 1978. *Man of Light in Iranian Sufism*. Boulder, CO: Shambala Press.
–. 1979. *Heavenly Earth, Celestial Earth: From Mazdean Iran to Shi'ite Iran*. Boston: Shambhala.
–. 2003. *Inside Iranian Islam: Spiritual and Philosophical Aspects, Volume II*. Trans, H. M. Van Woerkom: http://www.scribd.com/doc/9664772/Henry-Corbins-In-Iranian-Islam-Vol2, accessed July 12, 2011. This is an on-line-only translation of Corbin's work, published in Paris by Gallimard (1971).
Dobbs, B.J.T. 1975. *The Foundations of Newton's Alchemy*. Cambridge: Cambridge University Press.
Friedlander, Paul. 1969. *Plato: An Introduction*. Princeton, NJ: Princeton University Press.
Geraci, Robert. 2008. Apocalyptic AI: Religion and the promise of artificial intelligence. *Journal of the American Academy of Religion* 76 (1): 138-166.
Gleick, James. 2004. Isaac Newton's gravity: How a major new exhibition gets the scientist wrong: http://www.slate.com/id/2108438/ Thursday, October 21, 2004, accessed July 15, 2011.
Gödel, Kurt. 1955. Some basic theorems on the foundations of mathematics and their implications. In S. Feferman, ed. *Collected works / Kurt Gödel, Vol. III*. Oxford: Oxford University Press.
Haldane, J. B. S. 1924. *Daedalus: Or, Science and the Future*. London: Chatto and Windus.
Heisenberg, Werner. 1930. *The Physical Principles of Quantum Theory*. Translated by C. Eckart and F. C. Hoyt.Chicago: University of Chicago Press.
Herrin, Judith. 1987. *The Formation of Christendom*. Princeton, NJ: Princeton University Press.
Hopkins, Patrick D. 2005. Transcending the animal: How transhumanism and religion are and are not alike. *Journal of Evolution and Technology* 14 (1): 11-26.
Huff, Toby E. 2003. *The Rise of Early Modern Science: Islam, China and the West*. New York: Cambridge University Press.
Hughes, James. 2007. The compatibility of religious and transhumanist views of metaphysics, suffering, virtue and transcendence in an enhanced future: http://www.metanexus.net/magazine/tabid/68/id/9930/Default.aspx, accessed July 22, 2011.
Huxley, Julian. 1979 [1927]. *Religion without Revelation*. Westport, CT: Greenwood Press.

Josephson, John R., and Susan G. Josephson. 1994. *Abductive inference: Computation, philosophy, technology*. New York: Cambridge University Press.
Kant, Immanuel. 1999 [1781]. *Critique of Pure Reason*. Translated by P. Guyer and A. Wood.New York: Cambridge University Press.
Keynes, John Maynard. 1947. "Newton, the man". In *The Royal Society Tercentenary Celebrations 15-19 July 1946*, 27-34. Cambridge: Cambridge University Press.
Kurzweil, Ray. 2003. *Ray Kurzweil Reader*: http://www.kurzweilai.net/pdf/RayKurzweilReader.pdf, accessed July 12, 2011.
–. 2006. *The Singularity Is Near: When Humans Transcend Biology*. New York: Penguin.
Lowrie, Donald A. 1960. *Rebellious Prophet: A Life of Nicolai Berdyaev*. New York: Harper.
Lyons, Daniel. 2009. I, Robot. *Newsweek*, May 16: http://www.newsweek.com/2009/05/16/i-robot.html, accessed July 12, 2011.
Magnani, Lorenzo. 2000. *Abduction, Reason and Science: Processes of Discovery and Explanation*. New York: Springer.
Mehlman, Maxwell J. 2003. *Wondergenes: Genetic Enhancement and the Future of Society*. Bloomington: Indiana University Press.
Merchant, Carolyn. 1980. *The Death of Nature: Women, Ecology, and the Scientific Revolution*. New York: Harper Row.
Nasr, Seyyed Hossein. 1964. *Three Muslim Sages: Avicenna-Suhrawardi-ibn 'Arabi*. Cambridge, MA: Harvard University Press.
Nasr, Seyyed Hossein, and William C. Chittick. 2007. *The Essential Seyyed Hossein Nas*. Bloomington, IN: World Wisdom.
Netton, I. R. 1994. *Allāh Transcendent: Studies in the Structure and Semiotics of Islamic Philosophy, Theology, and Cosmology*. Surrey, UK: Curzon Press.
Ozdemir, Ibrahim. 2003. Toward an understanding of environmental ethics from a Qur'anic perspective. In R. C. Foltz, F. M. Denny, and A. Baharuddin, eds., *Islam and Ecology: A Bestowed Trust*, 3-38. Cambridge, MA: Harvard University Press.
Schimmel, Annemarie. 1975. *Mystical Dimensions of Islam*. Chapel Hill: University of North Carolina Press.
Shapin, Steven, and Simon Schaffer. 1985. *Leviathan and the Air Pump: Hobbes, Boyle and the Experimental Life*. Princeton, NJ: Princeton University Press.
Walbridge, John. 2001. *The Wisdom of the Mystic East: Suhrawardī and Platonic Orientalism*. Albany, NY: SUNY Press.
Ziai, Hossein. 1990. *Knowledge and Illumination*. Brown Judaic Studies No. 97. Atlanta: Scholars Press.
–. 1996. Suhrawardi. In S. H. Nasr and O. Leaman, eds., *History of Islamic Philosophy*, 434-64. London and New York: Routledge.

Transhumanism and the Orthodox Christian Tradition

Eugene Clay

From its very origins, as Hava Tirosh-Samuelson has shown in the first chapter of this collection, the modern Anglo-American transhumanist movement has generally regarded traditional Christianity with considerable suspicion and skepticism. Today, many of the most enthusiastic transhumanists, like their British forebears J.B.S. Haldane and J. D. Bernal, are emphatically atheistic; others, like the practicing Buddhist James Hughes, have heaped scorn on Christian ethical qualms about, for example, stem-cell research. Generally, transhumanists have failed to take Christian conceptions about humanity seriously: Julian Savulescu (2009) simply asserts, without discussion, that the concept of the soul is a "bad rationalization" (220); with ill-disguised contempt, Nick Bostrom (2009) ridicules the famous wager of Blaise Pascal (1623-62); and William Bainbridge (2005) dismisses Christian critics of transhumanism as venal enemies of progress and the Enlightenment. Transhumanists generally reject the idea of divine intervention and revelation, as recent surveys of the members of the World Transhumanist Association show (Hughes 2007). Transhumanist efforts to engage Christians have generally been feeble at best, motivated more by political expediency than by a real desire for intellectual exchange (Hughes 2009; Campbell and Walker 2005). As the transhumanist Eric Steinhart (2008) boldly puts it, "Since Christianity is an extremely powerful cultural force in the West, it is imperative for transhumanism to engage it carefully."

One need not dig deeply to find the reasons for transhumanist antipathy toward traditional Christian doctrines such as the existence of an almighty and just Creator-God, the immortality of the soul, or the resurrection of the body. God's commandments – and perhaps His very existence – place limits on human freedom; the concept of the soul is difficult, at the very least, to reconcile with mindless, purposeless Darwinian evolution; and belief in resurrection has led to a series of "superstitious" prohibitions on biological research. If human beings are to take control of their own evolution, say most transhumanists, they must put away childish fables about God and have the courage to place their own purposes into nature itself, embedding them in the very genetic codes of tomatoes, sheep, and human fetuses (Hughes 2004; Bostrom 2005; Bainbridge 2005; Sorgner 2009).

While dismissive of the Western Christian tradition, the Anglo-American transhumanists have completely ignored the theologians of the East. In sharp contrast, the Russian Transhumanist Movement, founded in 2003, has adopted the devoutly Orthodox Christian Nikolai Fedorovich Fedorov (1829-1903) as its inspiration. One of the most creative thinkers of the Russian religious renaissance, Fedorov drew upon Orthodox theology – especially the work of the brilliant theologian Maximos the Confessor (580-662) – to shape his vision of the nature and destiny of humanity. For both Maximos and Fedorov, human beings could freely and meaningfully participate in the divine work of redemption; for both philosophers, the ultimate end of salvation was deification (*theōsis*) – a radical transfiguration of the whole person, body and soul, and of the whole cosmos. By arguing that human nature was characterized by an autonomous will and a destiny of deification, Maximos laid the groundwork for Fedorov's speculative theology. Taking seriously Maximos's ideas about human participation in cosmic redemption, Fedorov contended that all humanity should unite in the common cause (*obshchee delo*) of raising the dead and regulating the universe through scientific means. In his posthumously published work *The Philosophy of the Common Cause* (1906, 1913), which might be considered the original transhumanist manifesto, Fedorov even called for enhancing the human body by adding wings, eliminating the alimentary canal, and making humans autotrophic – projects that anticipate James Hughes's *Citizen Cyborg* (2004) by over a century. But Fedorov was also a pious Orthodox Christian, a defender of autocracy (the Russian tsar was to rule the world!) and the agrarian way of life, deeply suspicious of Western technology (which made people "slaves of the factory"), firmly patriarchal, and convinced of Russia's divinely appointed messianic role in world history (Gacheva 2005; Sergay 2008; Semenova and Gacheva 1993; Tsiolkovskii 1925; Wiles 1965; Lukashevich 1977; Young 1979; Koehler 1979; Teskey 1982; Hagemeister 1989; Semenova 1990, 2004; Masing-Delic 1992; Gacheva et al. 1996; Lim 2006, 126-36; Bogdanov 2007).

Although not typically Orthodox, Fedorov's philosophy reflected centuries of Orthodox theological examination of human nature, destiny, and freedom. At its best, the transhumanism movement also engages these questions. This chapter seeks to spark a constructive conversation between transhumanism and the Orthodox theological tradition that will provide better and more considered answers to the challenges posed by new medical and genetic technologies. Largely ignorant of theology, transhumanists have struggled to develop useful ethical frameworks by which to judge and justify human enhancement (Caplan 2009). Too often, as N. Katherine Hayles (1999, 2008) has demonstrated, the transhumanists rely on rhetorical tricks, making assumptions about human nature that really need to be proven – or at least discussed – in argument. Hayles convincingly shows that the transhumanist vision rests on an impoverished view of humanity that privileges information flows over embodiment and regards consciousness as a mere epiphenomenon. By contrast, the two Orthodox theologians considered in this chapter, Fedorov and Maximos, offer a robust understanding of human nature, spiritual development, and human destiny that will enrich the discussion of the future of our species.

The Christian Roots of Transhumanism

The utopian transhumanist vision clearly derives much of its power from traditional Christian theology. Like transhumanism, Christianity looks forward to a transfiguration of the human species, most beautifully represented by the glorified Christ, who easily transcends the limits of both time and space. The transfigured Christ communes with the great prophets of old, Moses and Elijah; he passes through walls and appears in locked rooms (Matt. 17:2-3; John 20:26). Moreover, Christ's Resurrection is only the first fruits of the general resurrection. Every believer in Christ can anticipate the same kind of transfigured body that the risen Christ possesses. In writing about the resurrection, the Apostle Paul told the Corinthians, "As was the earthly man, so are those who are of the earth; and as is the man from heaven, so also are those who are of heaven. And just as we have borne the likeness of the earthly man, so shall we bear the likeness of the man from heaven" (I Cor. 15:48-49). Transhumanist dreams of transforming the body or of uploading consciousness and personality into supercomputers are secularized versions of the Christian promise of resurrection.

An even closer parallel to transhumanism is the ancient Christian doctrine of deification (*theōsis*). Around 180 CE, Irenaeus of Lyon wrote that the deification of humanity was the purpose of the Incarnation (*Adversus haereses.* 3.19.1; PG 7, cols. 939-40; ANF 1:448-49), and Athanasius of Alexandria (293-373) and Gregory of Nazianzus (329?–389) made similar statements in the fourth century (*Epistola ad Adelphium* 4; PG 26, col. 1077A; NPNF2, 4:576; *De incarnatione* 54.3; PG 26, col.192B; NPNF2, 4:65; *Orations* 29.19; PG 36, col. 100A; NPNF2, 7:308). The doctrine of the Incarnation – the idea that God took on flesh in the person of Christ and thereby transformed humanity itself – has had profound implications for the Christian understanding of human nature and its ultimate destiny. For these church fathers, Christian salvation was not simply an escape from eternal punishment, the consequences of sin, or even from sin itself; it was a profound transfiguration of the human species whose final, marvelous end could only be guessed (Russell 2004). "Dear friends, we are now children of God and *what we will be has not yet been made known.* But we know that when he [Christ] appears, we shall be like him, for we shall see him as he is" (I John 3:2, my emphasis).

Although certainly not absent from Western theology, reflection on deification has been especially rich in the Orthodox world. The Orthodox historian John Meyendorff (1973) has argued that the seven ecumenical councils recognized in the Orthodox Church represent primarily the working out of the doctrine of the Incarnation and its implications, including the idea of deification. In the last years of the Russian Empire, religious thinkers turned again to this doctrine as they sought to revitalize the moribund orthodoxy of the state church; in the emigration after 1917, Russian theologians, freed from ecclesiastical censorship, continued to develop these ideas and introduced them to a Western audience. Although it might come as a surprise to those who imagine that religion and science have always been in conflict, these religious philosophers had a profoundly positive influence on Russian and Soviet science. As Loren Graham and Jean-Michel Kantor (2009) have recently shown, the mystical theology of Father Pavel Aleksandrovich Florenskii (1882-1937) helped lead to a major advance in mathematical set theory and the concept of infinity. Likewise, Fedorov's writings about the Christian doctrine of the general resurrection and the destiny of the cosmos deeply affected the Russian scientists Konstantin Eduardovich Tsiolkovskii (1857-1935), the father of Soviet rocketry, and the biologist Vladimir Ivanovich Vernadskii (1863-1944), who developed the concept of the biosphere. Fedorov's conception of humanity was deeply rooted in the Orthodox tradition that had developed over several centuries.

Orthodox Conceptions of Human Nature and Human Destiny

Human nature represents a conundrum for transhumanists who claim to be heirs of the humanistic Enlightenment. Some transhumanists deny that human nature exists at all (Caplan 2009), while others insist that evolution has fashioned a common set of empirically verifiable characteristics broadly shared by the entire population (Pinker 2002). Some transhumanists, such as Julian Huxley, embrace the idea of human nature as a moral concept that includes the possibilities of transcendence: transhumanism means "man remaining man, but transcending himself, by realizing new possibilities of and for his human nature" (Huxley 1927 cited in Hughes 2004, 158). But other transhumanists are so anxious to transcend their own humanity that they strip human beings of the natural rights posited by Enlightenment thinkers such as Thomas Jefferson; instead, they argue that rights are part of personhood – a set of abstract characteristics that might include self-awareness and rationality – rather than human nature (Glenn 2003; Hughes 2004, chap. 7). Clearly, for transhumanists, "the very concept of human nature is confused" (Daniels 2009, 25); is it the moral foundation of the transhumanist enterprise, or is it something to be manipulated and ultimately discarded?

Consideration of Christian conceptions of human nature may provide some clarity in this ongoing debate. Three moments in Orthodox intellectual history are especially critical for understanding human nature, its destiny, and the challenges of transhumanism. First, in the fifth century at the Council of Chalcedon, the Church defined Christ as perfectly and eternally human. This definition naturally had a profound impact on later Christian discussions about the nature and destiny of humanity. Second, in the seventh century, the Byzantine monk Maximos the Confessor, against enormous political pressure, helped to define Orthodox anthropology through his insistence that human nature (*phusis*) included a free and autonomous will (*thelēma*) with its own operation or activity (*energia*). In particular, he held that Christ, as fully human, had to have a completely human autonomous will, separate and distinct from the divine will. Maximos's philosophical position – for which he suffered exile, the excision of his tongue, and the amputation of his right hand – allowed for human participation in God's work of redemption; it also made Christ, the perfect human, the model for such participation, a model that believing Christians could freely imitate. In Maximos's vision, human beings were God's partners, not just his subjects, freely choosing to obey their King, even as Christ, the God-Man, had done throughout his life (Balthasar 2003; Bathrellos 2004; Blowers 1991; Cooper 2005; Epifanovich 1996; Larchet 1996; Louth 1996; Maximus 1955, 1982a, 1991, 2003; Siecienski 2005; Törönen 2007).

Twelve centuries after Maximos, Nikolai Fedorov took this partnership a huge step further. As Anastasiia Gacheva (2005, 132) has written, Fedorov "demanded from humanity the fulfillment not only of the moral evangelical commandments, but also the ontological promises of Christianity – overcoming death, raising the dead, and transforming the entire universe into the Kingdom of God." For Fedorov, the Incarnation meant that God had delegated to humanity both the power and the responsibility to raise the dead and to renew the cosmos. This now became the "common cause" uniting all humanity. More radical than even the Anglo-American transhumanists, Fedorov demanded that the world end its senseless wars and devote all of its resources to reversing entropy and to rescuing the "fathers" from the land of the dead.

Human Nature and the Humanity of Christ

Orthodox Christology, which was hammered out in a series of ecumenical councils, had a great deal to say about human nature and its ultimate destiny. The doctrine of the Incarnation – the claim that Christ was truly God and shared the same substance or essence (*homoousios*) as God the Father – was affirmed at the First Ecumenical Council, held in Nicaea in 325. But if Christ was fully God, could he also be fully human? What did the doctrine of the Incarnation imply about human nature itself? One powerful theological line of thought, dominant in the preeminent school of Alexandria, Egypt, held that Christ's humanity – his human nature – had been swallowed up and overcome by his divine nature at the Incarnation. Archbishop Cyril of Alexandria (r. 412-44, d. 444) famously articulated this point of view in his formula that Christ had the "single incarnated nature of God the Word [*mia phusis tou Theou Logou sesarkōmenē*]." But for many Christians, including Pope Leo the Great (r. 440-61), Cyril's formula, wrongly interpreted, could make Christ something other than a human being. If Christ did not have a recognizably human nature, then he was no longer human, no longer "like his brothers in every way" (Heb. 2:17). In opposition to the Alexandrian monophysite (single nature, from the Greek words *monē*, "one," and *phusis*, "nature") position, Leo insisted that, even after the Incarnation, Christ continued to have two distinct natures, one divine and one human. Leo's dyophysite Christology was adopted in 451 at Chalcedon during the Fourth Ecumenical Council, which stated that Christ's two natures, although mysteriously joined in the Incarnation, remained "without confusion, change, division, or separation." The Incarnate Christ had and continued to have a fully human nature, with all the properties of that nature. He was, is, and will be "in every way like us, except for sin" (Tanner 1990, 86).

Although expressed in the abstruse language of fifth-century Greek philosophy, the resolution taken at Chalcedon had enormous implications for Christian anthropology. First, Chalcedonian Christology assumed that human beings shared a common human nature. The nature that God assumed in the Incarnation was common to all human beings, not just to the individual Jesus of Nazareth. Second, the council unequivocally affirmed the essential goodness of this common human nature. The eternal Incarnate Christ, who is God Himself, is also eternally human. Sin is *not* an essentially human characteristic, for Christ, the perfect human, never sinned; to err is *not* human, for Christ never erred. Sin is simply a deviation from the perfect: to be perfectly human is to be perfectly sinless. Third, Chalcedon pictured a partnership between God and humanity: Christ's human nature abides harmoniously with the divine nature; united together into a single person (*hupostasis*), these two natures accomplish the redemption of the entire cosmos. Moreover, such a partnership was not only possible but necessary for the divine act of salvation; human participation was vital to Chalcedonian soteriology. Finally, Chalcedon, without spelling it out explicitly, suggested a divine destiny for humanity, a destiny in which union with God was consistent with remaining human. Already in the second century, Irenaeus had made the Incarnation a model for the deification of the believer; Chalcedon indicated that, just as the Incarnation united the two different natures in Christ without destroying either one, so, too, could the believer strive toward a deification that would preserve his or her essential humanity. As Maximos the Confessor argued in the seventh century,

> God and man are paradigms one of another: God is humanized to man through love for humankind to the extent that man, enabled through love, deifies himself to God; and man … manifests God, who is invisible by nature, through the virtues. (*Ambiguum ad Iohannem* 10; PG 91, col. 1113BC; Cooper 2001, 161)

Will, Freedom, and Destiny

Maximos the Confessor defended the Chalcedonian affirmation of Christ's full humanity against political efforts to water it down. In particular, Maximos insisted that Christ possessed a fully autonomous human will that operated independently of his divine will. The Confessor faced considerable opposition and persecution from state authorities, who were trying to forge some compromise that would bring the non-Chalcedonians back into the imperial church; to defend his Christology, Maximos suffered imprisonment, exile, and savage dismemberment, which hastened his death (Allen 2002). For Chalcedon – and its violent implementation by Emperor Marcianus (r. 450-57), who repressed the monophysite party and burned its writings – it proved extremely costly for the Byzantine Empire. Most of Egypt – the empire's wealthy grain-producing region – refused to recognize Chalcedon, which was also rejected by Armenia, Abyssinia, and large numbers of Christians in Syria. From 451 to the Arab invasion in 641, monophysites led several rebellions against imperial rule, and Byzantine emperors sought some doctrinal compromise that would heal this politically dangerous schism. Indeed, some historians have ascribed the rapid Arab conquest of Egypt to the divisions engendered by Chalcedon.

Monotheletism and monoenergism represented two efforts at a theological compromise that would bring Egypt back into the Orthodox fold (Verghess 1980). Monotheletism held that, although Christ had two natures, he had but one will (*thelēma*); monenergism, that his two natures were so closely linked that they shared a "single theandric activity [*mia theandrikē energeia*]." But both compromises, in Maximos's view, represented a denial of Christ's full humanity. To be human was to have a human will that acted autonomously and independently of the divine will. As someone who was fully human, Christ throughout his earthly life always and in every circumstance bent his autonomous human will to the divine will. This spiritual feat of absolute obedience to the divine will was undertaken freely; and, through it, God saved the world. The struggle of the human will to obey the divine will is nowhere more clearly evident than in the Garden of Gethsemane, immediately before his arrest and execution, when Christ prayed, "Take this cup from me. Yet not what I will, but what you will" (Mark 14:36). Even when faced with his imminent suffering and death, Christ turns his human will to obey his divine will (*Opusculum theologicum* 7; PG 91, col. 80; Louth 1996, 186).

The existence of Christ's fully human will, with all the ethical struggles that such a will implied, was particularly important for daily Christian practice. Just as Christ submitted his will to the Father, so the monk, through his ascetic disciplines, submitted his will to God. Christ here served as the perfect example for the believer. To deny Christ a human will was to eliminate him as a model for the Christian struggling to turn his will Godward. It was also to deny the salvation of the will. Christ had to assume the human will so that it could be purified and saved – and so that humanity, and creation itself, could be deified, the ultimate end of salvation:

> A sure warrant for looking forward with hope to the deification of human nature is provided by the incarnation of God, which makes man god to the same degree as God himself became man. For it is clear that he who became man without sin will divinize human nature without changing it into the divine nature, and will raise it up for His own sake to the same degree as He lowered himself for man's sake. (Maximos 1981, 2:177-78, no. 62)

Human freedom was essential to Maximos's understanding of the purpose and nature of the universe. The Incarnation itself required Mary, the God-bearer (*theotokos*), to participate in salvation by giving his or her assent to give birth to Christ (Luke 1:38). Without freedom, humans could not *participate* in the divine activity of creation, salvation, and deification; and without that participation, God could not achieve his redemptive, salvific purpose to pervade and interpenetrate the cosmos, to redeem and deify his fallen creation. For God intends not simply to rescue his church from sin and hell, but to "restore everything" (Acts 3:21), "make all things new" (Revelation 21:5), and liberate creation itself from its bondage to decay (Romans 8:21). Maximos boldly declares the universal implications of deification:

> God made us so that we might become "partakers in the divine nature" (2 Peter 1:4) and sharers in his eternity, and so that we might come to be like him through deification by grace. It is through deification that all things are reconstituted and achieve their permanence; and it is for their sake that what is not is brought into being and given existence. (1981, 173, no. 42)

Maximos wrote extensively about this process of deification, in which, paradoxically, God becomes one with his creation even as he remains ontologically distinct from it. As Eric Perl puts it, "deified man is man by nature and God by grace and therefore both different from and identical with God" (1991, 142). For Maximos, this union of God and humanity is accomplished through participation and interpenetration (*perikhōrēsis*) – the same term used to describe the relationship among the three persons of the Trinity – pictured in the analogy of air thoroughly suffused by light or iron consumed by fire. In both analogies, two opposite substances interpenetrate one another yet retain their distinct natures. God's pervasive penetration of the believer is like that of the fire that causes iron to glow from within.

This deification is accomplished, at least in part, through the free participation of the believer in the sacraments, in works of kindness, and in acquiring virtue. The ascent to God is essentially a moral transformation in which the believer makes the invisible God visible through the practice of kindness, love, and mercy – the same love for humanity (*philanthrōpia*) that God expressed in his Incarnation (*Mystagogia* 24; PG 91, col. 713AB; Perl 1991).

Deification affects the whole person, transforming the senses (*aisthēsis*), reason (*logos*), and mind (*nous*). In deification, "the nature of the body is necessarily ennobled," Maximos declares (*Ambiguum ad Iohannem* 10; PG 91, col. 1113C; Cooper 2001, 162). "God alone is made manifest through the soul and the body, their natural characteristics [*phusika gnorismata*] being overwhelmed by the transcendence of glory" (*Capita theologica et oeconomica* 2.88; PG 90, cols. 1084-1173). As Adam Cooper notes, these "natural characteristics" refer "not to those marks that are proper to human nature by virtue of creation, but to the characteristic features of empirical life bordered by mortality and penetrated by corruption: sexual reproduction, passionate attachment, corruption, and death" (2001, 185). In other words, for Maximos, sex, passion, and mortality were not truly human traits; the new glorified and deified humanity, although corporeal, would be, like Christ, celibate, passionless, and immortal. Sexuality was a result of the fall; if Adam and Eve had never fallen, Maximos argued, God would have provided some means other than sinful sexual intercourse for reproduction (Meyendorff 1973, 107-8, 196-97; Maximus 1982b, 138-39, question I, 3; PG 90, col. 788B). The discipline of celibacy was one way in which the Christian could begin to cooperate with God in the grand transformation of humanity into its prelapsarian perfection.

Maximos, Transhumanism, and the Russian Religious Renaissance

Although steeped in a Neoplatonist worldview, Maximos's anthropocentric cosmic vision has several points of concordance with the Anglo-American transhumanist movement. First, as a defender of Chalcedon, Maximos firmly and positively affirms the essential goodness and potential of humanity. Second, Maximos, like the transhumanists, holds to a theory of progress in which humanity as a species has a glorious destiny. Third, as with the transhumanists, this glorious destiny depends on human action and choices. Humans have a significant and decisive role to play in their ultimate destiny. Fourth, Maximos's teleological anthropology foresees not simply a spiritual transformation of humanity but a corporeal one as well. Maximos values the body and sees it as central to deification, just as the transhumanists understand the body as the locus of the evolutionary change that will transcend humanity (Cooper 2005). Finally, both Maximos and the transhumanists understand the universe to have a purpose. For Maximos, this purpose is that of the Creator, whose love for his creation leads him to deify it through the Incarnation of Christ; for the transhumanists, this purpose originates in the mind and will of humanity, who, through the exercise of technology, can bend purposeless matter and energy to its desires and ultimately transcend human limits.

At the same time, of course, a vast gulf separates Maximos's theistic anthropology, with its speculative Neoplatonic metaphysics, from transhumanism, which largely denies or ignores God's role in the universe and grounds itself in contemporary science. First, Maximos's Christocentric theism is clearly alien to the transhumanist project, based, as it is, in materialist evolution. Second, transhumanists rely on empirical science; the Orthodox fathers, on a divine teleology. Certainly, this difference is clearly evident in their different approaches to defining human nature. Neither Maximos nor the six hundred fathers at Chalcedon bothered to conduct careful empirical observations of human societies to define human nature; unlike present-day evolutionary psychologists (Pinker 2002), they produced no list of empirically verified common human characteristics – other than the few sketched out in the creeds – that might serve as the beginnings of such a definition. Maximos would not have thought much of such an exercise, since even such empirically verifiable characteristics as sexuality are, in his view, not truly part of human nature but a result of the Fall. For Maximos, humanity is defined primarily teleologically – not empirically – through its relationship with God, its Creator, Redeemer, and Deifier. According to Chalcedon and Maximos, humanity is God's creation, corporal, mortal (although death will ultimately be overcome), limited, born in time, with a rational soul. Although transhumanists certainly would agree that humans have mortal bodies, they would agree with little else.

Moreover, contrary to the transhumanist vision, Maximos and Chalcedon see human nature as eternal. Although purified through the process of redemption and deification, humanity will remain eternally human even as it partakes of the divine nature. Humanity will never evolve into something else; in a Platonic sense, it will simply become what it truly is – what it was originally before the Fall and what God always intended for it. For transhumanists, followers of Darwinian evolution, such a belief in the immutability of a species is a grave error. However slowly, natural processes are already producing genetic changes in *Homo sapiens*, who will inevitably give rise to some new species. The only question before us, say the transhumanists, is whether we will use our technology to take control and direct this evolutionary process.

Theism versus atheism, teleology versus empiricism, the immutability of species versus Darwinian evolution. … Given the vast abyss that separates transhumanism from the Orthodox theology of the fifth through the seventh century, can the two engage in a productive dialogue? Does Orthodoxy have anything to say to transhumanism and vice versa? Perhaps the answer can be found in a later period of Orthodox thought. Maximos's positive vision of humanity, freedom, and deification helped lay the groundwork for the late imperial Russian "religious renaissance", whose major thinkers deliberately sought to bring Orthodoxy into a dialogue with Western science and philosophy – and who saw in their religion a divine warrant for significant human action (Evtuhov 1997; Kornblatt and Gustafson 1996; Valliere 2000; Zernov 1963). For Vladimir Sergeevich Solov'ev (1853-1900), Maximos, through his philosophical brilliance, had preserved Orthodoxy as a religion of Godmanhood (*Bogochelovechestvo*), in which fulfillment of the promises of scripture demanded a partnership between humanity and the deity. Solov'ev expanded on this idea in his 1891 lecture to the Moscow Psychological Association:

> The essential and radical distinction of our religion from other eastern religions, particularly Islam, is that Christianity as a religion of Godmanhood is predicated on divine action, but at the same time demands human action as well. From this perspective, the realization of the kingdom of God itself depends not only upon God, but on ourselves as well; for it is clear that the spiritual rebirth of humanity cannot occur independently of humanity, cannot be a merely external fact; it is a *cause* [*delo*] assigned to us, a *task* [*zadacha*] that we must fulfill. (1988, 2:339-40, emphasis in the original)

Solov'ev's vision of the "spiritual rebirth of humanity" had been deeply influenced by Nikolai Fedorov, whose philosophy provides perhaps the best possibility for a fruitful dialogue between transhumanism and Orthodoxy.

Nikolai Fedorovich Fedorov and the Science of Resurrection

One of the most original Christian thinkers of the late nineteenth century, Nikolai Fedorov, the illegitimate son of a Tambov nobleman, Prince Pavel Gagarin, sought to synthesize Orthodox teaching about the Incarnation and the resurrection with the modern materialist science of his day to solve the greatest of human problems – war, death, and natural disaster. The rambling title of his major work, written between 1878 and 1892 but published posthumously, gives some sense of his primary concerns: "The Question about Brotherhood or Kinship and about the Reasons for the Unfraternal, Unbrotherly, That Is, the Unpeaceful, Condition of the World, and about the Means to Restore Kinship" (Fyodorov 1965, 14). Fedorov attached cosmic significance to the Incarnation of Christ, which, in his view, had delivered divine omnipotence – and delegated the fulfillment of the divine promises – into human hands. Fedorov's deep Christian faith led him to a far more radical program than the Anglo-American transhumanists. He called on all humankind to end war and to unite as brothers in order to fulfill humanity's "common cause": the raising of the dead and the renewal of the cosmos, which Fedorov understood as no less than bringing in the kingdom of God. For Fedorov the entire universe was involved in a cosmic liturgy (*leitourgia* in Greek) – literally, service to the Lord God. As rational beings, humankind had to regulate nature and to fulfill the promises of scripture.

Although he lived in obscurity and published almost nothing in his lifetime, Fedorov was well acquainted with many members of the Russian literary and cultural elite. After working for nearly fifteen years, from 1854 to 1868, as a history and geography teacher in provincial district schools, Fedorov found employment as a librarian and cataloguer in the Rumiantsev Museum, the leading library of Russia. (Known in the Soviet period as the Lenin Library, it is now the Russian State Library, located next to the Kremlin.) His modest position and his ascetic lifestyle (he never married) allowed him to devote himself entirely to the pursuit of knowledge and to discuss his works with some of the library's patrons. The novelist Leo Tolstoy (1828-1910), for example, became acquainted with Fedorov in 1881 and, in a letter to one of his friends, wrote,

> He [Fedorov] has formulated a plan for the general affairs of all humankind, which has as its goal the resurrection of all people in the flesh. First of all, it's not as crazy as it seems. (Don't be afraid, I never did and do not now share his views, but I understand them so well that I feel myself able to defend them against the claims of all other beliefs having an external goal.) (1992, 63: 80-81; Wachtel 1992, 266-67)

After reading one of Fedorov's manuscripts, Vladimir Solov'ev wrote him:

> I accept your project [the raising of the dead] unconditionally and without hesitation. … Your project is the first movement forward of the human spirit on the path to Christ. For my part, I can only acknowledge you as my teacher and spiritual father. (Berdyaev 1950, 124)

Although Solov'ev, in fact, rejected significant parts of Fedorov's program, his letter – as well as Tolstoy's – indicates the deep respect that the librarian commanded from significant members of the Russian intelligentsia. Aware of the modest cataloguer's cultural importance, the famous artist Leonid Pasternak, father of the novelist and poet Boris Pasternak, surreptitiously sketched Fedorov's likeness, providing future generations with one of the few portraits of this remarkable philosopher.

Fedorov also extended his influence through his extraordinary personal generosity. Extremely ascetic, Fedorov gave away much of his tiny salary of 17.5 rubles per month to help others, his "stipend-recipients" (*stipendiaty*), one of whom, in 1873, was a sixteen-year-old mathematically gifted deaf student Konstantin Eduardovich Tsiolkovskii. Deeply impressed by Fedorov's project of raising the dead, Tsiolkovskii devoted his entire life to the exploration of the cosmos – a task inspired partly by Fedorov's grand vision of humanity's role as regulators of the universe and partly by the very practical need for new planets for the resurrected dead to colonize. By the 1890s, Tsiolkovskii had published works that laid out basic principles of rocket science, many of which are still foundational for rocket engineers. He calculated the relationship of the mass of the rocket to its fuel and argued that liquid was preferable to solid fuel. After the Russian Revolution, Tsiolkovskii became one of the founding figures of the Soviet space program; his students later launched the first artificial satellites and placed the first human being in orbit around the earth (Andrews 2009; Noble 1999, 121-22).

Despite these important personal ties, Fedorov's views gained wide circulation only after his death when his disciples Vladimir A. Kozhevnikov (d. 1917) and Nikolai P. Peterson (d. 1919) published a collection of his manuscripts in two volumes from 1906 to 1913 under the general title *Philosophy of the Common Cause* (Fedorov 1906, 1913). The editors died before they could publish the third volume that they had prepared (Koutaissoff 1984, 98). Obedient to their master's wish, the editors gave away these books for free to anyone who asked. Although the Stalinist secret police hunted down and executed many of Fedorov's disciples in the 1930s and 1940s, his works were widely discussed among Russian émigrés, and *Philosophy of the Common Cause* was reprinted in London in 1970. In the post-Stalinist USSR, a small group of influential thinkers continued to hold to Fedorov's philosophy, and in 1982, the Soviet Academy of Sciences published a new edition of his work – one of the rare occasions in which the officially atheist USSR gave its imprimatur to a Christian philosopher (Fedorov 1982). After the fall of the Soviet Union, Fedorov scholars issued a new, more complete edition of thinker's works in four volumes, with a supplementary volume of commentary (Fedorov 1995-2000). An abridged translation of his selected works is available in English (Fedorov 1990).

For Fedorov, God calls humanity to fulfill three major roles. First of all, human beings are all part of a single family, sons and daughters of their dead ancestors. This family relationship implies an obligation not only to the living – all war and conflict is fratricidal and contrary to God's law – but also to the dead, who must be rescued from their state of decay. Christ serves as the perfect model of this filial relationship. Like Christ, every person is the child of a father; just as Christ, the beloved son, obeys his father and does His will, so too all humanity must also do the will of the God of their fathers, to "reestablish the world to the blessed state of imperishability, as it was before the fall" (Fedorov 1995-2000, 1:401).

Second, God has destined humanity to triumph over death. This command flows naturally from the filial obligations that sons and daughters owe their parents, whom they must raise from the dead. Once again, Christ served as the model for this role; through his resurrection, he became victorious over death and made this triumph possible for all humanity. But Christ's resurrection was only the beginning of this conquest over death. Through the Incarnation, God had both given the power and delegated the responsibility for the resurrection of the dead to humanity itself:

> We must conceive of the resurrection as an unfinished work. ... Christ is the beginning of it; through us it continued, and it continues until now. The resurrection is not a thought only, but it is also not a fact; it is a project ... as something divine it is already decided, but as human it has still not been accomplished. (Fedorov 1995-2000, 1:142)

The general resurrection will require a united, global human effort that brought together all of the forces of humankind. Rather than battling one another, nations have to come together to make the promise of the resurrection come true:

> Christianity believes in the triumph over death; but this belief is dead, and that is why death exists; that belief will remain dead as long as it remains separated from all of mankind's other forces, that is, until all the forces of all people join together for the general goal of resurrection. (Fedorov 1970, 203-4; Wachtel 1992, 266)

The struggle against death was the primary means by which God educated humanity to bring about his kingdom. *Homo sapiens* was the only creature conscious of its own mortality, and "in the torments of the consciousness of mortality, the human soul was born" (Fedorov 1995-2000, 2:257). Scientific and technological progress resulted from this struggle against death, as naked, clawless, fangless humans fashioned tools to overcome their lack of natural defenses; art and literature, too, sprang from humanity's desire to become immortal. But through this terrible school of experience, God was transforming humanity – and through humanity, transforming nature itself.

> God is educating humanity by its own experience; He is the King, who does everything not only just for humanity but also through humanity. ... The Creator through us remakes the world, raises all that has perished; this is why nature has been left to its blindness, and humanity to its lusts. Through the work of resurrecting the dead, humanity, as a sui generis, self-made, free being freely ties himself to God by love. (Fedorov 1995-2000, 1:255)

Nature, in Fedorov's vision, is blind and purposeless, but people are purposeful and rational. The harsh struggle against death educates and sanctifies humanity's purposes, turning lusts into love, making humans into full partners with God: "Nature in us begins not only to recognize itself, but to direct itself" (Fedorov 1995-2000, 2:239).

In this way, God is preparing humans for their third great role – to become the governors of the universe, regulating and renewing the forces of nature. Again, Christ serves as the example: he stilled the seas, calmed the winds, healed the sick, and raised the dead. Moreover, he promised that his disciples would accomplish even greater works: "I tell you the truth, anyone who has faith in me will do what I have been doing. He will do even greater works than these, because I am going to the Father" (John 14:12). Overcoming the law of death, which reigns over all creation, means more than just raising the dead; it means overturning the Darwinian struggle for survival that characterizes all life; it means repealing the second law of thermodynamics and reversing entropy. Fedorov envisioned the literal fulfillment of Isaiah's prophetic promise:

> "The wolf and the lamb will feed together
> And the lion will eat straw like the ox,
> But dust will be the serpent's food.
> They will not harm nor destroy
> On all my holy mountain," says the Lord. (Isaiah 65:25; cf. Isaiah 11:6-9)

Fedorov's plans for the heavenly bodies were equally radical: "By their reason, the sons of man will direct the blind movement of the planets and the entire solar system" (Fedorov 1995-2000, 2:242). Earth itself would become a traveling spaceship, piloted by the united human race. (ibid., 2:240).

To realize these plans, human beings need to unite and redirect their resources toward these common goals. Armies would no longer fight one another but instead would direct their energies toward the regulation of nature, toward putting a final end to natural disasters, and toward reconstructing the individual lives and personalities of everyone who had ever existed, so that they could be raised back to life. As the major center of Orthodox Christianity, Russia would lead the way in this grand project – not by conquering other peoples but by providing a positive example through its patriarchal traditions, its agrarian economy, its right-believing tsar, and its culture of compassion, forgiveness, and love.

Despite these radical designs – which of the transhumanists has such bold plans to change the laws of physics? – Fedorov is in many respects conservative, opposed to both capitalist and socialist visions of progress offered during his lifetime:

> If the old tell the young, "You must grow, and I must diminish," then this is a kind wish, spoken by fatherly love. But if the young tell the old, "I must grow, and you must go off to the grave," then this is "progress", and hatred, not love, [that] is speaking – the hatred of the (of course) prodigal sons. In the absence of internal unification and of the external common cause of the entire human race, "progress" is a natural phenomenon, and until the human race is unified in the common cause for the transformation of the forces of death into the forces of life, humanity, like cattle, beasts, and soulless matter, will be subject to the force of nature. ... [Progress] is that sin that was punished by a confusion of tongues, which is similar to our own time, when people refuse all that is common and each one lives exclusively for himself to such an extent that people have ceased to understand one another. (1995-2000, 1:50-51)

Fedorov bitterly criticized both socialism and capitalism. While the socialists of his day claimed to stand for social justice, they did not care about the dead, "the most debased and mortally injured" of humanity (Fedorov 1995-2000, 4:431). Social justice needed to address not simply questions of wealth and poverty but of life and death. As for Western civilization, it was "created by the lusts of men to satisfy the lusts of women" – a civilization based on consumption and comfort, rather than on striving for truth and righteousness (Sergay 2008, 43). The greed of English capitalists had led to the creation of an anti-Christian international imperialist order that had "expropriated and expatriated" peasants from their land: "a dishonorable affair, separating the children from the dust of their fathers, depriving them of the possibility of fulfilling their filial duty" (Fedorov 1995-2000, 1:239).

In place of urban industrial capitalism, which he soundly rejected, Fedorov called for a return to the land. The patriarchal peasant commune (*mir*), characterized, as he thought, by fraternal love and the practice of mutual aid (*pomoch'*), provided a better foundation than did the city for raising the dead and regulating nature. Moreover, peasants, who depended on meteorological phenomena and natural forces, would much more easily understand and sympathize with his "common task" than deracinated city folk (Fedorov 1995-2000, 3:267-68).

Completion of the "common task" was necessary to avoid God's apocalyptic judgment, described in Christ's discourses on the Mount of Olives and in the Revelation to St. John. In perhaps his most original theological contribution to eschatology, Fedorov argued that the prophecies of the end of the world were only warnings, not certainties. If, in obedience to God's will, humanity turned from war and conflict to the great task of raising the dead, then God would spare the world the horrors of the Apocalypse. As Nicholas Berdiaev explained, Fedorov

> teaches that the apocalyptical prophecies are conditional, that they present merely a threat. If mankind does not unite for the common work of resurrecting deceased ancestors, the restoration of life of all mankind, then there will come the end of the world, the advent of Antichrist, the Last Judgment, and eternal destruction for many people. But if mankind lovingly unites for the common work and fulfills its duty with respect to deceased forefathers, if it does all it can for the cause of general salvation and resurrection, then there will be no end of the world, no Last Judgment, and no eternal destruction for anyone. This is a projective and active conception of the Apocalypse. It depends on man whether God's plan for the world will be successful. (1950, 129)

For Fedorov, humanity had rebelled against God not by eating of the forbidden tree of knowledge but by refusing to fulfill the very first divine commandment to subdue the earth and to have dominion over all creation (Genesis 1:28). Humanity's failure to regulate nature by reason condemned the universe to degeneration. Deprived of rational governance, nature became blind and corrupt. Only by uniting in this common cause can humanity obey its divine vocation (Russian Transhumanist Movement).

Although Fedorov is not well known outside Russia, some Anglo-American transhumanists have begun to embrace him – but not his Orthodox theological framework. In a blog dated August 4, 2009, on KurzweilAI.net, the Web site of the inventor and transhumanist Ray Kurzweil, one participant (who uses the pseudonym */:setAI*) writes, "I am pretty sure Fyodorv [*sic*] has been mentioned here – he really should be our 'mascot' – he had the basic mind-set we are trying to cultivate now – limitless knowledge / infinite existence / the ultimate fate of Life and Mind." The blogger's knowledge of Fedorov seems to be limited to the "Wikipedia" article that he cites.

Recently in a *Rolling Stone* interview, Kurzweil, who did not mention Fedorov at all, shared his hopes of raising his own father from the dead:

> Kurzweil's most ambitious plan for life after the Singularity, however, is also his most personal: Using technology, he plans to bring his dead father back to life. ... In a soft voice, he explains how the resurrection will work. "We can find some of his DNA around his grave site – that's a lot of information right there," he says. "The AI will send down some nanobots and get some bone or teeth and extract some DNA and put it all together. Then they'll get some information from my brain and anyone else who still remembers him."
>
> When I ask how exactly they'll extract the knowledge from his brain, Kurzweil bristles, as if the answer should be obvious: "Just send nanobots into my brain and reconstruct my recollections and memories." The machines will capture everything: the piggyback ride to a grocery store, the bedtime reading of Tom Swift, the moment he and his father rejoiced when the letter of acceptance from MIT arrived. To provide the nanobots with even more information, Kurzweil is safeguarding the boxes of his dad's mementos, so the artificial intelligence has as much data as possible from which to reconstruct him. Father 2.0 could take many forms, he says, from a virtual-reality avatar to a fully functioning robot. (Kushner 2009, 61)

Conclusion

The Anglo-American transhumanist movement offers a vision of a renewed humanity. At its best, transhumanism calls all people of the world to strive together toward a glorious destiny and to take responsibility for getting there. Transhumanists challenge the imagination and seek to break down artificial barriers to a better life.

The two Orthodox thinkers considered here openly invite a more extended conversation between Christianity and transhumanism. Both Maximos and Nikolai Fedorov also believe in a glorious destiny for humanity – a transfiguration that involves both body and the mind. Like the transhumanists, they both insist that human beings are, in large measure, responsible for their own destiny. Blessed by God with a free and autonomous will, humans can fulfill – or refuse to fulfill – the role that God has assigned for them. Both of them share a cosmic vision in which humanity as a species significantly participates in the divine transformation of the created order.

Unlike most transhumanists, however, Maximos and Fedorov understand the transformation of humanity as a fundamentally moral process, one that involves not just technical and material change but spiritual changes as well. For both thinkers, love is the key to this transformation. For Maximos, the Christian must increasingly and progressively be characterized by divine love in a mystical process of deification. The invisible God makes himself visible as Christians acquire and put into practice the divine virtues. For Fedorov, human beings form a single family, whose members share in the joys and obligations of kinship.

Of course, neither Maximos nor Fedorov offer ready-made answers to the challenges presented by recent advances in biotechnology. Contemporary American Christians are turning to Maximos for help in solving a number of practical questions about the Christian life, but I am unaware of any bioethicists who draw on Maximos (Bellini 2008; Siecienski 2005). Perhaps Adam Cooper's 2005 study of Maximos's theology of the body will have fruitful applications for bioethicists. As for Fedorov, many of the criticisms levied against the transhumanists can certainly also be levied against him as well. Fedorov is often impractical; he is unable to provide specific information or guidance about how to go about raising the dead; he ignores the laws of physics and wrongly imagines that it is possible to change them.

But both thinkers offer an optimistic Christian moral framework for discussing the transformation of humanity. Both thinkers give the lie to those scholars who imagine religion as uniformly pessimistic about human nature and the possibility of human transformation. Without such a moral framework, transhumanists are doomed to remain morally blind, incapable of answering their critics with anything better than epithets, such as "bio-Luddite" (Hughes 2004, 62-67).

But perhaps the most pressing questions for the contemporary debate about transhumanism are the political implications of a movement that so boldly calls for humans to evolve into something else, into a different and better species. Such a challenge rightly raises a host of alarms: the transhumanist project sounds too much like the eugenics movement of the early twentieth century, which, in the name of (pseudo-)science, sterilized those who were black and poor; it recalls, rightly or wrongly, the totalitarian horrors of National Socialism and the dream of a "master race." James Hughes believes that social democracy offers the best answer to the very practical political question about allocating the huge resources needed to direct the evolution of humanity; other transhumanists prefer a libertarian capitalist market system. Here the Orthodox tradition sounds a cautionary note. For Fedorov, the "common task" required the power of an absolute monarch. And when one of his disciples, the philosopher Aleksandr Konstantinovich Gorskii-Gornostaev (1884-1943), during the first of several arrests, was questioned in 1927 in the interrogation chambers of Soviet secret police, the Unified Main Political Admnistration (OGPU), he explained,

> Fedorov expressed the need for a strong power – a monarchy. This however did not constrain me to support autocracy. I understand this more broadly: in general terms, [Fedorov's project requires] a firm authority, a dictatorship, but not necessarily a monarchy. (Makarov 2002, 107)

Indeed, it is difficult to imagine that a democracy of equals could survive in the world envisioned by transhumanism, where the wealthy and powerful could enhance themselves and genetically pass down their advantages to their descendants (Wikler 2009). The revolutionary changes that transhumanism demands also suggest equally radical politics. What Valerian Nikolaevich Murav'ev (1885-1930), one of the Fedorovites, said about his own movement, might well be applied to the Anglo-American transhumanists: "We are much bigger Bolsheviks than the Bolsheviks themselves" (Makarov 2002, 99).

Maximos the Confessor also offers an important political lesson in the debate over transhumanism. Although a retired government official who had faithfully served his emperor, Maximos did not hesitate to defend the full humanity of Christ and the freedom of the human will even when he risked everything to do so. Maximos's willingness to sacrifice his own liberty – and even his life – to defend his vision of human nature and human dignity continues to testify to us about the importance of these issues. To be human is to have a human will and a divine destiny. Tongueless and dismembered, the Confessor still speaks from his exile in Lazica.

References

Allen, Pauline, ed. 2002. *Maximus the Confessor and His Companions: Documents from Exile.* New York: Oxford University Press.

Andrews, James. 2009. *Red Cosmos: K. E. Tsiolkovskii, Grandfather of Soviet Rocketry.* College Station: Texas A & M University Press.

ANF. 1969-73. *The Ante-Nicene Fathers: Translations of the Writings of the Fathers down to A.D. 325.* Edited by Alexander Roberts and James Donaldson. Grand Rapids, MI: William B. Eerdmans. Original edition, Edinburgh: T. and T. Clark, 1867-72.

Bainbridge, William Sims. 2005. The transhuman heresy. *Journal of Evolution and Technology* 14 (2): 1-10.

Balthasar, Hans Urs von. 2003. *Cosmic Liturgy: The Universe according to Maximus the Confessor.* Translated by Brian Daley. San Francisco: Ignatius Press.

Bathrellos, Demetrius. 2004. *The Byzantine Christ: Person, Nature, and Will in the Christology of Maximus the Confessor.* New York: Oxford University Press.

Bellini, Peter. 2008. Participation: An onto-epistemology for a theology of mission for the 21st century. PhD. diss.. Asbury Theological Seminary.
Berdyaev, Nicholas. 1950. N. F. Fedorov. *Russian Review* 9 (2): 124-150.
Blowers, Paul M. 1991. *Exegesis and Spiritual Pedagogy in Maximus the Confessor: An Investigation of the Quaestiones ad Thalassium*. Christianity and Judaism in Antiquity 7 Notre Dame, IN.: University of Notre Dame Press.
Bogdanov, V. V. 2007. Novoe o date rozhdeniia filosofa N. F. Fedorova. *Otechestvennye arkhivy* 6: 52-54.
Bostrom, Nick. 2005. A history of transhumanist thought. *Journal of Evolution and Technology* 14 (2): http://jetpress.org/volume14/bostrom.pdf, accessed July 12, 2011.
–. 2009. Pascal's mugging. *Analysis* 69: 443-45.
Campbell, Heidi, and Mark Walker. 2005. Religion and transhumanism: Introducing a conversation. *Journal of Evolution and Technology* 14 (2): http://jetpress.org/volume14/specialissueintro.html, accessed July 12, 2011.
Caplan, Arthur L. 2009. Good, better, or best? In Savulescu and Bostrom, eds., 199-209.
Cooper, Adam G. 2001. Maximus the Confessor on the structural dynamics of revelation. *Vigiliae Christianae* 55 (2): 161-86.
–. 2005. *The Body in St. Maximus the Confessor: Holy Flesh, Wholly Deified.* New York: Oxford University Press.
Daniels, Norman. 2009. Can anyone really be talking about ethically modifying human nature? In Savulescu and Bostrom, eds., 25-42.
Epifanovich, S. L. 1996. *Prepodobnyi Maksim Ispovednik i Vizantiiskoe Bogoslovie*. Moscow: Martis. First published Kiev: P. Barskii, 1915.
Evtuhov, Catherine. 1997. *The Cross and the Sickle: Sergei Bulgakov and the Fate of Russian Religious Philosophy*. Ithaca, NY: Cornell University Press.
Fedorov, Nikolai Fedorovich. (See also Fyodorov, Nicholas Fyodorovich). 1906. *Filosofiia obshchego dela.* Vol. 1. Edited by V. A. Kozhevnikov and N. P. Peterson. Vernyi: Semirechen. obl. pravl.
–. 1913. *Filosofiia obshchego dela.* Vol. 2. Edited by V. A. Kozhevnikov and N. P. Peterson. Moscow: A. Snegirevoi.
–. 1970. *Filosofiia obshchego dela*. London: Gregg.
–. 1982. *Sochineniia*. Moscow: Mysl'.
–. 1990. *What Was Man Created For? The Philosophy of the Common Task, Selected Works*. Translated by Elisabeth Koutaissoff and Marilyn Minto. London: Honeyglen Publishing/L'Age d'Homme.
–. 1995-2000. *Sobranie Sochinenii v Chetyrekh Tomakh*. 5 vols. Edited by Anastasiia Georgievna Gacheva and Svetlana Grigor'evna Semenova. Moscow: Progress Traditsiia.

Fyodorov, Nicholas Fyodorovich. 1965. The question of brotherhood or relatedness, and of the reasons for the unbrotherly dis-related, or unpeaceful state of the world, and of the means for the restoration of relatedness, trans. Ashleigh E. Moorhouse and George L. Klein. *Russian Philosophy* 3: 16-54.

Gacheva, Anastasiia Georgievna. 2005. Filosofiia istorii N. F. Fedorova. *Istoriia i istoriki* (1): 126-53.

Gacheva, Anastasiia Georgievna, Svetlana Grigor'evna Semenova, and M. V. Skorokhodov, eds. 1996. *Filosofiia Bessmertiia i Voskresheniia: Po Materialam VII Fedorovskikh Chtenii 8-10 Dekabria 1995 Goda, Moskva.* 2 vols. Moscow: Nasledie.

Glenn, Linda Macdonald. 2003. Biotechnology at the margins of personhood: An evolving legal paradigm. *Journal of Evolution and Technology* 13: http://www.jetpress.org/volume13/glenn.html, accessed July 12, 2011.

Graham, Loren, and Jean-Michel Kantor. 2009. *Naming Infinity: A True Story of Religious Mysticism and Mathematical Creativity*. Cambridge, MA: Harvard University Press.

Hagemeister, Michael. 1989. *Nikolaj Fedorov: Studien zu Leben, Werk, und Wirkung*. Munich: Verlag Otto Sanger.

Hayles, N. Katherine. 1999. *How We Became Posthuman: Virtual Bodies in Cybernetics, Literature, and Informatics*. Chicago: University of Chicago Press.

–. 2008. Wrestling with transhumanism. *The Global Spiral: A Publication of the Metanexus Institute:* http://www.metanexus.net/magazine/tabid/68/id/10543/Default.aspx, accessed July 12, 2011.

Hughes, James. 2004. *Citizen Cyborg: Why Democratic Societies Must Respond to the Redesigned Human of the Future*. Cambridge, MA: Westview Press.

–. 2007. The compatibility of religious and transhumanist views of metaphysics, suffering, virtue and transcendence in an enhanced future. *The Global Spiral*: http://www.metanexus.net/magazine/tabid/68/id/9930/Default.aspx, accessed July 12, 2011.

–. 2009. An epistle on H+ to the Italian Catholics: http://www.humanityplus.org/read/2009/09/an-epistle-on-h+-to-the-italian-catholics, accessed July 12, 2011.

Huxley, Julian. 1927. *Religion without Revelation.* New York: Harper and Brothers.

Koehler, Ludmila. 1979. *N. F. Fedorov: The Philosophy of Action.* Pittsburgh, PA: Institute for the Human Sciences.

Kornblatt, Judith, and Richard Gustafson, eds. 1996. *Russian Religious Thought.* Madison: University of Wisconsin Press.

Koutaissoff, Elisabeth. 1984. The philosophy of the common cause. *Slavonic and East European Review* 62 (1): 98-101.

Kushner, David. 2009. When man and machine merge. *Rolling Stone,* February 19, 57-61.

Larchet, Jean-Claude. 1996. *La Divinisation de l'Homme Selon Saint Maxime le Confesseur*. Cogitatio Fidei 194. Paris: Editions du Cerf.

Lim, Soojung. 2006. East Asia in Russian thought and literature, 1830s-1920s. PhD. diss., University of California, Los Angeles.

Louth, Andrew. 1996. *Maximus the Confessor*. New York: Routledge.

Lukashevich, Stephen. 1977. *N. F. Fedorov (1828-1903): A Study of Russian Eupsychian and Utopian Thought*. Newark: University of Delaware Press.

Makarov, V. G. 2002. Arkhivnye tainy: Filosofy i vlast'. Aleksandr Gorskii: Sud'ba, pokalechennaia 'po pravu vlasti'. *Voprosy filosofii* 8: 98-133.

Masing-Delic, Irene. 1992. *Abolishing Death: A Salvation Myth of Russian Twentieth-Century Literature*. Stanford, CA: Stanford University Press.

Maximos the Confessor. (See also Maximus). 1981. First century of various texts on theology, the divine economy, and virtue and vice. In *Philokalia: The Complete Text Compiled by St. Nikodimos of the Holy Mountain and St. Makarios of Corinth*, trans. and ed. G.E.H. Palmer, Philip Sherrard, and Kallistos Ware, vol. 2. London: Faber and Faber.

Maximus. 1955. *The Four Centuries on Charity*. Translated by Polycarp Sherwood. Ancient Christian Writers 21. New York: Newman Press.

–. 1982a. *The Church, the Liturgy, and the Soul of Man: The Mystagogia of St. Maximus the Confessor*. Edited by Julian Stead. Still River, MA: St. Bede's Publications.

–. 1982b. *Maximi Confessoris Quaestiones et Dubia*. Edited by José H. Declerck. Corpus Christianorum: Series graeca 10. Leuven: University Press.

–. 1991. *Maximi Confessoris Opuscula Exegetica Duo*. Edited by Peter van Deun. Corpus Christianorum: Series graeca 23. Turnhout: Brepols.

–. 2003. *On the Cosmic Mystery of Jesus Christ: Selected Writings from St. Maximus the Confessor*. Edited by Paul M. Blowers and Robert Louis Wilken. Crestwood, NY: St. Vladimir's Seminary Press.

Meyendorff, John. 1973. *Christ in Eastern Christian Thought*. Washington, DC: Corpus Books.

Noble, David F. 1999. *The Religion of Technology: The Divinity of Man and the Spirit of Invention*. New York: Penguin.

NPNF2. 1983. *A Select Library of the Nicene and Post-Nicene Fathers of the Christian Church, Second Series*. 14 vols. Edited by Philip Schaff and Henry Wace. Grand Rapids, MI: William B. Eerdmans. Original edition, New York: Christian Literature Company, 1890-1900.

Perl, Eric David. 1991. Methexis: Creation, incarnation, deification in Saint Maximus Confessor, PhD. diss., Yale University.

PG. 1857-66. *Patriologiae Cursus Completus, Series Graeca.* 161 vols. Edited by Jacques Paul Migne. Paris: Migne.

Pinker, Stephen. 2002. *The Blank Slate: The Modern Denial of Human Nature.* New York: Penguin.

Russell, Norman. 2004. *The Doctrine of Deification in the Greek Patristic Tradition.* New York: Oxford University Press.

Russian Transhumanist Movement: http://www.transhumanism-russia.ru/, accessed July 12, 2011 (in Russian).

Savulescu, Julian. 2009. The human prejudice and the moral status of enhanced beings: What do we owe the gods? In Savulescu and Bostrom, eds., 211-47.

Savulescu, Julian, and Nick Bostrom, eds. 2009. *Human Enhancement.* New York: Oxford University Press.

Semenova, Svetlana Grigor'evna. 1990. *Nikolai Fedorov: Tvorchestvo Zhizni.* Moscow: Sovetskii pisatel'.

–. 2004. *Filosof Budushchego Veka.* Moscow: Pashkov dom.

Semenova, Svetlana Grigor'evna, and Anastasiia Georgievna Gacheva, eds. 1993. *Russkii Kosmizm: Antologiia Filosofskoi Mysli.* Moscow: Pedagogika-Press.

Sergay, Timothy D. 2008. Boris Pasternak's "Christmas myth": Fedorov, Berdiaev, Dickens, Blok. PhD. diss., Yale University.

Siecienski, A. Edward. 2005. The use of Maximus the Confessor's writing on the *filioque* at the Council of Ferrara-Florence (1438-1439). PhD. diss., Fordham University.

Solov'ev, Vladimir Sergeevich. 1988. *Sochinenie v Dvukh Tomakh.* Edited by A.V. Gulyga and A. F. Losev. Moscow: Mysl'.

Sorgner, S. L. 2009. Nietzsche, the overhuman, and the transhuman. *Journal of Evolution and Technology* 20 (1): 29-42: http://jetpress.org/v20/sorgner.htm, accessed July 11, 2011.

Steinhart, Eric. 2008. Teilhard de Chardin and transhumanism. *Journal of Evolution and Technology* 20 (1): 1-22: http://jetpress.org/v20/steinhart.htm, accessed July 11, 2011.

Tanner, Norman, ed. 1990. *Decrees of the Ecumenical Councils.* Vol. 1. Washington, DC: Georgetown University Press.

Teskey, Ayleen. 1982. *Platonov and Fyodorov: The Influence of Christian Philosophy on a Soviet Writer.* Amersham, UK: Avebury Publishing.

Tolstoi, Lev Nikolaevich. 1992. *Polnoe Sobranie Sochinenii.* 91 vols. in 79. Edited by V. G. Chertkov et al. Moscow: Terra. Original edition, Moscow, 1928-64.

Törönen, Melchisedec. 2007. *Union and Distinction in the Thought of St. Maximus the Confessor.* New York: Oxford University Press.

Tsiolkovskii, Konstantin Eduardovich. 1925. *Monizm Vselennoi*. Kaluga: 1-aia gosudarstvennaia tipografiia.

Valliere, Paul. 2000. *Modern Russian Theology: Bukharev, Soloviev, Bulgakov: Orthodox Theology in a New Key*. Grand Rapids, MI: Eerdmans.

Verghess Paul. 1980. The Monothelete controversy: A historical survey. *Greek Orthodox Theological Review* 20: 196-211.

Wachtel, Andrew. 1992. Resurrection a la russe: Tolstoy's *The Living Corpse* as cultural paradigm. *PMLA* 107 (2): 261-73.

Wikler, Daniel. 2009. Paternalism in the age of cognitive enhancement: Do civil liberties presuppose roughly equal mental ability? In Savulescu and Bostrom, eds., 341-55.

Wiles, Peter. 1965. On physical immortality: Materialism and transcendence. *Survey: A Journal of Soviet and East European Studies* 56: 125-43; and 57: 142-–61.

Young, George M. 1979. *Nikolai Fedorov: An Introduction*. Belmont, MA: Nordland.

Zernov, Nicolas. 1963. *The Russian Religious Renaissance of the Twentieth Century*. Translated by George L. Kline. New York: Harper & Row.

"The True Dreams of Mankind"[1] Mircea Eliade's Transhumanist Fiction and the History of Religions

Steven M. Wasserstrom

> I should not speak so plainly of a gentleman, long since past answering, had not the pulpit, of late years, publicly owned his doctrine, and made it the current divinity of the times.
> – John Locke, *Enquiry Concerning Human Understanding*[2]

Mircea Eliade (1907-1986) was the twentieth century's most prominent historian of religions; indeed, he virtually created the field now known as "history of religions" in the United States. Up to the end of his life, he continued to be burdened with extraordinary honors: he was named the (honorifically titular) editor of the landmark *Encyclopedia of Religion*, lived to see a chair in his name established at the University of Chicago, and was deemed "the world's leading historian of religions" and a "cult figure on world campuses" (*People*), "by nearly unanimous consent the most influential student of religion in the world today" (*New York Times Book Review*), and even "the greatest humanistic scholar in the world" (Maritain 1985, 23).

Eliade was a *wunderkind* in his native Romania and became a leading man of letters in the interwar period, when he was still quite young (Wedemeyer and Doniger 2010). By the mid-1930s, he was publishing fiction, journalism, and political interventions in addition to his budding studies in religion. One thread running through his otherwise variegated writing was his so-called traditionalism. Traditionalism, deemed to be the heir of authentic Western esoteric traditions, was the product first and foremost of a writer of some genius, René Guénon (1886-1951).[3] Guénon's reactionary antimodernism impressed the young Eliade, who associated himself with its ideas and with its proponents. During World War II, Eliade served his country, among other things, as press and propaganda attaché in Lisbon. In a long postwar interval (1945-1955), he published several weighty tomes that earned him international acclaim. This fame led to his 1955 move to the University of Chicago, where he taught until his death in 1986. Throughout his adult life, he also published fiction with some frequency. Finally, he also

1 "My scientific books nearly all express the true dreams of mankind" (Lannes and Ferrier 1980, 27).

2 I am pleased to thank my student Michael Ostling for bringing this quotation to my attention. I thank Hava Tirosh-Samuelson for the invitation to participate in this volume. An earlier version of this paper was delivered as "Hedgehog's Lament: Notes on the Necessity and the Impossibility of Understanding Religion," The Jacob Perlow Lecture at Skidmore College. I thank Marla Segol for her invitation and her hospitality and Paul Flanders for his help bringing it to completion.

3 The standard work on traditionalism is Sedgwick (2004).

wrote his journals, which laid down yet another layer to his richly stratified biography. At his own insistence, this vast output is best understood as a whole, as an integrated singular corpus.

Eliade termed his postwar academic project "the History of Religions." This holistic, antireductionistic approach posited the irreducibility of religious reality, whose key manifestations he termed "hierophanies." Religious reality, also dubbed "the sacred," was treated always in dialectical interaction with "the profane." The sacred found its paradigmatic expression in prehistoric religion, in "Eastern" spiritualities, in Yoga, shamanism, alchemy, and other traditional and esoteric symbols. This approach to the sacred precluded social scientific explanations and rejected psychoanalytic and materialistic studies as being incapable of understanding "real" religion. As such, the history of religions was an interpretive strategy for understanding various symbols of ultimacy in the abstract, that is, out of their original social and psychological contexts. It is fair to say that this approach was normative in evaluation and antihistorical in methodology.

So what happens when perhaps the greatest living American filmmaker meets the man called the "the greatest humanistic scholar in the world?" The 2007 Francis Coppola film based on Eliade's 1978 novella *Youth without Youth* (henceforth *YWY*) answered that rhetorical question. The present study was stimulated by my perplexity at the seemingly inexplicable shortcomings of Coppola's film. Only after close analysis did I see that, as I shall try to show, the film failed because Coppola failed to see Eliade's deadly serious transhumanism in it. In my effort to understand Coppola's failure, I returned to *YWY*, which I had first read in 1992. I experienced the proverbial "aha!" moment when I suddenly realized that *YWY* was a kind of fictionalized version of *Morning of the Magicians* (henceforth *MM*). At the core of both *MM* and *YWY*, I realized, was precisely what Coppola missed – Eliade's traditionalist transhumanism.[4] Eliade's transhumanism grounded not merely his occasional writings but also his history of religions (to use the term he gave to his discipline). He praised this larger transhumanism in the 1920s and continued, in journals, fiction, and scholarship, to idealize it for over fifty years. It lies at the core of his ideal humanity, a humankind that transcends itself by following an avant garde of the few, the brave, the adepts. Coppola's misrecognition of this central theme in *YWY* led me, with appropriate circuitousness, to the present essay.

I shall proceed as follows. First, Eliade's novella *The Secret of Dr. Honigberger* (henceforth *SDH*) shows that his traditionalist transhumanism was in place already in 1940. His wartime *Portugal Journal* (henceforth *PJ*) continued,

4 For the purposes of this paper, I understand *transhumanism* to be the explicit motif running through all Eliade's works (journals, fiction, and scholarship) defined and exemplified in his words as a "transcending [of] the human condition" (see section 2).

in private, his ardent traditionalist transhumanism throughout the war years. In the 1960s, *Morning of the Magicians*, written by Louis Pauwels and Jacques Bergier, added a full-blown technosophy to his traditionalism and transhumanism. The fullest version of an occultist, traditionalist, and technosophic transhumanism, *MM* provided a template for Eliade's 1978 *YWY.*

1. Fictional Miracles

I shall try to show that three texts especially illuminate Eliade's transhumanism as it is found in the novella *YWY*. They are *SDH*, *PJ*, and *MM*.

In 1940, Eliade published the original Romanian version of *The Secret of Dr. Honigberger*, a story written earlier the previous year.[5] He published its English translation in 1970, as one of two *Tales of the Occult.*[6] *SDH* features a fictionalized version of the Indologist Johann Martin Honigberger (1795-1869) and his influence on a character identified by the initials "JE." As critics have noted, one "secret" of *SDH* is Eliade's relations with a real historical contemporary "JE," that is, Baron Julius Evola (1898-1974). Quite simply, *SDH* is fictionalization of Eliade's relations with Evola, an allegory of their shared dependence on the traditionalism of René Guénon. By 1939, when he wrote *SDH* "at a frenzied pace," the Eliade-Evola friendship was already well established, having started as early as 1927 (Ricketts 1988, 1299).

The plot of *SDH* culminates in Honigberger's revelations of the traditionalist theme par excellence, finding the hidden center of the world, called Shambala or Agarttha. *SDH* not only evoked Agarttha and Yogic initiation but dramatically invoked the radical antimodernism championed by the traditionalists Guénon and Evola in works of the immediately preceding years. The traditionalist themes in *SDH* include "impersonal consciousness" (118), "demonic forces unleashed since the Renaissance" (119), shifting of the world-axis (120), and the Kali-Yuga (120). *SDH*, originally published at the outset of World War II, concerns the quest for such a sovereign "Center of the World," Guénon's imperialistic watchword of the day. Godwin observes that

> the ideal of Shambala taken in its broadest sense [is] that of reverence for a center in the Orient from which comes the impulse for the imminent renewal of humanity, and to a Lord, King, or Ruler of the World who is neither Christ nor Lucifer. (1993, 103)

---

5 Written at a "frenzied pace" in the "winter of 1940," according to Ricketts 1988, 1091 (henceforth RR).

6 Eliade used this title in his introduction, though the publisher had changed it, as it appeared on the cover, to *Two Strange Tales*.

This Guénonian myth is also succinctly recapitulated in *MM:*

> The King-Giant, the Man-God concentrates in himself and directs the psychic forces of the community. He controls this network of radiations in such a way that the stars are maintained in their courses and the catastrophe staved off. This is the essential function of the giant-magician. To a certain extent, he keeps the solar system in its place. He is at the head of a sort of powerhouse of psychic energy; it is in this that his kingship resides. (Pauwels and Bergier 1968, 252)

Guénon concluded his *Lord of the World* with "prophecies" of Joseph de Maistre. "We must be ready for an immense event in the divine order *which we are travelling towards with an accelerated speed* that must astound all those who watch. Awesome oracles have pronounced already that the time is now" (Guénon 1983 [1927], 67, emphasis added). Near the end of *SDH*, the narrator states that Honigberger "was beginning to see more and more clearly the series of cataclysms which were to burst over Europe. This view is in agreement, by the way, with a whole series of prophecies, more or less apocalyptic in nature, concerning Kali-yuga, the 'dark age' whose end, we are told, *we are approaching with rapid steps*" (*SDH,* 120, emphasis added).

In the following fragment of *PJ* from 1941, published by Eliade in Portugal in 1943 and reprinted in English in 1985, Eliade described a painting of St. Peter as

> the true Cosmocrator ... the true ruler of the world, the Universal Monarch who imposes his laws and ordinances everywhere ... the archaic symbolism of Melchizedek, the Priest-King, the Universal Monarch, the Chakravartin who stand at the center of the earth and turns the wheel, and through whom all things are possible and obtain their being. (Eliade 1988b, 146, reprinted in *PJ* 244)

This description, like SDH, was transparently inspired by Guénon's 1927 Le Roi du Monde. The chain of associations – Universal Monarch / Melchizedek / Universal Monarch / Chakravartin who stand at the center of the earth and turns the wheel – unmistakably recapitulates the distinctively eclectic Guénonian blend of themes defining the so-called "Center of the World." Evola summarized Guénon's *Le Roi du Monde's* hyperimperialism:

> In his unique work entitled *Le Roi du Monde* (Paris, 1927), Guénon attempted to demonstrate the recurrence, in various and different traditions, of the idea of the "Universal Ruler" as well as its concretization as the idea of the one source of the forces which have traditionally ordained the greatest historical cycles. (Evola 1995a, 19)

"The Symbolism of the Center" subsequently comprised the theme of both Eliade's first Eranos lecture in 1951 – and the opening essay in his second postwar collection of essays, *Myths, Dreams, and Mysteries* (1960). With this "archetype," he proclaimed his dramatic debut on the stage of postwar international scholarship. These treatments of the "symbolism of the center" and its Universal

Ruler cover the same ground, on the basis of much the same sources, which he first published as *Cosmologie si alchimie bibiloniana* in Bucharest 1937. The author himself, late in life, stressed this point: "In this little book [*Cosmologie si alchimie bibiloniana*] are found, *in nuce*, all my interpretations relative to the symbolism of the center of the world" (*Autobiography, Volume II*, 8n2).[7] The "Symbolism of the Center of the World" also preoccupied Evola, especially in those crucial few years after 1937 – during which year Eliade introduced Evola to the Iron Guard strongman Corneliu Zelea Codreanu, when the latter visited Bucharest in 1937 (Sedgwick 2004, 114). In 1937, Eliade published *Cosmologie si alchimie bibiloniana*, and Evola published *The Mystery of the Grail* in Italian. In the latter work, we find key Evolian themes of the Center stated synoptically:

> [The Center is] a metaphysical kingdom, to which all dominators "from above" are related in a mysterious, objective, and ontological way; this is the case both with the real heirs of the primordial tradition and with those who reproduced more or less perfectly and consciously the primordial type of *regnum* in a given land and civilization. This is how the traditional notion of an invisible "king of Kings," or "Universal Ruler," or "King of the World," came to be associated with specific symbols. ... [T]hese are first and foremost symbols of *centrality*: the center, the pole, the region in the middle of the earth, the central stone of the foundation, the magnet. ... [T]he various traditions have foreshadowed this constant theme of the *regnum* and of the Supreme Center of the world, in itself or in its emanations and reproductions (Evola 1997, 18, emphasis in original).

Evola's footnote on this passage reads: "On this subject matter see René Guénon's *Le Roi du monde* (Paris, 1927) to which I will often refer in the course of this book" (18). Despite the fact that Guénon did not review Eliade's work positively at this time, it seems clear enough that Eliade's theory of the Center, articulated in *SDH* and *PJ*, from as early as 1937 derived from contemporaneous usages by Guénon and Evola. It is interesting to note that in *Patterns in Comparative Religion* (1958b) and elsewhere in the postwar work, Eliade consistently referred to "The Center" in quotation marks, presumably to mark it as a technical term, though without revealing to which technical lexicon it belonged.

Eliade's 1935 book review of Evola's *Crisis of the Modern World* affirmed their shared apocalyptic and initiatory themes, including those of Evola's programmatic *Pagan Imperialism*.[8] In other words, five years before his Evolan allegory in *SDH*, Eliade had already praised those very themes he would fictionalize half a decade later. We will see this pattern repeated when *YWY* fictiona-

7 Eliade wrote an essay on this subject which he republished at least four times.

8 I consulted the translation from Romanian into French by Faust Bradesco in *Les Deux Etendards 1* (1988), 42-43. Evola published an Italian book titled *Pagan Imperialism* in 1928. Its 1933 German version, according to Eliade in 1935, was a "politicized" version of the earlier book. The politicization is more fully described by Gregor (2005, 201-2).

lized the "nonfiction" themes of *MM*. In any case, for present purposes, *SDH* reveals an Eliade close to the traditionalism of Evola and Guénon and particularly to the occultist transhumanism favored by Evola.

The traditionalist dimension of Eliade's corpus can properly be considered transhumanist. Its esotericism was predicated on a cult of mastery, in which "masters" were superior men whose superiority alone revealed the ultimate mysteries of humanity. Yogis, shamans, and alchemists were models of this supremacy. Ascending to their rarified heights required a "break in plane," a breakthrough to "higher" realities. This ascendency was also seen as a breakthrough to higher "powers." For Eliade and his traditionalist associates, acquiring these "powers" resulted in "transcending the human conditions." Human frailties and limitations, human subordination to the dialectic of good and evil, even mortality itself, according to various forms of traditionalism, could be achieved – but only by masters, only by a few enlightened avatars. However, according to one scientific version of traditionalism, which first impressed Eliade in the 1950s and 1960s, these few masters were forerunners of a mutation in the human race. The race will eventually become superhuman, but only after an apocalyptic breakdown of civilization. It can be supposed that Eliade "knew" all this because he understood himself to be such a "master."

2. Transhumanist Themes in *The Portugal Journal* (1940-45)

A second stimulus for the current inquiry was the long-delayed posthumous publication of Eliade's *Portugal Journal* (*PJ*) in 2010. In his lifetime, Eliade published four volumes of his journals, covering the postwar years, as well as two volumes of autobiography, covering the years until 1945. There were other journals, however, that he chose not to publish. Preceded by publication of the original Romanian and by a Spanish translation, the 2010 English translation of *PJ* has not yet received much scholarly scrutiny (Eliade 2010). I will, therefore, largely allow it to speak for itself. I copy below some sections attesting to Eliade's transhumanism during World War II.

I should first note that *PJ* includes important events confirming Eliade's traditionalism – for example, Carl Schmitt, in Berlin 1942, telling an enthusiastic Eliade that "René Guénon is the most interesting man in the world" (32). This comment seems to echo what Eliade wrote about Evola in 1935, that he was "one of the most interesting spirits of the war generation."[9] In other words, *PJ* fully corroborates the worldview of *SDH*, and, as we shall see, of *YWY* as well:

9 Elide's review of Evola's *Crisis*, translated by Bradesco, 42. See note 8 above.

May 17, 1942
The elect man – and any man can become *elect* when he is infused with spirit – moves on another plane. … I learn essential things about the real man by following the reaction of the individual *vis-à-vis* the spirit; man *vis-à-vis* death, *vis-à-vis* love: *there* is an object for research! (emphasis in original)

June 10, 1943
But the *act* of creation, Eros, can unleash primordial *powers and visions of a force that far surpasses the contemporary mental horizon:* cf. the mystique of archaic origins, Dionysus, etc. The sentiment that he can *create*, the certainty that he *is life* and can *give birth to life transforms man into a vast, cosmic being.* … I'm attempting a grandiose thing: a new synthesis of world culture [and to] the spiritual meanings of the life long since superseded in the mental evolution of humankind.

January 3, 1945
I want to write a book challenging the modern world, an invitation to the *absolute freedom* which I decipher in certain myths and discover still in certain persons even in our age (yogins, mystics, the phenomenon of levitation, the incombustibility of the body, clairvoyance, prophecy, etc. which demonstrate the *autonomy of man from the laws of matter, the freedom that man could obtain.* (emphasis added)

April 16, 1945
In contrast to many, I do not believe that "civilization" necessarily annihilates man. If modern man is less healthy, is degenerate, neuropathic, without roots, etc., this is not due to the fact that he lives in an industrial society, that he resides in a metropolis, that he has a radio, motion pictures, etc. – but simply to that fact that man has *not yet succeeded in adapting to the new cosmic milieu created by his own discoveries and means of production.* (emphasis added)

August 16, 1945
[O]nly those who succeed in discovering and possessing themselves totally, who obtain a minimum of spiritual autonomy, who realize the grandeur of the human condition – only those can be called *mature*, grown-up, "full-sized" men. The rest … *can* be compared to the millions of herrings that perished soon after leaving the egg. The *idea must be made clear that only those mature examples constitute the species homo sapiens; that the millions of individuals who survive in subhuman modalities do not represent it and do not obligate it.* (emphasis added)

Eliade finds "grandeur" in millions of subhumans – who do not deserve to live because they are not really humans – dying so that the "elect," the "full-sized" humans can thrive. By contrast to this revulsion for the masses, the Romanian diarist identified with a certain elite, "men who could be your masters" (see September 1944 entry).

3. *Morning of the Magicians* (in French, 1960)

Man is not finished. He is on the brink of a formidable mutation which will confer on him the powers the ancients attributed to the gods. A few specimens of the New Man exist in the world, who have perhaps come here from beyond the frontiers of time and space. (Pauwels and Bergier 1968, 215)

Pauwels and Bergier's *Morning of the Magicians* weds traditionalism and transhumanism with their own distinctive technosophy. This marriage, as I shall show, is allegorized in *YWY*.

Eliade and Louis Pauwels (1920-1997) purveyed a peculiarly serious popularization of what may been called "esoteric Nazism." By "esoteric Nazism," I do not refer to what George L. Mosse has called "the mystical origins of National Socialism," which comprises a serious and reputable area of research and analysis (Mosse 1987, 197-214). Rather, I refer to an abstruse but nonetheless popular culture meme that portrays Nazism as being manipulated by a secret order. Such occultist Nazism found a classic expression in Trevor Ravenscroft's *Spear of Destiny* (1973), which has remained in print for over a generation (Godwin 1993, 99). Ravenscroft's association of ancient secret societies and Nazism is now a standard feature of certain occultist circles, not to speak of conspiracy theories and a numerous genres of popular culture. But the pioneering and most popular account of this meme was *MM* (ibid.).

A fermented mix of Nazi human experimentation, mystical vision, and hunger for total power, *MM* was originally a French bestseller in 1960. *MM* eventually became a foundational text of the international New Age movement and, more importantly for present purposes, a technosophic classic of prototranshumanism. Pauwels further popularized this worldview in his magazine *Planète* and other publications of "le mouvement *Planète*."[10] Eliade notably and repeatedly remarked at some length, in three public speeches, in the 1960s, '70s, and '80s, that *MM* and "le mouvement *Planète*" were of great cultural significance.[11] *MM* is a curious mélange of popular science, occultism, astrology, science fiction, and spiritual techniques. But it is more than that. It tacitly pretends to reveal numerous vital secrets – of our universe, of the Second World War, of lost civilizations, of Hitler's obsession with astrology, and so on. … [T]he reader is convinced that he is being given facts, or at least reasonable hypotheses – that, in any case, he is not being misled" (Eliade 1976, 9).

The third lecture of these three lectures, "*Homo Faber and Homo Religiosus*" (henceforth "HFHR") was published just a year before Eliade's death. It glamorizes and publicizes Pauwels, on an explicitly transhumanist note – that, thanks

---

10 For a study of the cultural impact and implications of *Planète*, see Jean-Bruno Renard, "Le mouvement *Planète*: un épisode important de l'histoire culturelle française," *Politica Hermetica* 10 (1996): 152-74. For a fuller discussion, see Stoczkowski (1999). I thank Dr. Daniel Dubuisson for directing me to this source.

11 "Cultural Fashions and the History of Religions" in 1967, reprinted in Eliade 1976; "The Occult and the Modern World," originally the Freud Memorial Lecture in 1974, republished in Eliade 1976; and "Homo Faber and Homo Religiosus," delivered in 1983 and published in Eliade 1985a.

to modern technology, we are "*condemned to immortality*" (Eliade 1985a, 9-11). Given his lifelong transhumanism, it should not be surprising that this final lecture is devoted to such heroes of transhumanism as Teilhard de Chardin, Arthur Clarke, Herman Kahn and ... Louis Pauwels (4-5). "HFHR" attributes to them, with no little enthusiasm, a scientific utopianism. Declaring nothing less than the "apotheosis of *homo faber*" traced back to alchemists' quest for immortality by means of matter, leading, indeed to "the perfection of man" (8), Eliade continues that "scientific and technological progress has made it possible to prolong and periodically regenerate human life" (9), concluding by citing an unnamed group of American scientific "Gnostics" who "believe in a future 'super-mankind'" (10). Ultimately, the aged historian of religions concludes "we are *condemned* to be immortal" (11, emphasis in the original).

Pauwels wrote to Eliade in April 1947, praising the French translation of *SDH*, "because you offer less for amusement than for meditation" (Eliade 1990a, 51). *MM* cites Eliade explicitly (344) and a second time implicitly.[12] One theme Eliade shared with *MM* put a mystical transhumanist spin on a fictional account of World War II. Pauwels, likewise, influenced by Guénon in *MM*, memorably articulated a notorious version of this equation: Nazism was "Guénonism *plus* tanks" (Bergier and Pauwels 1968, 259).

4. *Youth without Youth* (1978)

I turn now to Eliade's novella *Youth without Youth*, written in "November-December 1976" and published in Romanian in 1978. It portrays one Dominic Matei – alter ego both for Eliade and for Francis Ford Coppola ("I'm really a lot like the man in the movie," Coppola told A. O. Scott in the *New York Times*) – struck by lightning on his forehead, at midnight of Easter 1938 in Bucharest; he is rejuvenated, rendered omniscient, and temporally immortal, growing younger. The story of his subsequent life turns out to be, through a weird and fantastical tangle of strange events, ultimately reconnected to the "transfiguration" of 1938.[13] In *Images and Symbols*, Eliade's 1952 book (and his first essay collection published after the war) cited in *MM*, he suggested that "transcending the

12 The citation, cited verbatim but not attributed to Eliade in *MM*, is found in Eliade 1961 [1952], 12. The second citation, of an "anthropologist" at the 1956 parapsychology conference at Royaumont, concerns the powers of Siddhis. Eliade was at this conference, as he recalls in his entry for June 19, 1957, in *Journal* II, 166. Since Eliade wrote frequently on the powers of Siddhis, it is reasonable to surmise that he was that "anthropologist."

13 Orthodox Easter in 1938 was on April 11; Codreanu was arrested on April 16 and Eliade on July 14, 1938. The legionary revolt transpired January 21-23, 1941.

human condition" was physically achievable: "no one has yet given a satisfactory explanation of the astonishing *youthfulness* of some yogins' (Eliade 1961 [1952], 86n21, emphasis in the original). In the same book, he claimed that a "flash of lightning" puts the seer *beyond time* (ibid., 82), in what he elsewhere calls "lightning-flash kratophanies" (Eliade 1958b, 25). Just such a miracle blessed his alter ego Matei in a flash on Easter 1938.

MM contains numerous thematic links with Eliade's *YWY*, beyond the fact that *MM* quotes Eliade implicitly, as previously stated. These shared "initiatory" themes include alchemy (103-42), esoteric theories of history, popular literature as device, the idea of the perfect man having perfect memory, time travel, "pseudo-sciences under the Nazis," a Nazi doctor who commits suicide at war's end, and a central preoccupation with "fantastic realism" (*MM*, xxvi). Other points of common interest help explain Eliade's praises. Both dramatize the mystical meaning of the Dead Sea Scrolls (*MM*, 306-7; *YWY*, 78). Both glamorize a certain ontologically amphibian "fantastic reality" (*MM*) or what has been called "the function of the unreal."[14] The reality of levitation, appears in *MM* (369) where Pauwels cites the same obscure authority, Olivier Leroy, who is elsewhere invoked in this connection by Eliade.[15]

There's more than just similar motifs: there are similar plots and similar language. In *MM*, on meeting a youthful-looking old man at a café, the narrator "had the most recent contact imaginable with alchemy; a conversation in a *bistro* at Saint-Germain-des-Prés (*MM*, 103); in *YWY*, an alchemist, described as elderly but youthful-appearing, approaches the author seated at a café (*YWY*, 76-80). In his lecture largely dedicated to *MM*, Eliade describes it as emerging in a "cultural milieu … dominated by a few ideas and a number of clichés" associated not just with Paris but with Saint-Germain-des-Prés (Eliade 1976, 10). In the 1970 introduction to *SDH*, Eliade uses similar phrasing: "I have knowingly utilized a number of [occultist] clichés" (*SDH*, x). "It's only a metaphor. A metaphor that's become a cliché," he added. "You find it in all the so-called occultist pulp literature" (*YWY*, 79). The magician in the novel claims to have met or have known someone who met contemporary alchemists, including Fulcanelli and Eugene Cansiliet (*MM* 103, 118); Eliade names two contemporary alchemists whom he met, Fulcanelli and Cansiliet (Lannes and Ferrier 1980).

In the following, I will survey four transhumanist themes shared in *SDH*, *MM*, and *YWY*.

---

14 See Matei Calinescu, "The Function of the Unreal: Reflections on Mircea Eliade's Short Fiction," in *Imagination and Meaning: The Scholarly and Literary Worlds of Mircea Eliade*, edited by N. J. Girardot and M. L. Ricketts (New York: Seabury Press, 1982).

15 In the preface to the *Comentarii la Legenda Masterului Manole* (1943, 7), Eliade sets against the positivist methods of Tylor, Mannhardt, and Frazer those of "Olivier Leroy, Guénon, Evola, and Coomaraswamy". Cited in Spineto (2008).

A. The Doctrine of Awakening

One of the occult powers acquired in *SDH*, *MM*, and *YWY* is "waking sleep." This potentiality is presented in parallel extended soliloquies in a substantial section of *SDH* (87-101). Dr. Honigberger writes that "I *woke up sleeping*, or, more precisely, I woke up in *sleep*, without having fallen asleep in the true sense of the word" (98). Then the narrator comments that Honigberger explored this state of consciousness.

MM devotes four chapters to achieving the "Awakened State" (348-73). Pauwels and Bergier put on it a distinctly scientific transhumanist spin: "In proportion as technical progress will gradually allow men time to breathe, so will the quest for the 'third state' of awareness and lucidity take precedence over all other aspirations" (358-59). So too is an almost identical condition of the superevolved future human described in terms of waking sleep in Eliade's *YWY* (46-57): "[Matei] thought he was beginning to understand what had happened. The enormous concentration of electricity that, by exploding over him, had shot through him, had regenerated his entire organism and amplified all his mental faculties" (53).

B. Ontological Mutations

Nazi human experimentation haunts *YWY*, where some two-thirds of the book deals with this theme. Matei's rejuvenation by a lightning bolt is a miracle that attracts the attention of a Nazi scientist, one "Dr. Rudolf."

> Among the intimates of Goebbels there is an enigmatic and ambiguous personage, a certain Dr. Rudolf, who ... believes that electrocution by a current of at least a million volts could produce radical mutation in the human species. ... Some members of Goebbels's entourage are encouraged. ... The Gestapo has been given a free hand. (*YWY* 95)

Here, at the dark heart of his fantasy, Eliade presents Nazi doctors who perform human experiments designed to attain exactly the sort of immortalization enjoyed by his alter ego – in short, that the *Nazi scientists desire him and his secret powers*.

As we have seen, *MM* associates the imperative for the "mutation of the human species" with the experimental implementation of "esoteric Nazi philosophy." *MM*, in turn, imagines the application of millions of volts to make a Superman:

> an exceptional particle of fantastic energy (an energy of 10^{18} electron volts, whereas the fission of uranium produces only 2 x 10^8). Let us assume that *only once* in the history of the human race, such a particle came into contact with a human brain. Who knows if the enormous energy resulting therefrom might not have produced an activation inducing for the first time an "awakened" state in Man? ... It was perhaps exceptional cosmic "events" releasing fantastic energy, which turned Man into Superman. (372, emphasis in original)

MM and *YWY*, thus, specify an "eschatology of electricity" leading to nothing less than "the mutation of the human species." This idea is virtually the leitmotif of *MM*, the final section of which is titled "Some Reflections on the Mutants" (399-416). The protagonist in *YWY* also proclaims an incontrovertibly analogous worldview: "I'm a 'mutant'. ... I anticipate the post-historic existence of man. Like in a science-fiction novel', he added, smiling with amusement" (99). "I was gifted with a universal erudition such as will become accessible to man only many thousands of years from now" (104). "[T]he true meaning of the nuclear catastrophe can only be this: the mutation of the human species, the appearance of the superman. ... [O]f course only a few million individuals will survive. But they will constitute so many supermen" (124).

As noted above, Eliade was a source for *MM*. At this point, it becomes necessary to inquire into Eliade's sources for his theory of mutation. It is first important to emphasize how important "ontological mutation" was in Eliade's corpus. He invokes it as early as 1948.[16] He cites it in the very first article in the decade-long run of *Antaios* (*Antaios* 1, pp. 6 and 9, "*Wandlung*" in the German). The notion recurs in his widely read monograph *The Sacred and the Profane* (181) and in his 1953 "The Yearning for Paradise in Primitive Tradition,"[17] which was republished in Eliade 1960 (104, 108).

In addition to *MM*, there are several other likely sources for his usage of "ontological mutation." The Romanian author Lucian Blaga, whose "genius" Eliade admired, used the concept "ontological mutation."[18] But a more proximate source may be Julius Evola. In *Mussolini's Intellectuals*, James A. Gregor notes that Evola in 1941 elaborated a racialist theory of "'idiovariations' – unpredictable genetic mutations in hereditary transmission between generations – to make a case for the influence, from 'on high', of 'superbiological' and 'spiritual' forces in the shaping of races" (2005, 210). As we have seen, *MM* directly links just such a spiritual "mutation of the human species" with the experimental implementation of "esoteric Nazi philosophy." Like *YWY*, *MM* describes a Nazi scientist seeking the esoteric secret of energy. *MM* and *YWY*, strange as it sounds, *glorify the positive mutational potential of Nazi human experimentation.*

Furthermore, both *MM* and *YWY* go to some lengths to assert that Nazi horrors had a higher purpose. *MM* is explicitly and proudly reactionary and defends its

---

16 "Durohana and Waking Dream", reprinted in "Mutation" (Eliade 1960, 117).

17 *Diogenes* 1953, reprinted in *Daedalus* 88 (2), *Myth and Mythmaking* (Spring 1959): 255-67.

18 See http://books.google.com/books?id=1XgelhwJLXkC&pg=PA85&lpg=PA85&dq=ontological+mutation&source=bl&ots=AOuxYyEiTo&sig=65Cv0Fow8zSt09yWhFirlszfWEI&hl=en&ei=QwWZTJ6zNYWmsQPHwtSoDA&sa=X&oi=book_result&ct=result&resnum=1&ved=0CBIQ6AEwAA#v=onepage&q=ontological%20mutation&f=false, accessed July 20, 2011. In his *Portugal Journal* of April 22, 1943, Eliade confessed, "Nevertheless, I have admiration for Blaga's genius."

own politics at considerable length (64-65). It is apposite to note that Pauwels has been implicated in the early stages of French Holocaust Denial (Eatwell 1991, 122-23). Already in *MM*, Pauwels had said that "certain sessions of the Nuremberg Trial were meaningless. The judges could not possibly have any kind of communication with those who were really responsible, most of whom, in any case, had disappeared, leaving in the dock only the men who had been their instruments" (257). The Holocaust, according to *MM*, was in any case a mere melodrama of human sacrifice: "The gas ovens of Auschwitz? Merely ritual" (293).

"Dr. Rudolf", *YWY*'s Nazi mutation scientist, is arguably the central plot device of the novella. This subplot unfolds over roughly two-thirds of the book (*YWY*, 57-125). Its Nazis remain distant and mysterious: "someone on high up in the Gestapo decided to kidnap you" (58); Rudolf is "an enigmatic and ambiguous personage" (61).

Concerning attractive mysteries of a secret Nazi program of human mutation, *YWY* invokes a closely related variant of the version in the *MM*. *YWY* invokes the archetypally transhumanist "possibility of a human species superior to *homo sapiens*" (90). Thus, mutation through lightning in *YWY* was a transhumanism manifestly congruent with such claims made for electrocutional mutation in *MM*.

C. Immortality

Louis Pauwels and Jacques Bergier's successors to *MM*, *Impossible Possibilities* (1971) and *Eternal Man* (1972), read like precursors of contemporary transhumanist writing. These pop potboilers tout immortality perfected by technological advances. Such a vision remains strong in present transhumanism. See, for a reasonable summary of these aspirations, Bova (2000). The subtitle of Eliade's *Yoga* (1958a) is *Immortality and Freedom* – written before World War II and expanded to its final form after the war.

While the fictional Dr. Rudolf seeking the electrocutional secret of longevity works for Goebbels, the actual Nazi leader responsible for human experimentation was Heinrich Himmler. More generally, "Heinrich Himmler ... wanted to cultivate a new human type. . . .[:] '[W]e want to create an upper class for Germany, selected constantly over centuries, a new aristocracy, recruited always from the best sons and daughters of our nation, an aristocracy that *never becomes old.*'"[19] Eliade worked during the war effectively at one degree of separation from Himmler, through his contacts with Walther Wüst and other leaders of the Ahnenerbe.[20]

---

19 From Herbert F. Ziegler, *Nazi Germany's New Aristocracy: The SS-Leadership 1925-1939* (Princeton, NJ: Princeton University Press, 1989), 52 (emphasis added).

20 A point I hope to elaborate in my forthcoming *Political Mysteries*.

Eliade crafted *YWY* to echo not only key themes of *MM* but, I suggest, also the key themes of his own 1940 *SDH*. Both stories end in their final sentences with a metempsychosis – that is, a kind of immortalization – that of one "Stephen" in *SDH* and that of one Martin Audricourt in *YWY*. Moreover, in both cases, those who are reincarnated are apparently not given their "real" names. And, finally, the character "Stephens" of *YWY* points to the "Stephen" at the very end of *SDH*. All these, in turn, point to "Stefan," the protagonist of Eliade's major novel *The Forbidden Forest* (1978b).

D. The "Powers"

Before the young Romanian left for India in 1928, Baron Evola begged Eliade to report only eyewitness accounts of Yoga or "*Magic Powers*", as Eliade noted in *Journal III* (161). In the 1940 *SDH*, Honigberger seems to make just such a report: "For only after you acquire the first *powers* and the scales suddenly fall from your eyes do you realize how very great is man's ignorance" (*SDH,* 96, emphasis in original).

Thus, in his essay on "Powers and Holiness," Eliade spoke of the "paradox by which the human condition is surpassed" (Eliade1961 [1952], 150), while in *Yoga*, these "powers" gave the "elect" occultist capacities to "transcend the human condition." This theme of "Powers" pervades Eliade's work, as it does *MM*. Thus, we read in an interview given by Eliade in 1978, the same year in which he published *YWY*:

> For the SS, the annihilation of millions of people in the concentration camps *also had a meaning, even an eschatological one.* ... *It is possible to imagine* how those sick men, or *zealots*, or *fanatics* – those modern Manicheans – saw Evil as being embodied in certain races: the Jews, the Gypsies. *Sacrificing* them by the millions was thus *not a crime*, since they were the incarnation of Evil, of the devil. ... The Aztecs believed they were helping the sun god; the Nazis believed they were realizing their historical destiny. *And the same is true* for the Russians. (Eliade 1982b, 127, emphasis added)

To which one may compare parallel assertions in *MM*:

> Wolfram Sievers was appointed official executioner, a kind of ritualistic, sacrificial butcher [whose exterminations were] a means of overcoming the indifference of the "Powers" and attracting their attention. From the Mayas to the Nazis, this was the magic significance of human sacrifices. (283)[21]

21 For Eliade as for Pauwels, this "sacrifice" was nothing less than eschatological. In *Myths, Dreams and Mysteries*, originally published in French in 1957, four years before *MM* came out, the now-American historian of religions underscored this point: "The heroic duel is a sacrifice: war is a decadent ritual in which a *holocaust of innumerable victims* is offered up to the gods of victory" (1960, 200; emphasis added).

This usage of "Powers" in quotation marks, like Eliade's usage of "Center" in quotation marks, leads the reader to search elsewhere in *MM* for this technical usage. After invoking the Nazis's "coming race of Supermen which would result from mutations of the human species" (276), *MM* specifies the "Universe in which people like Himmler live [who are called on by the Powers] to liquidate a few million 'false' men'" (286). As for Hitler, *MM* drives home repeatedly his subservience to the Powers: "He thought that all he had to do was to make full use of his 'Powers'. But one cannot use such Powers; one can only serve them" (288). At this point, *MM* cites some unresearchable source to the effect that it is "difficult to say exactly when Hitler began to dream of biological mutations" (288). And *MM* goes on: "It is no longer a question of Germany the immortal or of a National-Socialist State, but of magical preparation for the coming of a Man-God, the New Man whom the Powers will establish on the Earth" (290); "The world is matter to be transformed to liberate the concentrated energy of the Wise Men – a psychic energy capable of attracting the Powers from Beyond" (292).

The protagonist of both *SDH* and *YWY* is a stand-in, an alter ego, for Eliade himself. The secrets of Eliade, sketched in confidence in his personal unpublished journals, shines through his fictional characters; like a ventriloquist, their speech is his speech, their dreams his dreams. *MM* recommends – to put it mildly – the experiences enjoyed by these Eliadean alter egos.

5. *Morning of the Magicians*: The SS Ahnenerbe and Nazi Occultism

> We are to radically liquidate the past and form a new species, [a mutation of a superior order] infinitely superior to the man of today.
>
> – YWY, 141

The four texts studied to this point present a fairly consistent transhumanism. I have shown that Eliade's early versions of this transhumanism were beholden to Evola and Guénon.

Evola aspired to work for the SS Ahnenerbe. The Ahnenerbe, according to *MM*, had "a magical conception of the world and of man, to which they had sacrificed all the youth of their country and offered to the gods an ocean of blood. They had done everything in their power to conciliate the Powers" (296). They were "militant monks who had signed a pact with the Powers" (296).

MM identified Friedrich Hielscher as the "spiritual mentor" and even "High Priest" of Wolfram Sievers at the Ahnenerbe (294-95). Hielscher was acquainted with Evola and a longtime friend of Ernst Jünger, as well as with Ahnenerbe leaders Sievers and Richard Wolfram. While the notoriously unreliable accounts in *MM* inflate his "spiritual leadership," it is clear from Hielscher's own account, corroborated in Jünger's wartime journals, that Hielscher saw himself as a of kind of cult leader.[22] Whether Hielscher directed a secret cult that exploited Sievers and the Ahnenerbe, as asserted by Pauwels in *MM*, he certainly was acquainted with and shared some of the mystically tinged religious inclinations of Eliade's friends Jünger and Evola, who were also his friends. This background, in short, suggests that the literary parallels concerning human experimentation in *MM* and *YWY* are not inconsistent with a certain historical context.

For a precious glimpse into this context, Eliade's journal entry for January 13, 1943, must be cited:

> *13 January 1943*
> I receive a letter today from the German Ambassador, Baron Hoyningen-Huene, by which he invites me, in the name of the Rector of the University of Münich [Walther Wüst, Kurator of the Ahnenerbe], to participate in the inauguration of the Sven Heddin Central-Asiatic Institute, which will take place in Münich, 14-20 January. ... The German government is bearing all travel expenses.
>
> Von Bredow telephones me in the evening, saying that I would leave on 18 January by plane. On the 19th I'll be at Stuttgart where someone will be waiting at the airport to accompany me by train to Münich. . . .
>
> I must go, even though the weather is infernal and an airplane trip in winter is rather risky. Last month, Cantemir tells me, two Lufthansa planes crashed. I think of myself as on military duty, and I'm going. (2010, 60)

For the German government to subvent Eliade's continental travel, on short notice, in the middle of the war, tells us something of his promising contribution to the intellectual mission of the Ahnenerbe – a standing of which the *PJ* seems to be proud. In *YWY*, an Ahnenerbe-like scientist similarly seeks to exploit Matei's secrets. Since Eliade retained the *PJ*, and so retained access to dates of his activities of 1943, the repetition of the tellingly identical date of January 20, 1943, can only have been intentionally specified. *January 20, 1943, the very date on which he actually was invited to a major Ahnenerbe event, was the date in YWY on which he was first "observed" to be a mutant.*[23]

Dr. Rudolf, inaccurately rendered odious by Coppola, resembles a prototypical Ahnenerbe scholar. Eliade enjoyed early and sustained favorable relations, both of a personal and a scholarly kind, with important Ahnenerbe scholars, as well as many Ahnenerbe associates of lesser importance. Therefore, Coppola has it precisely backwards, as a closer reading of *YWY* clearly bears out. The key point is that the transfiguration of Matei is virtually miraculous, unique, and desirable and, indeed, the prefiguration of a more potent human species of the future. Matei is sought by Rudolf because Rudolf wants the absolute human power to transcend ordinary human power; Matei is the avatar of transhumanism, and Rudolf wants

22 See now the Jünger-Hielscher letters.

23 This episode even includes, as in the real *PJ*, an airplane crashing in the Atlantic as a consequence (82).

a piece of his cosmological action. By any sensible and moral measure, Matei's transformation into a superman is portrayed as a thing of the greatest good, even if it must be kept hidden. The logic of the text is unmistakable. Rudolf, "a notorious Nazi" (*YWY,* 85) wants this truly great and good potency with which to perform human experimentation.

He was on the right track, scientifically, at least according to the logic of *YWY*. Eliade's actual associates in the Ahnenerbe belonged to an organization that implemented human experimentation, many of whom were directly and indirectly complicit in the conceptualization, mythologization, and implementation of SS genocide; many more were passive bystanders. The Shoah was overwhelmingly a project of the SS, and the Ahnenerbe was the official scholarly wing of the SS. The present work is not one of prosecution, and I am not pressing prosecutorial inquiries. My concern here is simply to demonstrate that Coppola's blunder ironically leads us to the revelation of Eliade's transhumanism. Eliade was proud of the fact that Matei, his alter ego, was sought by Dr. Rudolf, just as Eliade in his wartime diaries is proud to be invited to an Ahnenerbe event. Not to put too fine a point on it, Rudolf is playing on the right team, for the good guys. Nothing in the story suggests the contrary. Coppola didn't understand this, and so his cinematic version came out inevitably garbled.

6. Eliade's "Transcending the Human Condition" as Occultist Technosophy

In *YWY,* the elderly protagonist is struck "on the top of his head by lightning" (3). Subsequently, he learns of "the regeneration and rejuvenation of on old man who was struck by lightning. A significant detail: the lightning struck in the center of the cranial cap" (125). What is particularly notable in the scenario of *YWY, the striking of the cranial cap,* can be identified elsewhere in Eliade's scholarship with *brahmarandhra,* "the opening at the summit of the cranium" (Eliade 1960, 109n4).[24] As Eliade saw it, the personality, by means of precisely such extraordinary experiences, could breach the human condition, to attain a superlife. He understood that

> the joy that a *human being* has created, has imitated God's work, has been saved from a destined sterility, has breached those walls of impotence and finitude. On the one hand there is the formula "I am created by God," which inevitably arouses the consciousness of nothingness, of religious fear, of the taste of dust and ashes. On the other hand there is the statement "A human being, like

24 This is the theme of Eliade's contribution to the Gershom Scholem festschrift, which Eliade republished in 1985, the year before he died.

myself, has created, like God", which brings the joy that a fellow creature has imitated creation, has become a demiurge, a force in the creating. (Eliade 1982c, 8, emphasis in the original)

In October 1965, Eliade gave a lecture at the University of Chicago titled "Cultural Fashions and History of Religions." He published it as the lead article in *Occultism, Witchcraft, and Cultural Fashions. Essays in Comparative Religions* (henceforth *OWCF*) in 1976, the year he wrote *YWY*. *OWCF* deals with *Planète* in one essay and Guénon in another. He concluded the essay "The Occult in the Modern World" with a kind of transhumanist flourish, citing Stanley Kubrick's film *2001,* a key precursor of transhumanist futurology (*OWCF*, 68). The film *2001*, it will be recalled, concludes with, in effect, cosmic transcendence of the human condition.

At war's end, Eliade asked himself a question: "Why don't we take account of other men's capacity for freedom, of their creative will, of their possibilities for transcending "fallen man?" (*PJ*, January 2, 1945). In his first major book, *Yoga*, "transcending the human condition" was the leitmotif of his exposition:

> [A]s in other religious initiations, the yogin begins by forsaking the profane world (family, society) and, guided by his guru, applies himself to passing successively beyond the behavior patterns and values proper to the human condition. … [A]sana is distinctly a sign of transcending the human condition. … But their immediate purpose is even now obvious; it is to abolish (or to transcend) the human condition by a refusal to conform to the most elementary human inclinations. (1958a, 4)

In *Patterns in Comparative Religion*, another major book after the war, Eliade, proclaims the capacity "to transcend, by natural means, the human condition" (1958b, 383). In the widely read *The Sacred and the Profane*, he tells the reader that "religious man assumes a humanity that has a transhuman, transcendent model" (1959b, 99) and announces the "fundamental mystical experience – that is, transcending the human condition" (175). In *Shamanism*, a third big book before he found his position in Chicago, he invokes "transcending the profane human condition" (1964, 95). In *Images and Symbols* from early after the war, he asserts that transcending "pairs of opposites" results in "abolishing the polarity that besets the human condition" (1961 [1952], 84). A late statement of Eliade (which he purports to limit to an identifiable group from antiquity): "Through the possession of *gnosis*, the *pneumatikoi* consider themselves free from the human condition, beyond social rules and ethical interdictions" (*OWCF*, 109).

"The Symbolism of Ascent" was the very first article in the very first issue of *Antaios*, the journal Eliade coedited with Ernst Jünger. The *Antaios* German version, which had appeared in 1957 in French, was published simultaneously, in 1959, in an English version, in *Myths, Dreams and Mysteries*.[25] Ascending sovereigns "no

25 In the "Acknowledgments" to the English edition of 1960 (246), Eliade remarks on versions from 1948, 1950, and 1956.

longer participate in the human condition" (1960, 101); the shaman has "surpassed the human condition" (102); archaic man exhibits a "longing to go beyond and 'above' the human condition" (106); the *arhat's* flight "signif[ies] transcendence of the human condition" (109).

"Like a science-fiction novel, he added, smiling with amusement" (*YWY,* 68). Pauwels and Eliade proclaimed a distaste for science fiction, making an exception for Ray Bradbury and Arthur C. Clarke. The key to understanding their transhumanism is not science fiction, however. It is Teilhard de Chardin.

Pierre Teilhard de Chardin (1881-1955), whose transhumanism is addressed elsewhere in the present volume, was one of the few modern thinkers, outside of traditionalists, whom Eliade acknowledged as having achieved some genuinely profound insights. Chief among them, perhaps, was the prophecy of the Omega Point. Like the work of Eliade and the traditionalists, this positive apocalypticism was neither Catholic nor scientific, neither confessional nor orthodox. Rather, it was the quasi-prophetic product of the creative imagination of a single religious genius. The belief system of Teilhard, like that of Eliade, was a freelance creation. While Eliade implemented an academic history of religions and Teilhard practiced a scientific paleontology, both shared an ultimate interest in "planetary" thought, which was best expressed not rationally but rather "poetically." The unitive, transcendent, soteriological character of their "planetary" prophecies, however aesthetic in origin, predicted a qualitative "reintegration" of the human race. In both cases, then, their predictions of a transcendence of the human condition are closer to prophecy than they are to science. Their transhumanism, while free of confessional limitations, was nonetheless closer to religion than it was to science, even while in the guise of technosophy.

Eliade cites Teilhard in a vein of enthusiastic approval long before the writing and publication of *YWY*. He reports a conversation he had with him in 1950 (*Journal I*) and a dinner conversation he had about him in October 1962 (*Journal III*, 170-71). There are further favorable invocations of Teilhard in *The Forge and the Crucible* (1962), in the 1976 "Le Mythe de l'Alchimie," in his journals (May 17, 1963), and in interviews. Teilhard looms large in *MM*, too. Eliade affirmed this similarity: "Probably the readers of *Planète* and of Teilhard de Chardin are not the same, but they have many things in common" (*OWCF*, 11). *MM* gives the fullest and most direct statement of the transhumanism outlined in this paper, with reference to Teilhard; it is the epitome of occultist technosophy:

> Man can have access to a secret world – *see* the Light, *see* Eternity, comprehend the Laws of Energy, integrate within himself the rhythm of the Universe, consciously apprehend the ultimate concentration of forces, and, like Teilhard de Chardin, live the incomprehensible life that starts from "Point Omega," in which the whole of creation, at the end of terrestrial time, will find its accomplishment, consummation and exaltation. Man is capable of everything. (*MM* 341, emphasis in original)

7. Conclusion: Eliade's Technosophic Occultism

We would not dismiss a great mathematician's proofs because he beat his wife. The life is the life, and the work is the work. That being said, the case of Eliade's life versus his work demands a qualitatively different order of assessment *because he wanted all his various writings to be judged as a whole.* As he proudly proclaimed, "Seul l'ensemble de mes écrits *peut révéler la signification de mon activité* (Only the totality of my writing can reveal the significance of my activity).[26] I have tried to show that Eliade's unified lifework presents us with a thoroughgoing transhumanism. His grand opus consistently championed *techniques* dedicated to "transcending the human condition." What distinguishes Eliade's cultivation of so-called "Powers," a species of transhumanisim, from run-of-the-mill magic is his mix of genres that metaphysically amounts to a *technosophic occultism*.

Mircea Eliade's technosophic occultism had sources in *Naturphilosophie*, fantastic literature, Yoga, traditionalism; and these were further articulated in his fiction, his private journals, and, of course, in his scholarship. It was announced in his fiction of 1940 and again in 1978, and it was corroborated in closely related guise in *MM*. Eliade's sustained and multifarious connections to Ahnenerbe scholarship, finally, throw some dark light, as it were, on his proud transhumanism. Francis Ford Coppola construed *YWY* as being a fantastic tale redolent with nostalgia. This construal elided the audacity and primacy of Mircea Eliade's daring and disturbing transhumanist novella.

References

Bova, Ben. 2000. *Immortality: How Science Is Extending Your Life Span and the World.* Vol. 1. New York: Avon Books.

Eatwell, Roger. 1991. The Holocaust denial: A study in propaganda technique. In *Neo-Facism in Europe*, edited by L. Cheles, R. Ferguson, M. Vaughn, et al., 120-46. London: Longman Group Ltd.

Eliade, Mircea. 1958a. *Yoga: Immortality and Freedom.* Translated by W. R. Trask. New York: Pantheon Books.

–. 1958b. *Patterns in Comparative Religion.* Translated by R. Sheed. New York: Sheed and Ward.

–. 1958c. *Rites and Symbols of Initiation: The Mysteries of Birth and Rebirth.* Translated by W. R. Trask. New York: Harper and Row.

26 Eliade, cited in Marino (1980, 439). In his autobiography (v. 1), Eliade announced that "[n]early all the ideas that I expounded in the books published in France after 1946 are found *in nuce* in studies written between 1933 and 1939" (1981, 309).

–. 1959a. *Cosmos and History: The Myth of the Eternal Return*. Translated by W. R. Trask. New York: Harper/Bollingen.
–. 1959b. *The Sacred and Profane: The Nature of Religion*. Translated by W. R. Trask. New York: Harcourt, Brace.
–. 1960. *Myths, Dreams and Mysteries: The Encounter between Contemporary Faiths and Archaic Realities*. Translated by P. Mairet. New York: Harper and Row.
–. 1961 [1952]. *Images and Symbols: Studies in Religious Symbolism*. Translated by P. Mairet. New York: Sheed and Ward.
–. 1962. *The Forge and Crucible*. Translated by S. Corrin. London: Rider.
–. 1963. *Myth and Reality*. Translated by W. R. Trask. New York: Harper and Row.
–. 1964. *Shamanism: Archaic Techniques of Ecstasy*. Translated by W. R. Trask. New York: Bollingen Foundation.
–. 1965. *Two and the One*. Translated by J. M. Cohen. London: Harvill Press.
–. 1969. *The Quest: History and Meaning in Religion*. Chicago: University of Chicago Press.
–. 1972. *Zalmoxis: The Vanishing God: Comparative Studies in the Religious and Folklore of Dacia and Eastern Europe*. Translated by W. R. Trask. Chicago: University of Chicago Press.
–. 1976. *Occultism, Witchcraft and Cultural Fashions: Essays in Comparative Religions*. Chicago: University of Chicago Press. Cited as *OWCF* in text.
–. 1977. *No Souvenirs: Journal, 1957-1969*. Translated by F. H. Johnson Jr. New York: Harper and Row.
–. 1978a. *Youth without Youth*. Translated by Mac Linscott Ricketts. Chicago: University of Chicago Press. Cited as *YWY* in text.
–. 1978b. *The Forbidden Forest*. Translated by Mac Linscott Ricketts and Mary Park Stevenson. South Bend, IN: University of Notre Dame Press.
–. 1978c. *History of Religious Ideas, Volume 1. From the Stone Age to the Eleusinian Mysteries*. Chicago: University of Chicago Press.
–. 1981. *Autobiography, Volume I: Journey East, Journey West, 1907-1937*. Translated by Mac Linscott Ricketts. San Francisco: Harper & Row.
–. 1982a. *Imagination and Meaning: The Scholarly and Literary Worlds of Mircea Eliade*. Edited by N. J. Girardot and M. L. Ricketts. New York: Seabury Press.
–. 1982b. *Ordeal by Labyrinth: Conversations with Claude-Henri Rocquet*. Translated by D. Coltman. Chicago: University of Chicago Press.
–. 1982c. *Tales of the Sacred and the Supernatural*. Philadelphia: Westminster Press.

–. 1982c. *History of Religious Ideas, Volume 2. From Gautama Buddha to the Triumph of Christianity*. Chicago: University of Chicago Press.
–. 1985a. *History of Religions: Retrospect and Prospect*. Edited by J. Kitagawa. New York: Macmillian. Contains "*Homo Faber and Homo Religiosus*," cited as "HFHR" in text.
–. 1985b. *History of Religious Ideas: From Gautama Buddha to the Triumph of Christianity*. Translated by W. R. Trask. Chicago: University of Chicago Press.
–. 1986. *Two Strange Tales*. Boston: Shambhala. Original in Romanian, *Nopti la Semapore*, 1940. Cited as *SDH* in text (*Secret of Dr. Honigberger*).
–. 1988a. *Autobiography, Volume II: Exile's Odyssey – 1938-1969*. Translated by Mac Linscott Ricetts. Chicago: University of Chicago Press.
–. 1988b. *Symbolism, the Sacred and the Arts*. Edited by Diane Apostolos-Cappadona. New York: Crossroad.
–. 1989a. *Journal II: 1957-1969*. Translated by F. H. Johnson Jr. Chicago: University of Chicago Press.
–. 1989b. *Journal III: 1970-1978*. Translated by T. L. Fagan. Chicago: University of Chicago Press.
–. 1990a. *Journal I: 1945-1955*. Translated by Mac Linscott Ricketts. Chicago: University of Chicago Press
–. 1990b. *Journal IV: 1979-1985*. Translated by Mac Linscott Ricketts. Chicago: University of Chicago Press.
–. 2010. *The Portugal Journal*. Translated by Mac Linscott Ricketts. Albany: State University of New York Press. Cited as *PJ* in text.
Evola, Julius. 1983. *The Metaphysics of Sex*. New York: Inner Traditions.
–. 1992. *The Yoga of Power*. Translated by G. Stucco. Rochester, NY: Inner Traditions.
–. 1995a. *Revolt against the Modern World*. Translated by G. Stucco. Rochester, NY: Inner Traditions.
–. 1995b. *The Hermetic Tradition. Symbols and Teachings of the Royal Art*. Translated by E. E. Rehmus. Rochester, NY: Inner Traditions.
–. 1996. *The Doctrine of Awakening: The Attainment of Self-Mastery According to the Earliest Buddhist Texts*. Translated by H. E. Musson. Rochester, NY: Inner Traditions.
–. 1997. *The Mystery of the Grail: Initiation and Magic in the Quest for the Spirit*. Translated by G. Stucco. Rochester, NY: Inner Traditions.
Godwin, Jocelyn. 1993. *Arktos: The Polar Myth in Science, Symbolism and Nazi Survival*. Grand Rapids, MI. Phanes Press.
Gregor, A. James. 2005. *Mussolini's Intellectuals: Fascist Social and Political Thought*. Princeton, NJ: Princeton University Press.

Guénon, Rene. 1983 [1927]. *The Lord of the World/Le Roi du Monde*. Edited by S. D. Fohr. Translated by H. D. Fohr. Ripon, North Yorkshire, UK: Coombe Springs Press. This is a bilingual version.

Lannes, Sophie, and Jean-Louis Ferrier. 1980. A conversation with Mircea Eliade, on the pursuit of "the true dreams of mankind." *Encounter* 54.

Locke, John. 1980 [1690]. *Second Treatise on Government*. Indianapolis, IN: Hackett (1980). Text revised 1764.

Marino, Adrian. 1980. *L'hermeneutique de Mircea Eliade*. Paris: Gallimard.

Maritain, Jacques. 1985. In Jerald C. Brauer, "Mircea Eliade and the Divinity School." *Criterion* 24/23: 23-27.

Mosse, George L. 1987. *Masses and Man: Nationalist and Fascist Perceptions of Reality*. Detroit, MI: Wayne State University Press.

Pauwels, Louis, and Jacques Bergier. 1968. *The Morning of the Magicians*. New York: Avon. Cited as *MM* in text.

–. 1971. *Impossible Possibilities*. Translated by Andrew White. New York: Stein and Day.

–. 1972. *Eternal Man*. Translated by M. Heron. London: Souvenir Press.

Ravenscroft, Trevor. 1973. *Spear of Destiny*. New York: Putnam.

Rennie, Bryan, ed. 2008. *The International Eliade*. Albany: State University of New York Press.

Ricketts, Mac Linscott. 1988. *Mircea Eliade: The Romanian Roots*. 2 vols. New York: Columbia University Press.

Sedgwick, Mark. 2004. *Against the Modern World: Traditionalism and the Secret Intellectual History of the Twentieth Century*. Oxford: Oxford University Press.

Spineto, Natale. 2008. Mircea Eliade and Traditionalism. In Bryan Rennie, ed., *The International Eliade*, 131-49. Albany: State University of New York Press.

Stoczkowski, Wiktor. 1999. *Des hommes, des dieux et des extraterrestres*: *Ethnologie d'une croyance moderne*. Paris: Flammarion.

Wedemeyer, Christian, and Wendy Doniger, eds. 2010. *Hermeneutics, Politics, and the History of Religions: The Contested Legacies of Joachim Wach and Mircea Eliade*. Oxford: Oxford University Press.

Part II:
The Promise and Perils of Human Enhancement

What is Race?: Transhumanism and the Evolutionary Sciences

Brian Gratton

"Pardon him. ... He is a barbarian, and thinks that the customs of his tribe ... are the laws of nature!"

– G. B. Shaw, *Caesar and Cleopatra*

The intellectual and technical advances of evolutionary science in our time have inspired transhumanism. Upon that scientific foundation, transhumanists build their vision of how to create a better being. Hava Tirosh-Samuelson's essay in this volume (chapter 1) shows that transhumanism has links as well to the eugenics campaign of the early twentieth century, a movement built on the first flowering of evolutionary thinking. For most eugenicists, race mattered (Kevles 1985; Barkan 1992). Drawing from early evolutionary theory, they concluded that race and ethnicity had strong and differential effects on the characteristics of human beings, profoundly reinforcing a nonscientific belief in racial differences common among Western Europeans. Despite a similar reliance on the new evolutionary science, transhumanists exhibit no tendency toward racist or ethnocentric positions. Indeed, transhumanists draw the conclusion that we are all the same, driven by the same genetic forces, and trapped, body and mind, by the same selection history.

But like their predecessors, the eugenicists, transhumanists have no truck with nurture as the source of difference. They reject the social constructivist claim that race and ethnicity are ephemeral inventions, independent of genetics, and built by dominant groups for their advantage (Barkan 1992). Though cultures may adumbrate racial characteristics, ethnocentrism and racism are natural to human beings. Indeed, racism and ethnic conflict are among the bad human conditions that transhumanists plan to leave behind. Their program of improvement seeks to rid the transhuman of the psychological tendency to degrade the other. But insomuch as the transhumanist voyage succeeds, it will end in a better race or, more grandly, a superior species. Critics have posed a question about the likely effects of strong distinctions between human groups. Would they spark a conflagration between the human and the posthuman? To understand the transhumanist view of the issues that race and ethnicity present, we review first the conclusions drawn by the evolutionary sciences on which they depend, turning first to evolutionary biology and then to evolutionary psychology.

Evolutionary Biology

Recent discoveries in evolutionary biology have not led to a broad debate about the utility of racial categories for understanding differential human behavior. Evolutionary biologists recognize, like ordinary people do, the heritability of striking phenotypic differences. Still, most scientists consider such racial distinctions to have little to no consequence: the genetic blueprint is essentially the same for us all. This follows from the dominant assumption that, since the basic speciation of the modern human more than 100,000 years ago, "most of the behavioural changes seen since ... are cultural rather than genetic adaptations" (Renfrew 2010, 162). Evolutionary discoveries have, however, shifted once more the pendulum between nurture and nature toward the power of heritability, that is, one's nature as genetically determined, in explaining human behavior. In 1975, Edward O. Wilson's *Sociobiology* (1975) attacked the assumption common to nearly all social scientists that cultures and societies and families, rather than nature, made people act as they did. Even though Wilson had little to say about racial differences, Arthur Jensen did in his notable 1969 article on race and intelligence). The potential that a biological basis for human behavior might reinforce beliefs about racial differences (such as in intelligence) inspired a vigorous counterattack by prominent scientists including Richard Lewontin (1972) and Stephen Jay Gould (1996). Those in the debate had before them the breakthroughs of the new evolutionary theorists: the gene as the locus of selection for fitness, kin selection or inclusive fitness, reciprocity and altruism as evolutionarily reasonable, and the implausibility of group selection (Hamilton 1964; Trivers 1971; Dawkins 2006; Maynard Smith 1964).

For Lewontin, the science demonstrated that the social constructivists were right, not wrong: he famously demonstrated that there was, on average, much more variability between individuals of the same putative racial group as between the average of one race and another. Aware of the different expression of the same genes in different environments (epigenetics), Lewontin confirmed the social-constructivist view that race was culturally invented, a position his followers continue to maintain (Singh and Uyenoyama 2000; for a trenchant criticism, see Edwards 2003). Gould went still further, resisting any biological determination of distinctions by race in favor of cultural evolution.

This standard has been more difficult to carry into battle with the rapid advance of new evolutionary genetic science in the ensuing decades. First, the very high level of shared genetic code between humans and other primates (exceeding 98 percent) gives cold comfort to the notion that small levels of difference won't matter (though gene expression and regulation might), while passing the ammunition to primatologists who think chimp behavior has a lot to say about our own.

The common sense observation of striking phenotypic differences between groups leads to questions not about the 99.9 percent shared identity in DNA between two randomly selected individuals in the world population, but to the power of the remaining 0.1 percent, upon which sit several million points of difference.

Second, genetic distinctions among humans predict with near absolute accuracy conventional racial and ethnic categories (for a minority objection, see Hunley, Healy, and Long 2009). Noah Rosenberg and Jonathan Pritchard used "375 polymorphisms called short tandem repeats" in a highly diverse sample of one thousand persons. They could then distinguish five groups: "sub-Saharan Africans; Europeans and Asians west of the Himalayas; East Asians; inhabitants of Guinea and Melanesia; and Native Americans" (cited by Bamshad and Olson 2003; see Edwards 2003). They could also identify ethnicity within these larger groups. Nei and Roychoudhury (1993) also identified five major human groups by the common clades (their ancestors in evolutionary branches) of each: sub-Saharan Africans, Caucasians, Greater Asians, Australopapuans and Amerindians. Tang et al (2005) compared genetic markers with self-reported race and ethnicity, and using cluster analysis of the markers, found an 0.14 percent error rate among 3,636 respondents. These findings, largely on genetic sequences not related to skin color or other "superficial" traits, led to the conclusion that "populations do, generally, cluster by broad geographic regions that correspond with common racial classification (Africa, Europe, Asia, Oceania, Americas)" and that such categories correspond to self-identification and "continental ancestry" (Tishkoff and Kidd 2004, quoted by Wade 2004). Yang et al (2005) used "ancestry informative markers" through allele frequency differences (alleles being alternative forms of a gene) to identify admixture groups like African Americans, Mexicans, Mexican Americans, and Puerto Ricans. These corresponded with self-identified ethnicity at probability levels exceeding 99 percent.

Given the linkage between genetic predisposition to certain diseases found in races and ethnic groups, scientists point to the capacity of racial classification to raise the efficiency of estimating disease susceptibility among different individuals. Until the specific human sequence variation for individuals is available, ethnic and racial information provides useful information. Objecting strongly to medical literature that claimed there was no biological basis for race, Risch argued not only that there was such evidence but that, until we have a sequenced genome for each person, race and ethnicity remained indispensable to medical research and diagnosis (Risch et al 2002; Burchard et al 2003).

As a result, more scientists use the term *race* (e.g., *Science* 2008), a shift reflected in biology textbooks (Morning 2008). In doing so, they adhere to the concept of a *subspecies* in biology, a term they perhaps fear employing more than *race* (on the equivalence in terminology, and a denial that human subspecies exist, see the government Human Genome Project 2010). While there are arguments over what constitutes a subspecies, the general rule is that it is a group that is genetically isolated (usually geographically isolated so that interbreeding is rare; in human societies, stiff rules for endogamy can have the same effect as geographic distance) for long enough to present identifiable distinctions (such as spots or courtship behavior). Nonetheless, its members can and will mate successfully with those of other subspecies when the opportunity arises. Animal subspecies are not necessarily easier to identify, morphologically speaking, than human races (Sarich and Miele 2004). Moreover, *Homo sapiens* have greater diversity between groups than certain animals for whom subspecies are regularly employed. There is less genetic difference between *species* of the Canis genus, for example, than between "ethnic groups among human beings" (Serpell 1995). Such findings have led even some social scientists to agree that races are "genetic entities" due to differences in allele frequencies after "generations of reproductive isolation" (Van den Oord and Rowe 2000, 286).

But, as the response to this article proved, the primary reaction to racial categorization has been hesitant (Frank 2001). The growing number of evolutionary biologists who think race and ethnicity have a genetic component are cautious to ascribe deep import to the distinctions they discover, seeing them as minor variations on a largely common template, creating largely inconsequential traits. Highly esteemed scientists such as Luigi Luca Cavalli-Sforza (2000) object to any racial categorization or, rather, argue that it is futile. Cavalli-Sforza agrees that population isolation in human history led to genetic distance between human groups; indeed, such differences revealed the ancient migrations and settlements in our prehistory that Cavalli-Sforza enabled us to explore. Moreover, they often correlate well with linguistic and dialectical differences (Cavalli-Sforza 2004). He accepts that "races" exist, but points out that, were we to be so persnickety, we could define Florentines and Pisanos as different races (which, one guesses, each city's citizens have done). Using Cavalli-Sforza's methods, we could find genetic distance between them – the choice of where to draw the line makes any real definition pointless. Cavalli-Sforza, like many scientists, conceives of distinctions as occurring on a cline of gradual almost imperceptible change in allele frequencies across distance (for a recent confirmation, see Serre and Pääbo 2004). Similar views – accepting the genetic distinctions, but finding them largely unimportant – characterize the approach of many evolutionary biologists. Richard Dawkins's recent treatment of race speaks to the current, uneasy truce (2004). Differences exist, but drawing boundaries depends largely on cultural or social choices.

Still, a minority of evolutionary scientists see racial boundaries as both essential and crucial, signally striking differences in intelligence, sexual behavior, and even moral character. Geographical isolation and endogamy created divisions among humankind. *Homo sapiens* appeared perhaps 200,000 years ago, and the separation of Africans and non-Africans in the migration from that continent occurred less than 80,000 years ago, so these scholars tend to assert that fundamental evolutionary change can occur at relatively short temporal intervals. Physical and behavioral changes in foxes bred for dog-like qualities suggest rapid evolutionary cycles are possible in mammals (Jazin et al 2005). Among human beings, the rise of lactose tolerance in northern European and herding regions in Africa signaled a marked adaptation within less than 5,000 years, raising the possibility that geographically and culturally separate groups could evolve differently (Bersaglieri et al 2004; Tishkoff et al 2007). Similar short cycle evidence of positive selection can be seen in sickle-cell and other allele frequency shifts in response to malaria and in the pigmentation changes concordant with degrees of sunlight and warmth. While the promise of single gene markers has been largely unfulfilled, the known location of the genetic source for obsessive-compulsive disorder in dogs implies a world of possibility for why dogs, and people, act like they do. Research on genetic predisposition to alcoholism reports linkages to certain ethnicities with higher levels of alcoholism, implying a genetic basis for a social, and historically important, behavior (Edenberg et al 2006). Similar linkages show recent selection pressure differences in regulation of neural genes linked to receptivity to endogenous opiods that regulate perception, behavior, and memory (Rockman et al 2005).

Such findings have led to much more speculative exercises, such as the argument that prejudicial treatment in Eastern Europe resulted in adaptations that explain the high average levels of intelligence among Ashkenazi Jews (MacDonald 1994; Cochran and Harpending 2009). In still more extreme cases, proponents of a new, fully fledged racialized genetic theory propose distinctions in intelligence, morality, and sexual and family behavior (Levin 1997; Rushton 1980, 1995, 2005, 2010; Sarich and Miele 2004). Few mainstream evolutionary scientists agree with these propositions, and those who might entertain them clearly fear the effect on their reputations (Holloway 2008). Yet it is clear that most concur that race and ethnicity have biological markers and that behavioral distinctions they might create will once again be considered in evolutionary science.

Evolutionary Psychology

Social constructivists, inspired in part by antagonism to eugenicists' belief that race was essential and determinative, assert that races and ethnic groups are products of human invention. For sociologists, historians, and psychologists, racial traits were not primordial but instrumental, contingent, and dependent on hierarchies of power (an excellent summary of this position can be found in the 1998 statement on race by the American Anthropological Association). Indeed, for the majority, race and ethnicity are largely modern devices invented by the Nation State and its elites in order to gain power, and taken to extremes by Western imperialists. Ethnic conflict is, they argue, neither endemic in human cultures (many of which, they assert, exhibit cooperation and lack of prejudice) nor is it eternal (having risen primarily with the European Nation State). In large part, the history of race is a history of a Western European idea.

Among the new evolutionary fields, the most crucial to transhumanism is evolutionary psychology, and it sets itself in diametric opposition to this social constructivist view (for a straightforward summary and bibliography, see Cosmides and Tooby 1997; see also Buss 2005; Durrant and Ellis 2003; Pinker 2002). Ironically, the field begins by agreeing that there are no essential racial or ethnic *differences*. All human beings share in the "psychological unity of humankind," all read the same script scrawled on the Stone Age tablet. Yet nothing about racism and ethnocentrism is unnatural, invented, or the product of a particular, and particularly venomous, culture. They argue, in short, that although race and ethnicity are invented, racism and ethnocentrism are real. Evolutionary psychologists argue that much of the behavior of all human beings is laid out in the genetic blueprint we inherit from early *homo sapiens* hunter-gatherer groups who wandered the African savannah 100,000 years ago. We all possess an inbred tendency toward racism and ethnocentrism; we stand on a genetic foundation that prompts quick and violent expression of ethnic and racial convictions. One might rephrase Leda Cosmides and John Tooby and say we share in the "psychotic unity of humankind." Evolutionary psychologists see us as hunter-gatherers still. Our need to protect or seize resources, to engage in "coalitionary strategies," implies that our capacity to categorize in-groups and out-groups has been imprinted in a common psychology. The "computational counterpart to the human genome" governs our tendency to demonize the other, and our weakness in resisting that urge: "Because we are unaware we are in a theater, with our roles and our lines largely written for us by our mental programs, we are credulously swept up in these plays (such as the genocidal drama of us versus them" (Tooby and Cosmides 2009, 70). They concur in an opinion advanced by other social scientists, that "ethnocentrism is a universal syndrome" (Shaw and Wong 1989, 44).

This primordialism places evolutionary psychologists in stark opposition, however, to the dominant view among social scientists, especially among those studying ethnic conflict, who see ethnicity and ethnocentrism as instrumental, ephemeral traits, culturally created for specific strategic purposes (as a leading example, see Laitin 2007). Opposing the apotheosis of culture in archeology, Taylor finds that all the evidence points to common and violent behavior. All cultures "have ways of being that are … lethally enforced at a local level. … Out groups (whether a different ethnicity, class, sexuality, creed, whether being one of twins, an albino, someone disabled, or an unusually talented individual) are suspect and challenging in their abnormality. Categories of special difference are typical foci for sacrifice, banishment, and ridicule" (Taylor 2009). The evidence for the primordial nature of conflict based in ethnic or racial distinctions is drawn from three sources linked to the Pleistocene era in which modern humans first emerged: (1) ethological studies of primates with whom we share much of our lineage and which, presumably, operate like hunter-gatherer societies; (2) anthrohistorical studies of a fairly numerous set of previous human hunter-gatherer groups and of the few still surviving and possibly not culturally contaminated; and (3) slim evidence based on experimental studies of contemporary human beings. The last is the deficiency most often noted in critiques of evolutionary psychology.

Observations of other primates provide considerable evidence for the innate character of group violence, particularly among chimpanzees, with whom we share nearly all our DNA. Franz de Waal, the most prominent evolutionary ethnologist, discards the euphemistic "coalition strategy" for male chimpanzee group behavior, preferring to describe it as "coalitionary killing" (de Waal 2005). Field evidence reveals not simply conflict between groups but actions that would be considered genocidal in the human context. De Waal and other leading students of primate behavior have no compunction in linking chimpanzee violence and human warfare and genocide (de Waal 2005; Wade 2004), and this has led some to argue that they also form ethnic allegiances: "like humans, they are highly ethnocentric-cum-xenophobic" (van der Dennen 2004). If we assume that the common ancestor of people and chimps had chimp-like social traits, there is reason to believe that humans harbor strong inclinations toward "male kin bonding and lethal territorial aggression." De Waal cites anthropological evidence to show concordance between chimpanzee and human behavior, using anthropological studies of the small number of hunter-gatherer groups still extant. He reports that the Yanomamo tribe endures a 30 percent male death rate from aggression, a rate equal to that among Gombe chimps (2005), and findings of male-led conflict and death are repeatedly reported for other hunter-gatherer societies (Bowles 2006; Gat 2009). De Waal is at pains to argue that we also share tendencies toward empathy with our primate cousins (2005, 2006) – the bonoboos featured especially in these claims – but even empathy is linked to the murderous group inclination itself. He is not romantic about the capacity of culture to change behavior. He despairs that captive chimps are "just as xenophobic as those in the wild." His and other primatologists' research also indicates that those who know each other and got along might then form other coalitions and attack their former friends. For de Waal, this suggests an evolutionary basis to social constructions, explaining how among Hutus and Tutsis and Serbs and Muslims, "ethnic groups that used to get along reasonably well may all of a sudden turn against each other" (2005, 135).

Mark Schaller has been especially prominent in providing experimental results for innate tendencies toward racism and ethnocentrism: "[C]ertain prejudicial ways of thinking and acting may have conferred adaptive benefits within ancestral environments, and now – even though contemporary environments are very different in very many ways – those prejudicial ways of thinking and acting may persist" (Schaller, Park, and Faulkner 2003, 111). Schaller bridges the divide between the African savannah and his campus in Vancouver by asserting that the "reciprocal relations between cognition and culture" mean that cognitive mechanisms both encourage and are encouraged by "cultural norms." Racial and ethnic identifications, linked to the deeply coded traits of all human beings, make xenophobia and racism not simply common but genetically predetermined. The regular experimental results by other researchers showing that very young children – indeed, infants – quickly apply in- and out-group racial and ethnic categories reinforce this reading (Castelli, De Amicis, and Sherman 2007; Bloom 2010), as does a potential biological component for this tendency toward racial categorization (Santos, Meyer-Lindenberg, and Deruelle 2010). Schaller and his colleagues trace these traits not to coalition building but to disease avoidance (Faulkner et al 2004) – one fascinating finding in this research is that xenophobia based on fear of disease is not present when foreigners come from a familiar immigrant group.

Still, these various findings pertain to intimate interpersonal relations between individuals or within small bands. Few successfully elaborate the process by which Pleistocene hunter-gatherer conflicts (involving about 150 members in each clan if equivalent in number to the few remaining hunter-gatherer societies and to the larger chimpanzee communities) became ethnic and racial conflicts encompassing millions of persons. As central evolutionary texts demonstrate, inclusive fitness and reciprocity theory indicate how members of very small groups have mutual interests, the first by broadening the calculable fitness of a gene from the individual to more distant members of a family, who carry some portion of it, and the second by placing altruism between unrelated persons within a similarly rational fitness strategy. One of the most innovative contributors to evolutionary theory on such altruistic cooperation, Robert Axelrod (Axelrod and Hamilton 1981), uses game-theory simulations to argue that the roots of ethnocentrism lie in evolutionary predispositions to favor in-groups (Hammond and Axelrod 2006). While altruistic acts based in inclusive fitness and reciprocity are adaptive only at the familial or small-group level, they are powerful enough in larger societies to trigger costly allegiance to ethnic groups, leading to cooperation and ethnocentrism outside the realm of selection. Thus, as others remark, conflict and hostility are the other side of cooperation and altruism.

Axelrod is attentive to the Hamiltonian view that group selection cannot occur, but others, such as Peter Richerson and Robert Boyd (2001), contend with the problem of the expanding scale of coalition, from hunter-gatherer band to village to tribe to nation, by turning to group selection, which proposes there can be evolutionary advantages to larger coalitions (for the most recent effort to assert this possibility, see Wilson and Wilson 2007). In these, even sacrificial altruists might not only survive but prosper and raise the average fitness of the group in contrast to other clans or groups. The appeal of group selection can be seen at the dawn of evolutionary theory. Charles Darwin noted that "a tribe including many members who, from possessing in a high degree the spirit of patriotism, fidelity, obedience, courage, and sympathy, were always ready to aid one another, and to sacrifice themselves for the common good, would be victorious over most other tribes; and this would be natural selection" (quoted in Richerson and Boyd 2001, 192). For Richerson and Boyd, group selection becomes an odd argument for the joint evolution of genes and culture, with "social selection against genotypes that are ill adapted to cultural institutions" (196). As in most accounts that make the leap from inclusive fitness to altruism, reciprocity and coalitions on a huge scale, the point of departure deserves scrutiny: "Evolutionary theory predicts that altruism should be stronger within ethnic groups than between them" (Salter 2004, 6). So also Samuel Bowles contends that what he calls "parochial altruism" – that is, which extends to ethnic or racial groups beyond those served by inclusive fitness or reciprocity – could be evolutionarily successful, using simulated evolutionary histories for groups as well as estimates of genetic variation and conflict in the archeological and anthropological record for hunter-gatherer groups. Like others, he sees this broader group selection (leading to the extinction of less altruistic competing communities) as the source of the murderous conflict he identifies as a fixed part of human relation with human. While Bowles believes cultural evolution has a role as well, he chains "modern nationalism" to what he observes in "ancestral humans" (Bowles 2006, 2008; Choi and Bowles 2007).

In contrast, Shaw and Wong (1989), more attentive to the standard rejection of group selection, base their argument on kin selection and inclusive fitness: "tight-knit kin groups" or "nucleus ethnic groups" expand (somehow) to generalized "phenotypic matching" (38-39). Essentially, ethnic group members are fooled into thinking that a largely unrelated person with the same phenotype is family. In a similar take, Salter (2004), who misuses the magisterial Horowitz (2000) to argue that ethnicity is built on family resemblance, tries a wide inclusive fitness line to create ethnicity, finding that "it might be adaptive for an individual to make sacrifices for a large number of co-ethnics" (6). In early attempts to understand ethnicity (and violence), Daly and Wilson (1988) and van den Berghe (1981) stressed the resemblance of family ties to ethnic ties and the biological connectedness of both family and ethnic group members (cf. Rushton 2005 and Salter 2003, for estimates of the cousin-like attachment of random pairs of ethnic group members). Van den Berghe observes that the attachments individuals make to ethnic groups are similar to those they make to family members and are, therefore, likely to have a common base. As familial features become part of the myth of ethnic group, actual relatedness becomes less relevant and, genetic proximity no longer holds and cannot explain ethnic attachments and the cooperative ties of ethnic group members. So, ethnocentrism appeals to sentiments that have an evolutionary basis in much smaller groups; in larger ones, while less effective, it can function if the ethnicity has a credible descent group (van den Berghe 1981).

David Goetze has ethnicity both ways, primordial and instrumental, arguing that "high kinship values make group attachments intense and durable, while high functional values tend to make assertions of ethnic identity responsive to the resource opportunities of the moment" (1998, 60). In this stance, he mirrors a very recent argument by the political scientist Henry E. Hale (2008), who accepts a genetic basis for group behavior and misbehavior but finds that self-interest and material gain are necessary for mass ethnocentric action. For Goetze, a group-selection principle appears in that groups which created intense ethnic attachment may have been more reproductively successful than those who relied on other methods, like paying Hessians to fight for them.

Robert Kurzaban, John Tooby, and Leda Cosmides have taken up the perilous question of race and propose a neat device for removing race from the equation. They point out that our ancestors, the hunter-gatherers, would rarely, if ever, have "encountered a person of a different race, so natural selection could not have favored brain mechanisms designed to notice and remember a non-existent dimension of ancestral social life" (2001, 15387). Instead, these ancestors developed a skill we possess, that of detecting coalitions. They would have profited from "being equipped with neurocognitive machinery that tracked these shifting alliances" (ibid.). As many social psychologists point out, visual cues that allow discrimination among people are highly useful, so in this scenario, color is just a very useful datum for the mental machinery seeking cues. It can, therefore, be got rid of.

Transhumanism

Although transhumanism borrows much of its spirit from new evolutionary science, it has little to say about race and ethnicity, except to declare stridently that the movement is "antiracist." A search of writings by leading figures, like Nick Bostrom, uncovers few references to race or ethnicity – indeed, the fiercest attacks on transhumanism rarely mention racial implications (see Wolfe 2009;

Graham 2002; Badmington 2004; Dinello 2005). Attentive to evolutionary biology, transhumanists know that racial differences can be traced to genetic differences and almost never argue for the social construction of race (for an exception, see Overall 2009). Still, they appear content with the majority view that these genetic distinctions are small and inconsequential and do not mention the growing uncertainty in the field over the meaning of race.

Where transhumanists speak about these subjects, the text is formulaic, employing the mildly Left rhetoric characteristic of their public statements. Bostrom's "Table of Transhumanist Values" lists among the movement's necessary virtues that of "[d]iversity (species, races, religious creeds, sexual orientations, life styles, etc.)" and, as is common in other manifestos, declares that "[r]acism, sexism, speciesism, belligerent nationalism and religious intolerance are unacceptable" (2005b). H+ or humanity+ (formerly, the World Transhumanist Association) declares that "Racism in all forms, including specieist human-racism, must be opposed" (Humanity+ 2010; World Transhumanist Association 2008). The Transhumanist Association openly condemned racism in 2002, as incompatible to its humanist and tolerant roots. Bostrom pointed out that persons with "nonstandard lifestyles," including the disabled, homosexuals, and, one presumes, racially marginalized persons, are a lot like transhumanists and should be brought into the fold. The THA web page profiles a section on transhumanism and people of color (Center for Genetics and Society 2010). The party line is repeated at other major transhumanist centers, such as Extropy! (2005): "The philosophy of extropy is fundamentally opposed to any form of racism or other judgment of individuals based on similar specious groupings." Uneasiness with social constructivist rather than scientific views on race follows in that their position is not based on "[a]ny kind of post-modernist 'politically correct' cultural relativism," but on the arrival of rational human civilization with the "18th century Enlightenment."

Why are transhumanists stridently antiracist, given their debt to eugenics and their close reading of the new evolutionary sciences? On the surface, they present themselves as supremely confident of the rule of law and the ascendancy, and correctness, of antiracist views in the liberal, democratic regimes in which they live (Bostrom 2005a; see Agar 2007). They appear convinced that these civic rules will spread across the world (Bailey 2005). Anders Sandberg (2010) expresses this conceit neatly, showing how the ideal transhumanist society would, among its merits, oppose racism: a "modern western liberal democratic welfare state, with a commitment to equalization of opportunity through voluntary treatments and a certain level of income redistribution, basic guaranteed minimal income and medical treatments and culturally dominated by ideas of tolerance, cooperation and the rights of minorities."

Aside from these sentiments, transhumanist reticence about the meaning of race and regular rejections of racism reflect a strategic response to a historical problem. One of the chief tasks of those who wish to advance transhumanism is to reject any connection with its infamous grandfather, eugenics. Leading transhumanists exert considerable energy in explaining why eugenics, which sought state control over the reproduction of less-gifted human beings, cannot be equated with transhumanism, which seeks the individual's right to control his or her replication. Bostrom, for example, states that "it would be ethically unacceptable, as well as potentially very dangerous, to have the state impose a one-size-fits-all formula on what kind of people should exist in the next generation," even as he accepts the marginally limited rights, even duty, of parents to improve the genetic characteristics of their children. In the same interview, David Pearce strongly seconds his views (Lomeña 2007). Nicholas Agar (2004) describes this twist as "liberal eugenics"; transhumanists regularly trace their ancestry not to evolutionary science but to the Enlightenment and to Renaissance humanism, to individual rights and to a pluralistic conception of human improvement (Sandberg 2010). As Agar argues, "an evil doctrine" is thus made into a "morally acceptable one" (2004, 135). Extropians clearly recognize the strategic issue: opposing racism is essential because the "transhumanist agenda" is "sometimes confused in public discourse with primitive notions of racialist eugenics." Much of the liberal, "antifascist," antiracist stance of the transhumanists stems from a strategy, best expressed by James Hughes in the essay "The Politics of Transhumanism" (2002). In this paper, Hughes attacks "Eugenicus," who had claimed the mantle of transhumanism but also approved of evolutionary scientists like J. Phillipe Rushton who link intelligence to race (Grubach 2000). In his argument, Hughes is at pains to emphasize the "public relations disaster that could result if Nazism was associated with transhumanism."

But ultimately, transhumanist antiracism represents a strategy for the future. Transhumanists regularly attack the "human-racists" or "human racist bio-conservatives" who criticize their agenda. In the list of evilisms, the new entry *speciesism* betrays their belief that the posthuman will be not only racially distinct but species distinct. Given their belief that they will be a superior race (not just an artificially different category) or a truly different (and superior) species, opposition to such a transformation must be labeled as racist or speciest (Savulescu 2009a). Bostrom signals this need to oppose racism because of the utility of a nonracist ideology: "In order to prepare for a time when the human species may start branching out in various directions, we need to start now to strongly encourage the development of moral sentiments that are broad enough [*sic* to] encompass within the sphere of moral concern sentiences that are constituted differently from ourselves" (2005b).

In a recent piece on "Beyond the Human Race – and 'Human-Racism'," Hughes expands the attack by promoting a still broader tolerance. Revealing an understanding of recent evolutionary science, he argues that our genetic commonality with other primates and even with Neanderthals proves the fallacy of the demand that we defend the purity of the human type (2010). Since, according to Hughes, "apes ... use language, transmit culture, and understand abstract ideas like death and morality," they are much like us and should possess rights. Hughes argues that human morality could encompass "gorillas, cyborgs and mutants." David Pearce (2007) calls for the abolition of all suffering in all species (partly through abstaining from meat eating, partly through rewriting of the genome). He decries the fact that our "our anthropocentric bias is deeply rooted."

Deep tolerance appears unlikely in the genocidal scenario envisioned by the critics of transhumanism. Using the *Gattaca* critique, named after a film that featured the clash of ordinary man with a genetically enhanced group, Francis Fukuyama expresses the fear that "[i]f we start transforming ourselves into something superior, what rights will these enhanced creatures claim, and what rights will they possess when compared to those left behind?" (2004). George Annas and colleagues carry this anxiety out to its logical possibility: "The posthuman will come to see us (the garden variety human) as an inferior subspecies without human rights to be enslaved or slaughtered preemptively. It is this potential for genocide based on genetic difference, that I have termed 'genetic genocide,' that makes species-altering genetic engineering a potential weapon of mass destruction" (Annas 2001; Annas, Andrews, and Isai 2002). Agar, contemplating the transhumanist belief that the posthuman might be a species apart, considers how its repulsion for ordinary men and women might be "much more profound than that resulting from the racist thinking to which humans seem susceptible" (2007, 13).

Most transhumanists calmly dismiss these doomsday predictions. Bostrom (2005a) and Ronald Bailey (2005) take comfort in their favored liberal democratic regimes and the laws these regimes maintain. Bostrom does not shrink from the challenge that more privileged persons might eventually enhance "themselves and their offspring to a point where the human species, for many practical purposes, splits into two or more species" (2003). He justifies species differentiation first on the fact that inequality is not always a bad thing and may bring benefits not only to posthumans but to the lower orders. Second, he suggests that "social policies" can provide others access to genetic benefits and otherwise placate them. Third, he moves toward a position much closer to eugenics than usual in transhumanist prose: "we might as well make some enhancements obligatory for children ... requiring genetic enhancements for everybody to the same degree." Hughes (2004) has taken the potential for conflict most seriously, committing considerable effort to devices that might contain disputes between humans and posthumans. He describes a "democratic transhumanism," in which subsidies and other programs could ameliorate stark distinctions.

The optimistic take on what might happen if a superior race or distinct species arose sits uncomfortably with transhumanists' straightforward agreement with evolutionary social psychology: ethnocentrism is resident in the human psyche. Indeed, they see the propensity to form violent coalitions as one of the vile human characteristics they seek to transcend. Savulescu critiques the end result of evolution: "limited altruism, limited co-operative instincts" and the possibility of "annihilation by our own design," making our basic psychology corrupt and limited (2009b). In his *A Darwinian Left: Politics, Evolution, and Cooperation* (2000), the controversial and renowned philosopher Peter Singer also underlines the biological tendency toward selfishness and hierarchy. In order to achieve the conventionally leftist moral positions he has staked out (e.g., redistribution of wealth), that nature must be undone. Like the transhumanists, he advocates the exploitation of genetic science to reshape human nature, reducing conflict and increasing cooperation. Pearce carries this argument to celestial heights. It is true that humans are racist, ethnocentric, and violent, but the posthuman might become "saints and angels … with a richer capacity for empathetic understanding of other sentient beings" (Lomeña 2007). Despite a rich understanding, and dislike for what makes the human tick, transhumanists condemn prejudice against nonconsequential racial distinctions but are eerily sanguine about the consequences of the powerfully consequential ones they hope to achieve.

Conclusion

Evolutionary scientists remain uncertain about the meaning of race and ethnicity, but the pendulum now swings inexorably from nurture toward nature. Among evolutionary biologists, it is becoming impossible to claim that race and ethnicity do not exist as genetic entities, though what consequences such differences have remain undetermined. Transhumanism adopts the older position on the pendulum, ignoring the most recent findings. Their antiracist line, though not social constructivist, fits well with their liberal sentiments. But most important, it fits their need to deflect attention from their connection to the racist agenda in eugenics and their hope to defuse objections that the future might feature clashes between the human and the posthuman.

How deep the opposition to racial thinking lies within the transhumanist ideology is anyone's guess. Given their commitment to new evolutionary theory and technique, they must be aware of the shifting ground on what race is and what it means for human behavior. An occasional reference suggests that they may not be as resistant to racial distinctions as they proclaim. H+ does attack eugenics, but in part because that approach works too slowly. Should evolutionary biology discover deep racial and ethnic differences in substantive traits such as intelligence, transhumanists might seek to advance toward the posthuman through the best of the human races and avoid the lesser types. In this case, the DNA of eugenics embedded in the movement is likely to reemerge. As Michael White's essay in this volume suggests, distinctions among human beings may be seized on by those intent on building a better person (Agar 2004 considers racial characteristics in this light). Still, this is speculation, and the current record on race among transhumanists is, while thin, conventionally opposed to racial prejudices.

What they have expressed most clearly is their belief that, in the future, should their efforts be successful, there will be distinct races, perhaps even different species of humankind. By their very nature, these new groups will have consequential genetic differences, making one group vastly superior in intelligence, longevity, and even character. One aspect of the ordinary human that transhumanists intend to eradicate comes from their understanding of evolutionary social psychology: an innate tendency toward ethnocentric views about others. They find deplorable the harm caused by unimportant markers, by those who falsely think themselves superior. Yet they believe no harm will result when there are beings who rightly think of themselves as being a higher order of humanity.

References

Agar, Nicholas. 2004. *Liberal Eugenics: In Defence of Human Enhancement.* Oxford: Blackwell.

–. 2007. Whereto transhumanism? The literature reaches a critical mass. *Hastings Center Report* 37 (3): 12-17.

American Anthropological Association. 1998. Statement on race: http://www.aaanet.org/stmts/racepp.htm, accessed July 13, 2011.

Annas, George J. 2001. Genism, racism, and the prospect of genetic genocide. Paper for the World Conference against Racism, Durban, South Africa: http://www.gjga.org/conference.asp?action=item&source=documents&id=19, accessed July 13, 2011.

Annas, George J., Lori B. Andrews, and Rosario M. Isai. 2002. Protecting the endangered human: Toward an international treaty prohibiting cloning and inheritable alterations. *American Journal of Law and Medicine* 28 (2-3): 151-78.

Axelrod, Robert, and William D. Hamilton. 1981. The evolution of cooperation. *Science*, n.s. 211(4489): 1390-96.

Badmington, Neil. 2004. *Alien Chic: Posthumanism and the Other Within.* New York: Routledge.

Bailey, Ronald. 2005. *Liberation Biology: The Scientific and Moral Case for Biotech Revolution*. Ann Arbor: University of Michigan Press.

Bamshad, Michael J., and Steve E. Olson. 2003. Does race exist? *Scientific American* 289 (6): 78-85.

Barkan, Elazar. 1992. *The Retreat of Scientific Racism: Changing Concepts of Race in Britain and the United States between the World Wars*. Cambridge: Cambridge University Press.

Bersaglieri, Todd, et al. 2004. Genetic signatures of strong recent positive selection at the lactose gene. *The American Journal of Human Genetics* 74 (6): 1111-20.

Bloom, Paul. 2010. The moral life of babies. *New York Times Magazine*, May 9, MM44: http://www.nytimes.com/2010/05/09/magazine/09babies-t.html?ref=magazine, accessed July 13, 2011.

Bostrom, Nick. 2003. Human genetic enhancements: A transhumanist perspective. *Journal of Value Inquiry* 37 (4): 493-506: http://www.nickbostrom.com/ethics/genetic.html, accessed July 13,2011.

–. 2005a. In defense of posthuman dignity. *Bioethics* 19 (3), June: 202-14.

–. 2005b. Transhumanist values. *Review of Contemporary Philosophy* 4 (1-2): 87-101: http://www.nickbostrom.com/ethics/values.html, accessed July 13, 2011.

Bowles, Samuel. 2006. Evolution of human altruism: Group competition, reproductive leveling, and the evolution of human altruism. *Science* 314 (5805): 1569-72.

–. 2008. Being human: Conflict: Altruism's midwife. *Nature* 456 (7220), November 20: 326-27.

Burchard, Esteban G., et al. 2003. The importance of race and ethnic background in biomedical research and clinical practice. *The New England Journal of Medicine* 348 (12): 1170-75.

Buss, David M. 2005. *The Murderer Next Door: Why the Mind Is Designed to Kill*. New York: Penguin Group.

Castelli, Luigi, Leyla De Amicis, and Steven J. Sherman. 2007. The loyal member effect: On the preference for ingroup members who engage in exclusive relations with the ingroup. *Developmental Psychology* 43 (6): 1347-59.

Cavalli-Sforza, Luigi L. 2000. *Genes, Peoples, and Languages* New York: North Point Press.

–. 2004. A scientific adventure: A fifty years' study of human evolution. In *The Evolution of Population Biology*, edited by R. S. Singh and M. K. Uyenoyama. Cambridge: Cambridge University Press.

Center for Genetics and Society. 2010. About race and human biotechnology: www.geneticsandsociety.org/article.php?list=type&type=105, accessed July 13, 2011.

Choi, Jung-Kyoo, and Samuel Bowles. 2007. The coevolution of parochial altruism and war. *Science* 318 (5850): 636-40.

Cochran, Gregory, and Henry Harpending. 2009. *The 10,000-Year Explosion: How Civilization Accelerated Human Evolution*. New York: Basic Books.

Cosmides, Leda, and John Tooby. 1997. Evolutionary psychology: A primer: http://www.psych.ucsb.edu/research/cep/primer.html, accessed July 13, 2011.

Daly, Martin, and Margo Wilson. 1988. Evolutionary social psychology and family homicide. *Science* 242: 519-24. (See *Science* (1989) 243: 462-64 for ensuing debate.)

Dawkins, Richard. 2004. *The Ancestor's Tale: A Pilgrimage to the Dawn of Evolution.* New York: Houghton Mifflin Co.

–. 2006. *The Selfish Gene*, 30th Anniversary Edition. Oxford: Oxford University Press.

De Waal, Frans B. M. 2005. *Our Inner Ape: A Leading Primatologist Explains Why We Are Who We Are*. New York: Penguin.

–. 2006. *Primates and Philosophers: How Morality Evolved.* Edited by S. Macedo and J. Ober. Princeton, NJ: Princeton University Press.

Dinello, Daniel. 2005. *Technophobia! Science Fiction Visions of Posthuman Technology*. Austin: University of Texas Press.

Durrant, Russell, and Bruce J. Ellis. 2003. Evolutionary psychology. In *Comprehensive Handbook of Psychology, Volume Three: Biological Psychology*, edited by M. Gallagher and R. J. Nelson, 1-33. New York: Wiley and Sons.

Edenberg, Howard J. et al. 2006. Association of alcohol dehydrogenase genes with alcohol dependence: A comprehensive analysis. *Human Molecular Genetics* 15 (9): 1539-49.

Edwards, Anthony W. F. 2003. Human genetic diversity: Lewontin's fallacy. *BioEssays* 25 (8): 798-801.

Extropy. 2005. Transhumanist FAQs. *Extropy Institute*: www.extropy.org/faq.htm#5.9, accessed July 13, 2011.

Faulkner, Jason, et al. 2004. Evolved disease-avoidance mechanisms and contemporary xenophobic attitudes. *Group Processes & Intergroup Relations* 7 (4): 333-53.

Frank, Reanne. 2001. The misuse of biology in demographic research on racial/ethnic differences: A reply to van den Oord and Rowe. *Demography* 38 (4): 563-67.

Fukuyama, Francis. 2004. Transhumanism. *Foreign Policy* 144: 42-43.

Gat, Azar. 2009. So why do people fight? Evolutionary theory and the causes of war. *European Journal of International Relations* 15 (4): 571-99.

Goetze, David. 1998. Evolution, mobility, and ethnic group formation. *Politics and the Life Sciences* 17 (1): 59-71.

Gould, Stephen J. 1996. *The Mismeasure of Man*. 2d ed. New York: Norton.
Graham, Elaine L. 2002. *Representations of the Post/Human: Monsters, Aliens and Others in Popular Culture*. Manchester, UK: Manchester University Press.
Grubach, Paul. 2000. On the biological meaning of race: http://www.euvolution.com/articles/race03.html, accessed July 13, 2011.
Hale, Henry F. 2008. *The Foundations of Ethnic Politics: Separatism of States and Nations in Eurasia and the World*. Cambridge: Cambridge University Press.
Hamilton, William D. 1964. The genetical evolution of social behavior. *Journal of Theoretical Biology* 7 (1): 1-16.
Hammond, Ross A., and Robert Axelrod. 2006. The evolution of ethnocentrism. *Journal of Conflict Resolution* 50 (6): 926-36.
Holloway, Ralph L. 2008. The human brain evolving: A personal retrospective. *Annual Review of Anthropology* 37 (1): 1-19: http://www.columbia.edu/~rlh2/2008humanbrain.personalretro.pdf, accessed July 13, 2011.
Horowitz, Donald L. 2000. *Ethnic Groups in Conflict*. Berkeley: University of California Press.
Hughes, James H. 2002. The politics of transhumanism. Version 2.0. Originally Presented at the 2001 Annual Meeting of the Society for Social Studies of Science, Cambridge, MA: http://www.changesurfer.com/Acad/TranshumPolitics.htm, accessed July 13, 2011.
–. 2004. *Citizen Cyborg: Why Democratic Societies Must Respond to the Redesigned Human of the Future*. Cambridge, MA: Westview Press.
–. 2010. Beyond the human race – and "human-racism": http://ieet.org/index.php/IEET/more/hughes20100512/, accessed July 13, 2011.
Human Genome Project. 2010: http://www.aaanet.org/stmts/racepp.htm, accessed July 13, 2011.
Humanity+. 2010: http://humanityplus.org, accessed July 13, 2011.
Hunley, Keith L., Meghan E. Healy, and Jeffrey C. Long. 2009. The global pattern of gene identity variation reveals a history of long-range migrations, bottlenecks, and local mate exchange: Implications for biological race. *American Journal of Physical Anthropology* 139 (1): 35-46.
Jazin, Elena, et al. 2005. Selection for tameness has changed brain gene expression in silver foxes. *Current Biology* 15 (22): 915-16.
Jensen, Arthur R. 1969. How much can we boost IQ and scholastic achievement? *Harvard Educational Review* 39 (1): 1-123.
Kevles, Daniel J. 1985. *In the Name of Eugenics: Genetics and the Uses of Human Heredity*. New York: Knopf.
Kurzaban, Robert, John Tooby, and Leda Cosmides. 2001. Can race be erased? Coalitional computation and social categorization. *Proceedings of the National Academy of Sciences* 98 (26): 15387-92.

Laitin, David D. 2007. *Nations, States and Violence*. Oxford: Oxford University Press.

Levin, Michael E. 1997. *Why Race Matters: Race Differences and What They Mean*. Ann Arbor: University of Michigan Press.

Lewontin, Richard C. 1972. The apportionment of human diversity. *Evolutionary Biology* 6: 391-98.

Lomeña, Andrés. 2007. Interview with Nick Bostrom and David Pearce about transhumanism, originally in *Cronopis* 27 December: http://sexgenderbody.com/content/interview-nick-bostrom-and-david-pearce-about-transhumanism, accessed July 13, 2011.

Macdonald, Kevin. 1994. *A People That Shall Dwell Alone: Judaism as a Group Evolutionary Strategy*. New York: Praeger.

Maynard Smith, John. 1964. Group selection and kin selection. *Nature* 201: 1145.

Morning, Ann. 2008. Reconstructing race in science and society: Biology textbooks, 1952-2002. *American Journal of Sociology* 114 (1): 106-37.

Nei, Masatoshi, and Arun K. Roychoudhury. 1993. Evolutionary relationships of human populations on a global scale. *Molecular Biology and Evolution* 10: 927-43.

Overall, Christine. 2009. Life enhancement technologies: Significance of social category membership. In *Human Enhancement*, ed. Julian Savulescu and Nick Bostrom. Oxford: Oxford University Press.

Pearce, David. 2007. The abolitionist project: http://www.abolitionist.com/, accessed July 13, 2011.

Pinker, Steven. 2002. *The Blank Slate: The Modern Denial of Human Nature*. New York: Penguin Group.

Renfrew, Colin. 2010. Archaeogenetics – Toward a "New Synthesis". *Current Biology* 20 (4): 162-65.

Richerson, Peter J., and Robert Boyd. 2001. The evolution of subjective commitment to groups: A tribal instincts hypothesis. In *Evolution and the Capacity for Commitment*, ed. Randolph M. Nesse. New York: Russell Sage.

Risch, Neil, et al. 2002. Categorization of humans in biomedical research: Genes, race and disease. *Genome Biology* 3 (7): 1-12.

Rockman, Matthew, et al. 2005. Ancient and recent positive selection transformed Opioid *cis*-regulation in humans. *PLoS Biology* 3 (12): 2208-19: http://www.ncbi.nlm.nih.gov/pmc/articles/PMC1283535/pdf/pbio.0030387.pdf, accessed July 11, 2011.

Rushton, J. Phillipe. 1980. *Altruism, Socialization, and Society*. New York: Prentice Hall.

–. 1995. *Race, Evolution, and Behavior: A Life History*. Ann Arbor: University of Michigan Press.

–. 2005. Ethnic nationalism, evolutionary psychology, and genetic similarity theory. *Nations and Nationalism* 11 (4): 489-507.
–. 2010. Web page for race evolution and behavior: www.charlesdarwinresearch.org/reb.html, accessed July 13, 2011.
Salter, Frank K. 2003. *On Genetic Interests: Family, Ethnicity, and Humanity in an Age of Mass Migration*. New York: Peter Lang Publishing.
–. 2004. Introduction. In *Welfare, Ethnicity and Altruism: New Findings and Evolutionary Theory*, ed. Frank K. Salter. London: Frank Cass.
Sandberg, Anders. 2010. Humanism as a core value of transhumanism: http://www.tecnoumanisti.org/sandberg.htm, accessed July 13, 2011.
Santos, Andreia, Andreas Meyer-Lindenberg, and Christine Deruelle. 2010. Absence of racial, but not gender, stereotyping in Williams syndrome children. *Current Biology* 20 (7): R307–R308.
Sarich, Vincent, and Frank Miele. 2004. *Race: The Reality of Human Differences*. Boulder, CO: Westview Press.
Savulescu, Julian. 2009a. The human prejudice and the moral status of enhanced beings: What do we owe the gods. In *Human Enhancement*, ed. J. Savulescu and N. Bostrom. Oxford: Oxford University Press.
–. 2009b. Genetically advance humanity or face extinction. Video of presentation at Festival of Dangerous Ideas: http://www.humanityplus.org/read/tag/video/, accessed July 13, 2011.
Science. 2008. 322 (5903) November 7. Special issue on "Genetics of Behavior".
Schaller, Mark, Justin H. Park, and Jason Faulkner. 2003. Prehistoric dangers and contemporary prejudices. *European Review of Social Psychology* 14: 105-37.
Serpell, James, ed. 1995. *The Domestic Dog: Its Evolution, Behaviour and Interactions with People*. Cambridge: Cambridge University Press.
Serre, David, and Svante Pääbo. 2004. Evidence for gradients of human genetic diversity within and among continents. *Genome Research* 14: 1679-85: http://genome.cshlp.org/content/14/9/1679.abstract, accessed July 13, 2011.
Shaw, R. Paul, and Yuwa Wong. 1989. *Genetic Seeds of Warfare: Evolution, Nationalism, and Patriotism.* Winchester, MA: Unwin Hyman.
Singer, Peter. 2000. *A Darwinian Left: Politics, Evolution, and Cooperation*. New Haven, CT: Yale University Press.
Singh, Rama S., and Marcy K. Uyenoyama, eds. 2000. *The Evolution of Population Biology*. Cambridge: Cambridge University Press.
Tang, Hua, et al. 2005. Genetic structure, self-identified race/ethnicity, and confounding in case-control association studies. *American Journal of Human Genetics* 6 (2): 268-75.
Taylor, Timothy. 2009. Culture: http://www.edge.org/q2009/q09_1.html#taylor, accessed July 13, 2011.

Tishkoff Sarah A., and Kenneth K. Kidd. 2004. Biogeography of human populations: Implications for race and medicine. *Nature Genetics*, Supplement 1: S21-27.

Tishkoff, Sarah A., et al. 2007. Convergent adaptation of human lactase persistence in Africa and Europe. *Nature Genetics* 39 (1): 31-40.

Trivers, Robert L. 1971. The evolution of reciprocal altruism. *The Quarterly Review of Biology* 46 (1): 35-37.

Tooby, John, and Leda Cosmides. 2009. The great pivot: Artificial intelligences, native intelligences, and the bridge between: http://www.edge.org/q2009/q09_11.html#tooby, accessed July 13, 2011.

Van den Berghe, Pierre L. 1981. The Ethnic Phenomenon. Westport, CT: Elsevier.

Van Den Oord, Edwin J.C.G., and David C. Rowe. 2000. Racial differences in birth health risk: A quantitative genetic approach. *Demography* 37 (3): 285-98.

Van der Dennen, Johan M. G. 2004. Selfish co-operation, loyalty structures, and proto-ethnocentrism in inter-group agnostic behaviors. In *Welfare, Ethnicity and Altruism: New Findings and Evolutionary Theory*, ed. F. Salter, 195-231. London: Frank Cass.

Wade, Nicholas. 2004. Articles highlight different views on genetic basis of race. New York Times, October 27: http://www.freerepublic.com/focus/f-news/1259269/posts, accessed July 13, 2011.

Wilson, David S., and Edward O. Wilson. 2007. Rethinking the theoretical foundation of sociobiology. *The Quarterly Review of Biology* 82 (4): 327-48.

Wilson, Edward O. 1975. *Sociobiology: The New Synthesis*. Cambridge, MA: Harvard University Press.

Wolfe, Cary. 2009. *What is Posthumanism?* Minneapolis: University of Minnesota Press.

Wade, Nicholas. 2004. Articles highlight different views on genetic basis of race. *New York Times*, October 27: http://www.nytimes.com/2004/10/27/science/27race.html, accessed July 13, 2013.

World Transhumanist Association. 2008. Anti-racists: http://www.transhumanism.org/index.php/WTA/communities/antiracists/, accessed July 13, 2011.

Yang, Nan, et al. 2005. Examination of ancestry and ethnic affiliation using highly informative diallelic DNA markers: Application to diverse and admixed populations and implications for clinical epidemiology and forensic medicine. *Hum Genet* 118 (3-4): 382-92.

In Sickness and in Health: The (Fuzzy) Boundary between "Therapy" and "Enhancement"

Kenneth L. Mossman

Drugs and medical devices to improve performance and enhance the human condition are among the most exciting, intriguing, and important outcomes of emerging NBIC technologies (nanotechnology, biotechnology, information technology, and cognitive science). NBIC technologies have opened up all sorts of possibilities for enhancing our minds and our bodies. Are NBIC technologies the gateway to a posthuman world in which the very nature of being human is threatened? Inexpensive and readily accessible enhancement technologies might lead to transhumanism – a transition process from the present-day human to a more evolved posthuman characterized by improved physical and mental performance. With these possibilities, what does it mean to be human?

The unlimited possibilities of NBIC technologies has generated considerable debate about whether we should go forward to develop the full potential of these technologies or move at a much slower pace to anticipate and respond better to technological risks and threats. Major positions were framed in 2002 with the publication of Francis Fukuyama's *Our Posthuman Future* and Gregory Stock's *Redesigning Humans*. Social philosopher Fukuyama takes a decidedly bioconservative view and argues that biotechnology and the ability to manipulate our DNA threatens the human species and what it means to be human. Uncontrolled tinkering with the healthy brain could lead to a threat on the essence of being human. The result is that posthumanism is essentially the absence of humanism. From a social perspective, Fukuyama predicts that unchecked technologies will have profound effects on the foundations of liberal democracy because human beings are equal by nature, and not everyone may have equal access to the benefits of enhancement technologies. Gregory Stock, a biophysicist and biotech entrepreneur, is unabashedly a techno-optimist. He believes that redesigning humans is going to occur despite any government resistance or other efforts to ban technology. Technologies to transform humans are already here, and progress will be hard to stop. Enhancement technologies are a global pursuit because potential benefits are too great. Even if these technologies are banned in some countries, other nations will aggressively pursue research and development.

Other prominent futurists and philosophers have also weighed in. Technoutopians like Ray Kurzweil believe these emerging technologies will solve almost every social problem, including eliminating poverty and abolishing suffering

(Kurzweil 2005, e.g., 241, 259, 371-72). But others are not so enthusiastic and are concerned about potentially serious technological harms. Environmental ethicist Bill McKibben opposes further development of technologies partly because of worries about distributive justice (2003, 37-40). Others like philosopher Nick Bostrom (2002) recognize that commercial potential will be an unstoppable driver for technological development and will provide real benefits for the advancement of the human condition but warns that some of these technologies could pose existential risks.

Understanding the challenges of human enhancement has become an issue of growing importance in the national consciousness. What distinguishes current technologic enhancement from historical uses of natural enhancers (such as caffeine and tobacco) is the specificity of enhancement technologies and their greater effectiveness. One only need look at the ongoing national debate on anabolic steroid use in Major League Baseball or the alarming use of neuroenhancement drugs by students to appreciate the social impacts of enhancement technologies.

This chapter addresses a fundamental aspect of the enhancement technology debate – the fuzzy boundary between treatments and enhancements. Enhancement and treatment are at opposite poles of the medical–intervention spectrum. Prophylaxes, or medical interventions that reduce or eliminate disease risk, are somewhere in between. Where on the spectrum a particular intervention falls depends on medical status (i.e., how we define *normal*, *presence*, or *absence of disease*) and the goals of the intervention. *Therapy* is generally defined as the management of disease. In the curative sense, therapy is the return to normal structure and function. *Enhancement* is defined as the alteration of characteristics, traits, and abilities beyond what is considered to be normal. The distinctions between therapy and enhancement rely on notions of disease, normalcy, nature, and naturalness. There is no bright line that separates therapy from enhancement. What is enhancement for one may be therapy for another. Not surprisingly, enhancement technologies have emerged as a natural outgrowth of medical advances for the diagnosis and treatment of established diseases. Drugs such as Adderall and Ritalin are commonly used to manage attention deficit and related disorders but can also be used to enhance normal cognitive functioning. Because "therapy" and "enhancement" may be difficult to separate, the justification and acceptability of enhancement cannot be easily uncoupled from concepts of health and therapy. When the boundary between enhancement and therapy is unclear, as in many behavioral disorders, opportunities for enhancements expand.

This chapter also explores the real and potential social consequences of uncontrolled uses of emerging technologies for nonmedical purposes. The demand for cognitive-enhancing drugs, particularly among high school and college students, is already alarming and raises serious questions about individual harms and long-term social costs. Technologies that are inherently desirable and beneficial can get out of control. In the face of unbounded demand, can the distribution and uses of enhancement technologies be controlled? If not, can runaway technologies lead to a posthuman world? The risks of that are nearly impossible to assess because both the probability of creating a posthuman world and the consequences of a posthuman world are essentially unknown and may never be knowable. Nevertheless, transhumanism has generated serious discussion among philosophers and futurists like Bostrom, Fukuyama, and Kurzweil. Are we already developing technologies that will be the gateway to transhumanism and a posthuman world? If a posthuman world is in our future, what will it look like? How will we know if we are there?

Medical enhancement raises issues about our ability to shape human nature through technological advancements. The social demand for enhancement technologies raises serious questions about how enhancements are used and how they are distributed in society. What are the costs and benefits of enhancements? Will human enhancement help everyone or only those who can pay for it? If unregulated, will enhancement technologies result in the creation of new social classes defined by those that benefit from technology and those that do not?

Distinguishing Enhancement from Therapy

To this point, discussions of the enhancement-therapy distinction have focused primarily on the ethical dimensions of the problem. Bioethical arguments raise serious questions about implementation of enhancement technologies but fall short of providing a clear, practical distinction between enhancement and therapy. Part of the difficulty is that therapy and enhancement share several common goals including fulfilling human desires and easing suffering (Sandel 2004, 2009). Sandel attempts to draw a line between therapy and enhancement based on the view that enhancement represents a desire to master nature and that no such desire exists for treatment. Kamm (2005, 2009) argues that any moral distinction must be based on the claim that therapy has inherently positive attributes that enhancement lacks, assuming that those who would benefit from treatment are worse off than those who would benefit from enhancement; she also argues that Sandel does not adequately defend his distinction based on mastery of nature. Schwartz (2005) questions Kamm's assumption that people benefiting from treatment are worse off than those benefiting from enhancement. Whether bioethical arguments can influence public opinion depends on social demand and acceptability of the enhancement technology. Bioethical concerns are not likely to be important drivers if the social benefits of the technology are perceived to be greater than the risks, including economic costs. Further, laws to restrict or ban enhancements would be difficult to establish and enforce if society believes that such enhancements are ethical or advantageous, as Gary Marchant and Alexandra López argue in this book (chapter 9). In the end, the decision to use enhancements boils down to the usual choices regarding what people are willing to risk to attain a particular benefit.

In this chapter, the therapy-enhancement distinction is discussed in the context of health, disease, and normal functioning. Any discussion of the distinction between therapy and enhancement must focus on what is "normal" and what is "disease." Enhancement requires understanding of what is normal. Otherwise, what is the basis for the claim that a particular medical intervention improves or enhances the individual? To enhance or improve on some characteristic, it is necessary to know what is in the norm or the average for that characteristic (Fitzgerald 2008).

A distinction based on what is normal has wide appeal in a medical-practice and medical-insurance context. But the line between enhancement and therapy is difficult to draw, and it does not provide a boundary between what is obligatory and nonobligatory in medical interventions. Further, difficult cases (e.g., behavioral disorders) make the distinction seem arbitrary (Daniels 2000). Chadwick (2008) argues there are difficulties in trying to explain enhancement as beyond therapy. If the therapy–enhancement distinction is to have utility, it needs to be able to differentiate, for example, between therapeutic and enhancement uses of cosmetic surgery. Chadwick suggests an alternative approach by distinguishing enhancement from improvement. Whereas enhancement is to add to, improvement is to make better. Accordingly, enhancing an individual with respect to a particular characteristic does not necessarily mean the individual is better overall. However, as a decision rule, an enhancement–improvement distinction lacks sufficient objectivity to have broad applicability.

The distinction between enhancement and therapy is not trivial and raises fundamental questions about the meaning of the term *disease*, about normal variations in human anatomy and performance, and about the safety and efficacy of enhancement technologies. First, the emergence of powerful enhancement technologies raises the requirement to distinguish between going beyond our human physiological capabilities and going beyond our current abilities to treat disease and illness. Second, does every human imperfection require medical intervention? Is society going down the slippery slope of medicalizing normal variations, e.g., seeing short stature or unusual behaviors and other normal human deviations as diseases that require medical management? Third, almost all the available enhancement technologies were developed first as treatment of diseases, and risks were evaluated in the context of the diseases being treated. Are the risks the same when these technologies are used to enhance otherwise healthy individuals? Is the science supporting safety and efficacy of enhancement technologies robust? Fourth, where do we draw the line between treatment and enhancement? Medical interventions for the management of disease are generally acceptable and desirable. Under what circumstances are enhancement technologies also acceptable and desirable? Should society pursue research on enhancement technologies as vigorously as it does for disease management? Should enhancement technologies be held to the same standards of safety as therapies?

Nothing New

Human enhancement is not new. For thousands of years, humans have used natural products such as caffeine and tobacco to change moods and behaviors and to improve cognition (Jung 2001, 4-21). Today, technological advances in biomedicine and bioengineering are available to enhance appearance, behavior, cognition, military-combat effectiveness, and physical performance. Surgical procedures to enhance physical appearance are a multibillion-dollar business in the U.S. Rhinoplasty, breast augmentation, face lifts, and liposuction are some of the more popular elective surgical procedures used to enhance appearance.

Mood and behavioral enhancers like alcohol, cocaine, amphetamines, opiates, and marijuana have been around for centuries. As we continue to learn more about brain chemistry, powerful drugs are being developed to stimulate imaginations and expand creativity. These mood enhancers work by modifying brain chemistry, particularly levels of neurotransmitters such as serotonin, dopamine, and norepinephrine. Drugs to improve cognitive abilities are now everywhere and can be easily obtained even by school children. Millions of middle-school and high-school students use Ritalin and other stimulants without prescription. Amphakines are a new class of enhancement drugs that improve alertness and memory by increasing glutamine neurotransmitter activity in the brain (Mehlman 2009, 16-19).

It should not be surprising that the largest source of funding for enhancement drugs is the U.S. military. A major goal of biomedical research funded by the military is improving combat effectiveness. Current research focuses on maintaining long-term peak performance, sustaining alertness, and enhancing sensory acuity. One product in development is a megaenergy pill that would sustain high-peak performance and cognitive functioning for several days without the need for calories. The benefits of military research have already spilled over to the public domain. A common eye surgical procedure to improve visual acuity called Lasik was first developed in the military (Mehlman 2009, 19-22).

No enhancement technology has generated more public interest and concern than drugs to improve physical performance, particularly in competitive sports. During the nineteenth century, athletes resorted to stimulants such as cocaine and amphetamines. Today, beta blockers are commonly used as a calmative by reducing blood pressure and heart rate. Blood doping and erythropoietin or EPO (a hormone produced by the kidney to boost red-blood-cell production) have been used by athletes to increase energy levels and endurance. Anabolic steroids and human growth hormone increase muscle mass and strength (Mehlman 2009, 10-12).

Antiaging methods, reproductive technologies, and genetic manipulation have also been considered as types of enhancements (Mehlman 2009, 22-33). However, it is unclear how these technologies per se actually improve function. For example, recombinant DNA technology to produce synthetic erythropoietin in large quantities is an example of genetic manipulation; but it is the EPO, not the technology that produces it, that enhances function. Reproductive technologies such as preimplantation genetic diagnosis (PGD) are actually selection methods, not enhancements.

What's Normal?

The distinction between therapy and enhancement centers on the inherently complicated idea of normality. What makes the enhancement-therapy distinction so difficult is that normality and, by extension, disease (i.e., an abnormal anatomical or physiological state) are moving targets. The differences between healthy and sick, fit and unfit, are bound up in personal and community views of what is normal because it reflects cultural and social dimensions of disease that transcend a strictly quantitative and objective description of disease. The distinction between normal and certain psychiatric and behavioral disorders illustrates the difficulties in distinguishing what is normal from disease that may require treatment. Psychiatric and behavioral disorders can be particularly difficult to diagnose because disease boundaries are somewhat fluid. Not only is it problematic to distinguish borderline conditions from normal but distinguishing closely related diseases such as autism and Asperger's syndrome can also be challenging. The reasons for the diagnostic difficulties are complex, but one important factor is that diagnosis relies almost exclusively on symptoms (surface appearance and behavior). Most other diseases in medicine are diagnosed based on quantitative clinical tests and an understanding of biological mechanisms. Currently, there are no simple blood tests or imaging procedures to diagnose psychiatric and behavioral disorders. There are a few exceptions like Down syndrome for which the genetic cause (an extra copy of chromosome 21) is well known and can be easily tested for.

Without clear, objective diagnostic criteria, it is challenging to distinguish between variations in normal from pathologic conditions and to distinguish closely related pathological conditions from one another. If a drug like Paxil is proven to be effective in patients with shyness, then shyness becomes a disorder (social anxiety) requiring treatment. The discovery of a remedy establishes the disease. Because of the uncertainties in diagnoses, the listing of mental disorders in the *Diagnostic and Statistical Manual of Mental Disorders* (the primary diagnostic manual in psychiatry) is constantly changing. The first manual (1952) listed 106 mental disorders, the second (1968) listed 182 and removed homosexuality as a disorder, the third edition (1980) lists 265, the revised third edition (1987) lists 292, and the current fourth version (1994) has identified 297 disorders (Mayes and Horwitz 2005). A fifth version of the manual is in preparation and is expected to be published in the next few years. It would be surprising if the number of disorders does not change again.

Normative standards are established through assessment of objective and subjective biometric criteria in a well-defined sample population assumed to be representative of the whole population. Intrinsic physical and behavioral traits (e.g., blood pressure, height, IQ) are normally distributed (bell-shaped curve) where most people are clustered around the mean value and relatively few people are at the tails with values that are either significantly higher or lower than the mean. Standards are often expressed as a range of values inclusive of the population average. The range of normal values reflects the natural variations of the trait in the population. The wider the range, the greater is the natural variation of the trait. But should the population average always function as a norm? Normative standards are based on a statistical analysis of the bell-shaped distribution or by a comparison of measurements in individuals with and without disease. Mental retardation is an example of a human disease that is defined by the statistical distribution of a biological characteristic. IQ is an intelligence metric that is normally distributed in the population with a mean value of 100. Individuals with measured IQs one or more standard deviations below the mean (below 85 IQ points) are considered to have below-average intelligence. Blood pressure is also normally distributed, but the range of normal is based primarily on measurements associated with blood-pressure-related diseases (e.g., coronary artery disease or stroke).

Individuals near the lower end of the normal distribution for a particular characteristic may be considered disadvantaged for that trait and, therefore, unhealthy in comparison with others. But the average may equally regard themselves as disadvantaged with regard to those who are above average or at the upper end of the distribution. In which cases of traits distributed "normally" should the average also function as a norm, or is the norm itself appropriately subject to alteration? Is it therapy to give growth hormone to a genetic dwarf but not to a short fellow who is just unhappy to be short (President's Council on Bioethics 2003, 18).

Many biological traits vary with age and gender, so different normative standards may apply. Normal testosterone levels refer to what is normal for men in their twenties. But even among younger men, testosterone levels can vary markedly over the course of a day. Many men in their sixties have testosterone levels below presumed normal levels but do not experience signs or symptoms that would justify hormone-replacement therapy (Groopman 2008). A statistical approach to normality avoids subjective assessments of normality but cannot distinguish between what is truly abnormal from what is unusual or rare (athletic talents good enough for a professional career are unusual but not abnormal).

Distinguishing states or conditions that occur as a result of natural variations from those due to pathology can be difficult. When biological traits are continuous variable (like blood pressure and height), the presence of disease may not depend solely on abnormal parametric values but on contributions of predisposing (genetic) factors and environmental risk factors. In such cases, setting standards of normality is difficult because standards are subject to environmental or social circumstances; normal function can also be relative to individuals and circumstances.

Disease may be defined as a collection of signs and symptoms that reflect a physical or mental state judged to be abnormal. The key word is "judged." What is considered normal in one community may be considered abnormal in another. Whether an individual has disease depends on the normative standards established in the community. In the deaf community, an individual with nerve deafness is considered normal and part of the deaf community. The same person is viewed as sensory deficient in the hearing world. For some in the deaf community, cochlear implants to correct nerve deafness is an affront to their culture, which, as they view it, is a minority threatened by the hearing majority. The deaf community feels its way of life is fully functional, and using American Sign Language instead of oral English gives them no disadvantage in society. On the other hand, the hearing community considers deafness a social disadvantage and a quality-of-life issue; the sensory deprivation needs to be corrected in order to be fully functional in society.

Ultimately, our visceral sense of what is normal depends on what we experience and what we become used to. Poor dental hygiene is the statistical norm in the United Kingdom (UK), but it is an abnormal condition (Lewis 1993). Our concept of normal changes as technology evolves because technology impacts our experiences and our expectations. Eyeglasses have been around for centuries; so many people now wear eyeglasses that it is no longer considered unnatural. In fact, for some celebrities like Elton John eyeglasses are part of their personal identity (Marx 2010).

Culture and Medicine

The notion that medicine is international and knows no borders has become almost commonplace. Throughout the world, the medical profession has roughly the same principles and speaks to some extent the same clinical and scientific *lingua franca*. The diagnosis and treatment of most diseases, including appendicitis, pneumonia, and rheumatism, are similar in different countries, and therapeutic success depends on the skill of the healthcare provider and the cooperation of the patient. Nevertheless, it is a gross oversimplification to assume that the practice of medicine is at all homogeneous in the Western world (Dunlop and Inch 1972). Even within the U.S., the use of diagnostic tests, especially imaging studies, varies considerably from one region of the country to another, with higher costs but no better patient outcomes associated with the highest-use regions (Gillik 2009).

Disease and what we consider to be normal are culturally and socially constructed but are also deeply rooted in a mechanistic and systems perspective of human function. The biomedical model emphasizes disease as physical or mental states that are quantifiable and objective deviations from homeostasis. The body is treated as a collection of parts, and diagnoses and treatments are focused on specific tissues, organs, and organ systems. The goal of therapy is to return homeostatic parameters (e.g., red-blood-cell count, blood pressure, blood glucose levels) to values within the normal range. Support by the patient's family is recognized as important to the overall success of therapy but is not central in many instances to diagnosis and management strategies. The cultural model argues that disease and its diagnosis and treatment represent more than alterations in specific body tissues and systems. Instead, medicine is a holistic art and science that involves the whole person both spiritually and physically. The disease boundary extends well beyond the patient to include the immediate family and extended social networks. The cultural model views the broader socioenvironmental contexts in which health, disease, health-related behavior, and normal development are embedded. For example, cancer patients often experience workplace stigmas where co-workers believe cancer reduces worker productivity and is a death sentence (Nessim and Smith 2002). Patients with the same disease are likely to be treated in much the same way under an evidence-based biomedical model but may be treated and managed quite differently under the cultural model. Consequently, a disease in one culturally and socially defined community may be viewed differently in another community with different social and cultural perspectives. Although American medicine is still based primarily on the biomedical model, the importance of cultural and social dimensions of health and disease is increasingly recognized.

Medicine is shaped by its specific cultural or national setting. Cultural influences are pervasive and involve every aspect of healthcare, including public health and prevention, disease diagnosis, and disease management. The behaviors of patients and healthcare providers are influenced in particular by local organizations such as hospitals and clinics, malpractice lawyers, and imaging centers. These are, in turn, influenced by institutions in the larger society, including the media, healthcare plans, and the government (Gillik 2009). National cultures are keys to understanding normality and disease and why a condition in one country is a disease requiring treatment but in another is a variation of normal. The same disease in France, Germany, the UK and the U.S. may be managed in an entirely different way because of different cultural norms (Payer 1996).

The line separating health and disease can be easily blurred. Among the Navajo for whom the prevalence of congenital hip disease is relatively high, treatment is not seen as necessary. Although the disorder may eventually become painful, the condition is not viewed as significant. Resulting limps carry no stigma for the Navajo, but they do for American society in general. Ideas about the visible signs of health also differ. American women strive for thinness, while, in Jamaica, a plump body is much more appealing (Loustaunau and Sobo 1997).

Perceptions of disease risk factors also differ culturally and socially. In Fiji, fat bodies signify social connections, financial resources, and, thus, "health" (Loustaunau and Sobo 1997). In the U.S., obesity is viewed as a clear sign of unhealthy living – public-health messages link obesity to cancer, diabetes, heart disease, and early mortality.

Differences in national culture provide important perspectives on the dynamic relationship between health and disease. Within the structure of the National Health Service, British doctors attempt to do less. They take fewer X-rays and prescribe fewer drugs than their American counterparts. Accordingly, the British patient is less likely to be labeled as sick and require treatment. In Britain, society's traditional and conventional wisdom is that "if you feel well, you are well." In the U.S., a wellness model of healthcare management is promoted by many healthcare insurers and, as a consequence, the "well-person" examination is encouraged. American physicians are more thorough in the search for disease (Marsh et al. 1976). But, excessive use of diagnostic and screening tests can have negative consequences; if you search long and hard enough, you are bound to find something untoward. Recent analyses of breast-cancer screening protocols in the U.S. illustrate how screening tests can lead to overdiagnosis and unnecessary treatment and other costs. The value of mammography as a breast-cancer screen is questionable in women younger than fifty years because screening costs (including pain, discomfort, and unnecessary additional diagnostic testing and treatments) greatly exceed the probability of early breast-cancer detection (Mandelblatt et al. 2009).

Medical management of blood pressure is an example of how normal is interpreted in different countries. Hypotension (low blood pressure) is a German disease. It is not considered a disease in the U.S. and is viewed by some American healthcare professionals as advantageous for long life. American physicians would treat low blood pressure if it resulted in serious signs and symptoms (e.g., vital signs in a medical emergency, fainting because of orthostatic hypotension), but Germans treat hypotension in asymptomatic patients. Hypertension or high blood pressure, on the other hand, is aggressively treated in the U.S. Americans with a diastolic blood pressure greater than 90 mm Hg are likely to be treated, but diastolic pressure would probably need to exceed 100 mm Hg to warrant treatment in the UK (Payer 1996, 86-90).

The liberal use of technology in the U.S. for diagnosis and disease management is encouraged by the healthcare system whereby invasive procedures are reimbursed at a higher rate than less aggressive alternatives. The threat of malpractice also contributes to excessive diagnostic testing and invasive treatments. American physicians tend to give higher doses of medications and perform more surgeries. Doses of psychotropic drugs in the U.S. tend to be higher than elsewhere. American physicians perform more diagnostic tests than physicians in the UK or Europe. For diagnostic-challenging diseases such as behavioral disorders, medical management is uncertain and opens the door to overdiagnosis and unnecessary treatment. Interestingly, technology-intensive approaches to medical care provide no clear advantages and are not associated with marked improvements in survival (Van de Werf et al. 1995). Therapeutic success for cancer and heart-disease management is no better in the U.S. than in France or Germany. When national healthcare effectiveness is measured by avoidable mortality from serious diseases such as bacterial infections, treatable cancers, diabetes, cardiovascular and cerebrovascular disease, and complications from surgical procedures (i.e., preventable deaths by access to appropriate healthcare interventions), the U.S. compares poorly among nineteen developed countries in the Organization for Economic Cooperation and Development (OECD). In an analysis of year 2000 OECD healthcare data, France was ranked first with the lowest rate of avoidable deaths, and the U.S. was ranked last with the highest rate (Nolte and McKee 2008). That is a severe indictment of the healthcare system in the wealthiest and most technically advanced country in the world.

Therapy or Enhancement?

What does *enhancement* mean? In therapy, the goals of intervention are clear – the patient is cured of the disease and returned to normal function, or signs and symptoms of the disease are reduced to conserve quality of life when cure is not possible. Because enhancement goes beyond normal function, what should the goals of enhancement technologies be? Can such goals even be defined?

When medical goals are unclear, the distinction between enhancement and therapy gets blurred. Is breast-reconstruction surgery enhancement or therapy when completed long after breast-cancer surgery? Is the breast reconstruction considered part of the cancer treatment or an enhancement to produce a more desirable cosmetic result? Is use of orthodontic appliances to straighten crooked teeth or to correct malocclusion enhancement or therapy in patients with cardiovascular disease? Dental appliances result in a more attractive smile but also may reduce the risk of periodontal disease, a serious comorbid condition that can exacerbate cardiovascular disease. Gastric-bypass surgery is a radical procedure and the most drastic means currently available for weight reduction. Physicians recommend the procedure because of patient health concerns, but the social stigma attached to obesity is what drives many patients to the operating table. Is gastric-bypass surgery therapy? The surgery removes no disease and repairs no defect or injury. Its purpose is to control a person's appetite by rearranging the digestive tract (Groopman 2008).

The enhancement-therapy boundary also gets fuzzy when an intervention is used to make up for a condition or disease instead of treating it. Mehlman (2009) refers to such interventions as "compensatory enhancement." Visually impaired persons taking cognitive-enhancing drugs or paraplegics strengthening their arms with anabolic-steroid injections are enhancement-like because they improve the person's capabilities without directly affecting the disease state or condition, but they are also therapeutic because they mitigate the effects of the person's disability (Mehlman 2009, 9).

Although therapy and enhancement interventions have different goals and objectives, they are inextricably linked in two ways. First, the technologies that serve the medical-enhancement and medical-therapy communities are the same. Enhancement drugs represent off-label uses of drugs approved for the treatment of specific diseases. Psychostimulant drugs like Adderall and Ritalin were developed to treat attention deficit and hyperactivity disorder (ADHD) and related abnormal behaviors, but these same drugs are also used as cognitive enhancements in normal people. These drugs likely function in the same way in patients and normal individuals, but no one knows for sure because long-term drug-safety and efficacy studies in normal volunteers have not been carried out. Second, physicians are the gatekeepers for the proper medical uses of drugs and medical devices. The public relies on the physician's professional judgment regarding proper dispensing of medicines for diagnostic, therapeutic, or prophylactic purposes. Physicians have an almost complete monopoly over the prescription and administration of drugs.

But there are difficulties when medical practice moves beyond therapy into the realm of enhancement. The path is clear when the doctor is treating disease. There is a well-defined target, and most treatment complications are known and can be anticipated. But a physician prescribing cognitive-enhancing or other medical interventions for goals beyond therapy is in unknown territory. Specific goals in terms of desired outcomes and expectations are not well-defined.[1] What defines interventional success or failure? How effective can doctor-patient communication and the informed consent process be when available medical options are not clearly delineated because health risks and benefits are not fully understood and cannot be explained adequately (Mehlman 2009, 99-120).

There is a serious danger that the rapid growth and availability of enhancement interventions (e.g., steroid drugs in athletic competitions and cognitive-enhancement drugs in academic settings) may lead to medicalization – the transformation of activities, behaviors, or conditions as disorders or diseases that require medical intervention. This revolution stems from the growth in medical knowledge and competence; the expanding domain of psychiatry, the "doctoring of the psyche"; increased success using medical interventions; and rising patient expectations of cure, relief, and salvation coming from healthcare professionals. As new drugs and other technologies with enhancement utility become available, there will be an increased tendency toward viewing everything in human life through the lens of disease and disability (President's Council on Bioethics 2003, 334-48).

Marketing demands for medical interventions is purpose-driven. Unlike enhancements, the market demand for therapies is limited to narrowly defined disease characteristics such as signs and symptoms. Drugs used for enhancement were initially developed to treat disease but have widespread demand that extends beyond disease boundaries. Dual use of technology makes enhancements attractive to people who are not sick but who would use them to look younger, perform better, or feel happier.

What is considered "normal" distinguishes enhancement from therapy. The therapy-enhancement dynamic shifts according to culturally determined norms. Aggressive therapy as practiced in the U.S. leads to the availability of medical interventions for enhancement purposes. The diagnosis of ADHD is higher in the U.S. than in other countries (McCabe et al. 2005). In fact, there is widespread concern that ADHD is seriously overdiagnosed; children who may not need them are prescribed stimulants. American consumption of psychotropic drugs for treating ADHD (and other mental disorders) and for enhancement of cognitive function far exceeds use in other countries (Berbatis et al. 2002; McCabe et al. 2005; International Narcotics Control Board 2009).

---

1 Cosmetic dentistry and surgery are exceptions. Although cosmetic interventions may be therapeutic, much of it is enhancement that addresses the patient's personal or professional needs or desires. Computer simulations can provide the doctor and patient with virtual outcomes, so the patient has realistic expectations and the physician has goals to shoot for. Although no specific result can be guaranteed, success can be evaluated by comparison of actual with expected outcomes.

The Drug Problem

Illegal drug use remains a serious and growing problem for two major reasons. First, a large fraction of the American population uses alcohol and tobacco. In a 2005 survey assessing the frequency of heavy drinking and binge drinking in the population, about 22 percent of persons aged twelve or older participated in binge drinking (i.e., five or more drinks on the same occasion on at least one day in the past thirty days, including heavy use at least once in the thirty days prior to the survey). Heavy drinking (i.e., five or more drinks on the same occasion on each of five or more days in the past thirty days) was reported by 6.6 percent of the survey population aged twelve or older (Substance Abuse and Mental Health Services Administration 2006, 27). Approximately 20 percent of the U.S. population aged eighteen years and older smoke cigarettes (American Cancer Society 2009, 47-48). These drugs are widely considered to be "gateway" drugs that may lead to subsequent as well as concurrent use of illicit drugs. Some children are abusing drugs by age twelve or thirteen, usually by starting with tobacco, alcohol, inhalants, marijuana, and psychotherapeutic drugs (Jung 2001, 3; National Institute of Drug Abuse 2003, 10). Second, multichannel access makes illicit drug distribution difficult to control. The alarming increase in the use of neurostimulant drugs in the U.S. is a powerful example of how readily available potentially dangerous drugs can be when social distribution of drugs is unregulated and uncontrolled. The problem is particularly worrisome for behavioral disorders because disease characteristics are vague and diagnosis may be difficult to make. The distinction between enhancement and therapy is challenging in these cases. In the face of diagnostic uncertainty, an aggressive, conservative medical model can lead to overdiagnosis.

Schedule II stimulants such as Adderall and Ritalin are prescribed for the treatment of ADHD. These drugs are listed under Schedule II of the U.S. Controlled Substances Act because they have a high potential for abuse, they have a currently accepted medical use in treatment in the U.S., and abuse of the drug may lead to severe psychological or physical dependence. Ritalin is the main central-nervous-system stimulant listed on Schedule II (International Narcotics Control Board 2009). Adderall and Ritalin improve the ability to focus mentally for considerable periods of time and, in an otherwise normal individual, can enhance cognitive functioning. Adderall is available only by prescription. It is not unheard of that students will fake symptoms of ADHD to get an Adderall prescription to improve academic performance (Talbot 2009). In a 2001 survey of about 11,000 students from 119 U.S. colleges, 7 percent of students admitted using prescription stimulants for nonmedical purposes (McCabe et al. 2005). In a recent *Nature* poll of 1,400 readers from sixty countries, 20 percent of respondents claimed to have used drugs for nonmedical reasons to stimulate their focus, concentration, or memory; one-third of the drugs used for nonmedical purposes were obtained over the Internet (Maher 2008). Psychotropic substances may be used in certain countries for different treatments or in accordance with different medical practices (International Narcotics Control Board 2009). In the U.S., illegal Schedule II drug use may result in a stiff monetary fine and/or imprisonment, depending on the nature and severity of the crime.

Distribution channels that are otherwise legal are often manipulated to acquire controlled-substance prescription drugs for illegal purposes, including drugs to enhance cognitive functions. Negligent or intentional overprescribing by physicians or other practitioners and doctor shopping (the practice of obtaining the same prescription medicines from different physicians) are common methods of controlled-substance prescription fraud. The fact that ADHD and related behavioral disorders can be difficult to diagnose facilitates fraudulent prescription practices because the diagnosis has high uncertainty. Prescription drugs can also be obtained illegally through online pharmacies, theft, and burglary (from residences, pharmacies, etc.), stereotypical drug dealing (selling pills to others), and receiving drugs from friends or family.

The Future Is Now

As long as market demand is sustained, there will always be questions about the value and proper place of enhancement technologies in society. Most of the performance-enhancing technologies of the future, like those in use today, will likely be developed to diagnose and treat disease. From a medical-management perspective, the complex character of many diseases like behavioral disorders offers a surprising advantage. Disease complexity provides more opportunity to manage the disease. As a consequence, psychotropic drugs have broad utility, and that makes them readily adaptable for off-label uses.

Market demand for enhancement drugs is driven primarily by well-known benefits of drug use, including superior athletic performance, longer and more intense focus on task, improved academic performance, and enhanced cognitive functioning. But current experience with enhancement technologies particularly in athletic competitions and academic settings raises serious questions about safety when the drug is used for off-label purpose (Appel 2008; Greely et al. 2008; Maher 2008). Drug safety is not unique to enhancement technologies. It is central to the U.S. Food and Drug Administration (FDA) drug-approval process and to diagnostic and therapeutic decision making.

No biological agent powerful enough to produce major changes in the body or the mind, including functional enhancement, is likely to be entirely without side effects. In therapeutic applications, complications lead to signs and symptoms related to the pharmacologic actions of the drug. Some cancer chemotherapeutic agents, for example, cause lethargy and susceptibility to infections because the drugs suppress bone-marrow function. Chronic anabolic-steroid use is associated with serious kidney damage (Herlitz et al. 2010). Drugs used for enhancement may be associated with a different set of complications related to the enhancement itself. Anabolic steroids are used to improve muscle strength and physical performance. If the resulting muscle improvements are unbalanced (e.g., not all muscle groups are enhanced to the same degree), tendon and ligament damage attached to inferior muscle groups may result. These types of drug complications are the unintended consequences of seeking enhancement benefits.

The decision to use drugs or medical devices is based on consideration of personal benefits and risks. In therapeutic interventions, risks and benefits are usually known well enough to make a decision with some degree of confidence. The amount of risk the patient is willing to tolerate or to accept depends on the benefits of the intervention. In cancer therapy, many chemotherapeutic agents have severe side effects, but these risks are acceptable because the drugs are life-extending or life-saving. Higher risks are acceptable as perceived benefits increase. Even very small risks are not acceptable if there is no perceived benefit.

The risk-benefit calculus is considerably different for enhancement interventions. The benefits are superior performance or other enhancement beyond normal function. Whereas therapeutic benefit can be measured in terms of cure or palliation, benefits of enhancement, especially for cognitive enhancements, may be much more difficult to measure. Enhancement decisions are made almost completely on the basis of perceived benefits with considerable discounting of risks. Risks associated with enhancement drugs are evaluated in the context of use as therapeutic interventions and not for enhancement purposes. Enhancement interventions are off-label applications of specific therapeutic uses as approved by the FDA. The FDA drug-approval process focuses only on safety and efficacy of the drug for a specific medical purpose. Risks of FDA-approved drugs for off-label (e.g., enhancement) purposes are not evaluated. The risks of neuroenhancement drugs are not fully known. What are the risks of stimulants such as Adderall and Ritalin in otherwise healthy individuals (e.g., college students)? Do these drugs lead to excessive alcohol consumption and alcohol poisonings? No one seems to know. What about long-term complications of drug use? Can chronic use of neuroenhancers lead to arrhythmias and other potentially fatal cardiac problems later in life? Individuals with undiagnosed bipolar disease may be at particular risk of potentially devastating effects of neuroenhancers. These drugs can trigger severe mania and depression in at-risk individuals taking these drugs in an uncontrolled manner. Cognitive enhancements result in biochemical changes in the brain, and the risk of unintended complications, particularly as a result of long-term use, is, therefore, both high and consequential.

Drug safety in children is of particular concern. Their brains may be particularly sensitive to drug effects because they are still in development. Depression can now be diagnosed in children as young as three years old. Depression at such a young age does not appear to be developmentally transient but instead demonstrates chronicity and recurrence (Luby et al. 2009). If these children are prescribed psychotropic drugs, what are the long-term consequences? Risks have not been adequately evaluated and are poorly understood in children. Equally troubling is the perception, particularly among teenagers and young adults, that controlled substances are safe even when used "recreationally." Abusers of controlled drugs are using these medicines in a manner for which they were never intended. This practice, coupled with the distorted perception of safety, makes these medicines much more dangerous. Teenagers and young adults taking ADHD drugs to get high or to enhance cognitive functioning may not realize that misuse can lead to serious medical complications. Often, drug abusers mistakenly equate FDA approval with drug safety. In one study, calls to poison-control centers about teens abusing attention-deficit drugs increased 76 percent over eight years – sobering evidence of the dangers of prescription-drug misuse. This increase parallels a near-doubling of prescription rates for Adderall and related medications from about four million eight years ago to eight million now (Setlik et al. 2009).

The availability of psychotropic-stimulant drugs as cognitive enhancers has reached alarming levels particularly in the U.S. (International Narcotics Control Board 2009). The problem is clearly the ease by which enhancement drugs are distributed within the normal population. The uncontrolled uses of enhancement technologies emerged from legitimate uses of drugs in medicine treatments. Two key factors seem to be in play. First, some drugs like Schedule II psychotropic stimulants have a high probability of abuse and dependency, and drug use can easily get out of control. Second, some diseases are not clearly definable, and diagnoses can be uncertain. The result is that diseases like ADHD are overdiagnosed. Further, it may not be clear when treatment of disease should be terminated or modified and when continued drug use is no longer treatment but a transition to off-label enhancement.

Unless effective controls for distribution and use are put in place, these disruptive and potentially harmful technologies could become so widespread that a profound effect on human social life could result. One obvious possibility is the emergence of a wealthy, privileged, and advantaged social class created by unbalanced opportunities and resources for enhancement technologies. Fukuyama has suggested the establishment of a regulatory framework and new laws to protect against the harms of unrestrained biotechnological enhancement (2002, 202-16).

A successful federal regulatory program to control distribution and use will be a challenge because of the pervasiveness of the drug-enhancement problem and the fact that it is essentially one involving control of personal behaviors. Marchant and Lopez (in this volume) argue that regulations to control use and distribution of enhancement technologies will be very difficult to implement and enforce particularly if society sees a value in the technology and if risks are acceptable. Mehlman suggests the most effective way to address health concerns of biomedical enhancements without compromising benefits is by improving drug safety and efficacy rather than regulating personal behaviors. One obvious way is by tightening FDA regulations (Mehlman 2009, 203-10).

If regulations to control personal behaviors are not likely to be effective, is there any other way to control distribution and use of drugs? Market forces will be a strong driver for consumption. As long as society views enhancement technologies as more beneficial than risky and enhancements are perceived to be inherently good, it will be difficult to keep them out of the hands of consumers. Even in the absence of a formalized legal regulatory framework, the medical community has the capacity and professional responsibility to society to control distribution of enhancement technologies. Physicians control prescription-drug use. Self-regulation can take the form of guidelines, policies, or recommendations established by professional medical organizations. Self-regulation does not have the force of law but, nevertheless, serves as the basis for professional standards of conduct. Violations of established professional standards can lead to reprimands or more serious consequences, including suspension or revocation of licensure.

The biomedical community has successfully self-regulated when challenged with risk uncertainties or unbridled growth of new technologies. The 1975 Asilomar Conference brought together leading molecular biologists to establish guidelines for the control of newly introduced recombinant DNA technology. The main result of the conference was a voluntary ban until the risks of recombinant DNA could be more fully evaluated. The conference also led to the establishment of a National Institutes of Health Recombinant DNA Advisory Committee that issued guidelines for all NIH-funded scientists, restricting how recombinant DNA organisms could be used (Fukuyama 2002, 196). More recently, the medical imaging community has issued guidelines in response to the astounding growth in diagnostic CT and nuclear-medicine studies in the U.S. The number of computerized-tomography (CT) studies has skyrocketed from about three million in 1980 to seventy million in 2007; the number of nuclear-medicine studies has also increased significantly from three million exams in 1980 to more than twenty million in 2007. In 2007, the American College of Radiology published guidelines for referring physicians, radiologists, and other healthcare professionals to better control patient radiation exposures and the number of repeat studies and clinically unnecessary studies without compromising medical care and diagnostic efficacy (Amis et al. 2007).

Perhaps the most effective strategy to control enhancement-drug distribution and use is the establishment of a national drug database to track personal drug inventories. The physician would establish a patient-specific inventory limit based on the patient's medical condition and treatment requirements. Once the limit is exceeded for a particular drug or class of drugs (e.g., Schedule II stimulants), no further prescriptions would be written or filled. A database system like this would effectively address the doctor-shopping problem. Doctor shopping is an easy way to stockpile prescription drugs. Unless a national database is established to track prescriptions, there is no way any one physician can know a patient's current drug inventory. Obviously, serious privacy and other legal issues in establishing this information network system need to be resolved. But a personal drug database would be instrumental in controlling illegal drug use and distribution. Maintaining an accurate and current personal drug inventory will require the cooperation of doctors, patients, and pharmacists. Physicians are key because they are the gatekeepers to medications and control proper use and dosages.

Public education to increase understanding of enhancement technologies and potential risks of chronic use of prescription medications for nonmedical purposes is clearly important. Public education is a powerful risk-management tool. Public messages can work; cigarette consumption rates in the U.S. decreased after dissemination of the U.S. Surgeon General's report on smoking and health in 1964. Messages would need to be carefully crafted to address the specific needs of adult and younger audiences. For example, pre-high-school, high-school, and college students have perceptions about disease and mortality risks that are different from adult views. Young people view themselves as immortal and immune from chronic health risks (Collins et al. 2004). Information pamphlets and other media could be provided to the public by physicians, teachers, health clinics, and employers in a way similar to current distribution programs about smoking and nutrition. Educational programs at the family, school, and community levels are critical to the success of drug-abuse-prevention programs (National Institute of Drug Abuse 2003).

Enhancement: A Gateway to Transhumanism?

The agenda of transhumanists is to eliminate disease, improve our physical capacities, enhance intelligence, improve our emotional condition, create a happier society for all, and ultimately eliminate aging. What's wrong with the pursuit of health and happiness? Why should there be limits on a human's ability to improve his or her intelligence and expand lifespan (Kristol and Cohen 2002)?

Programs to control use and distribution of enhancement drugs will have to overcome competitive impulses and the economic incentives that will drive people to use enhancement technologies. In reality, these pressures may be too difficult to overcome. What then? Anabolic steroids and cognitive enhancements are already widespread. Uncontrolled uses of enhancements and ready distribution of technologies may lead to transhumanism – a transition process from the present-day human to a more evolved posthuman characterized by improved physical and mental performance. Transhumanism in operational terms is the *process* whereby humans become posthumans, and the end state of the transhumanism process is the posthuman. Posthumans are individuals whose basic capacities greatly exceed the natural limits attainable by present human beings; as a consequence, their nature has radically changed. Bostrom defines the posthuman as having one or more of the following general capacities: (1) health span and the capacity to remain fully healthy and active and productive both mentally and physically, (2) cognition and the capacity for intellect such as memory and deductive and analytical reasoning, and (3) emotion and the capacity to enjoy life and to respond appropriately to life situations and other people (Bostrom 2008). What distinguishes posthuman states is the degree to which acquired capacities have exceeded what is considered normal for present-day humans.

The transhuman process relies on advanced technologies including genetic manipulation of cells and organisms through engineered viruses, neural interfaces, and other types of machine-computer-human coupling, memory-enhancing drugs, cognitive techniques and bioengineering for development of prostheses. The resulting posthuman depends on the technologies employed. For example, society in Aldous Huxley's *Brave New World* (1932) and the Crakers in Atwood's *Oryx and Crake* (2003) is the product of genetic manipulation through cloning technology. The transhumanism phenomenon starts with enhancements at the individual level and progresses to enhancements of the entire species or at least a very large population. Transhumanism processes can take on any of a number of possible configurations. In the simplest transhumanism scenario, current medical and pharmaceutical technologies become widely distributed and accessible to nearly everyone. These technologies, including cognitive-enhancing drugs, would modify human physiology to enhance physical and mental functioning. Neuroenhancement technologies might lead to novel ways humans communicate with each other and, as a result, establish powerful cognitive networks. The product might be a society of posthumans who are still considered human but have extraordinary capabilities beyond what normal humans have. The social consequences could be highly beneficial, including better health, longer lives, greater intelligence, and higher productivity. But consequences could also be highly detrimental. Posthumans might be considered a "superior race," with access to resources and social privileges unavailable to the unenhanced.

The most extreme transhumanism configuration is a fantastic, science-fiction scenario described by a posthuman world in which humans don't exist as humans at all. Instead, the physical body has been discarded; higher-order cortical functions, including language, intelligence, and consciousness, have been digitized and uploaded into machines that function as a sort of software resident intelligence for as long as a source of energy is available. This might be accomplished by scanning the neuronal and synaptic architecture of the brain at a sufficiently high resolution by means of nanotechnology. Physical embodiment would no longer be needed in this ultimate transhumanism world. Conscious machines would talk to other conscious machines, share ideas, and build other conscious machines. Another scenario might involve reshaping humankind with the help of germline modifications. Unlike somatic gene therapy in which only the genetic material of somatic cells is modified, germline modifications can be passed on to the next generation, and all the offspring's cells would contain the genetic changes. If germline modifications are performed consistently through successive generations, a genetically modified posthuman species might emerge (Gordijn and Chadwick 2008).

Huxley's *Brave New World* describes a transhumanism society and what society might look like if enhancement technologies develop in an unchecked and uncontrolled way. His world is a dystopia several hundred years into the future. There are no longer any diseases. Wars and aggression and suffering no longer exist, and psychotropic drugs are abundant (Kass 2002). People in this society "get what they want, and they never want what they can't get. … And, if anything should go wrong , there's *soma*." (Huxley 1932, 220). But there are serious problems. Human cloning technology is central to Huxley's world and has created a society characterized by homogeneity and mediocrity devoid of love, emotion, and all human virtues. Margaret Atwood's *Oryx and Crake* (2003) also describes a frightening dystopia, featuring the Crakers created by Crake, a talented molecular biologist, who wants to create a better world for humans. The world of *Oryx and Crake* does not depend on the availability of new scientific advances as in *Brave New World* but relies instead on taking already established technologies such as xenotransplantation and extending them unrealistically to a radical ending. The *Brave New World* and *Oryx and Crake* scenarios do not seem very likely. Although cloning technologies are available today, success in cloning higher-order mammals has been exceedingly difficult to achieve. Technical problems have yet to be resolved, public demand for cloning is extremely low, and most people are decidedly against it (Kass 2009). Stories like Huxley's and Atwood's pose the same question: how do humans differ from nonhumans, or, more directly, what does it mean to be human?

Enhancement technologies as a gateway to transhumanism should not be considered lightly. Enhancements are derived from therapeutic uses, and when the boundary between therapy and enhancement is uncertain (as in the case of many behavioral disorders), the opportunity for enhancement expands. What begins as a quest to treat disease may end up as a "compassionate" effort to stamp out disease itself (Cohen and Kristol 2002). Cognitive enhancement is one area where there can be a truly global experience by distributing drugs. Expansion is accelerated when there are limited or no controls on distributions and benefits are perceived to be greater than risks. Experience with psychostimulant drugs illustrates how rapidly off-label uses of prescription drugs can be exploited in the general populations.

Transhumanism could occur in a fairly short time (perhaps a few decades) once enabling technologies become readily available. Given these technologies are likely to be developed in the clinical setting to treat disease, those technologies involved in diseases for which diagnostic criteria are difficult to establish are likely to transition over to enhancements first and most easily. The introduction of enhancement technologies will depend on the perceived benefits and risks of the technology and monetary costs. If enhancements have little or no perceived risks, there would be minimal restrictions on uses. Safety, or the acceptability of risks, is socially determined, and society is likely to take advantage of emerging technologies if the perceived benefits outweigh risks.

What determines whether a particular technology has worthwhile benefits and reasonable costs boils down to personal choices. If the technology has questionable benefits or is too expensive, it is not likely to see widespread social acceptance. Neuroenhancements are likely to lead the way because enhanced cognitive abilities are attractive to everyone. Athletic enhancements are also attractive, but wholesale availability and use are restricted because of undesirable impacts on competition. The public is interested in high-level athletic performance but wants it based on natural athletic talents rather than enhanced by artificial means. Winning and athletic records have a different meaning when enhancements are involved.

What counts for transhumanism and a posthuman world? Will we know it when we get there? We may already be entering our posthuman future, and it may look very much like our own but characterized by better health, longer lives, more intelligence, and a higher level of performance. The introduction of cell phones, other communication devices, and the Internet has enhanced human capabilities in ways that could not have been predicted just a few decades ago. The social consequences have been profound. People interact and behave differently because of the unique avenues of communication opened by the new technologies. Has human nature been altered by the social introduction of these technologies? How would we know? And unregulated technologies come with unintended consequences. Talking or text messaging on a cell phone while driving has led to an increase in traffic accidents and deaths. Many jurisdictions have put laws into place to control this risky behavior (Mossman 2006, 167-81). Huxley's *Brave New World* presents an even more drastic outcome in a competitive and hierarchical posthuman world in which the notion of a "shared humanity" may be lost (Fukuyama 2002, 217-18).

Fear of what a posthuman world might bring should not deter society from pursing enhancement technology for the benefit of humankind. We ought to develop and use NBIC technologies to the fullest extent possible. But our enthusiasm to improve ourselves, our society, and our environment should be tempered by consideration for equitable resource access and unintended consequences and concerns for risks and burdens to future generations. Scientists and engineers at the forefront of technology development paint a rosy picture of a future world and tend to downplay risks. But scientists' views are not necessarily congruent with public perceptions. In a 2009 report from the Woodrow Wilson Center, the public is concerned about risks of synthetic biology, and the path from the lab to novel life forms is likely to be controversial (Hart Research Associates 2009). Where emerging technologies ultimately lead us is anyone's guess. But whatever the path, public acceptance of emerging technologies will depend on the capacity of the science and engineering community to have an honest and open conversation with the public about what they are doing and why it is important.

References

American Cancer Society. 2009. *Cancer Facts & Figures – 2009.* Atlanta: American Cancer Society, Inc.: http://www.cancer.org/Research/CancerFacts Figures/cancer-facts-figures-2009, accessed July 14, 2011.

Amis, E. Stephen, Priscilla F. Butler, Kimberly E. Applegate, et al. 2007. American College of Radiology white paper on radiation dose in medicine. *Journal of the American College of Radiology* 4: 272-84.

Appel, J. M. 2008. When the boss turns pusher: A proposal for employee protections in the age of cosmetic neurology. *Journal of Medical Ethics* 34: 616-18.

Atwood, Margaret. 2003. *Oryx and Crake.* New York: Anchor Books.

Berbatis, Constantine G., V. Bruce Sunderland, and Max Bulsara. 2002. Licit psychostimulant consumption in Australia, 1984-2000: International and jurisdictional comparison. *Medical Journal of Australia* 177: 539-43.

Bostrom, Nick. 2002. Existential risks: Analyzing human extinction scenarios. *Journal of Evolution and Technology* 9 (1): http://www.nickbostrom.com/ existential/risks.html, accessed July 14, 2011.

–. 2008. Why I want to be a posthuman when I grow up. In *Medical Enhancement and Posthumanity*, ed. B. Gordijn and R.Chadwick, 107-36. Amsterdam: Springer.

Chadwick, Ruth 2008. Therapy, enhancement and improvement. In Gordijn and Chadwick, eds., 25-37.

Cohen, Eric, and William Kristol. 2002. Cloning stem cells and beyond. In Kristol and Cohen, eds., 297-305.

Collins, Kristina M., Marilyn Dantico, Nelma B.C. Shearer, and Kenneth L. Mossman. 2004. Heart disease awareness among college students. *Journal of Community Health* 29: 405-20.

Daniels, Norman. 2000. Normal functioning and the treatment-enhancement distinction. *Cambridge Quarterly of Healthcare Ethics* 9: 309-22.

Dunlop, Derrick, and R. S. Inch. 1972. Variations in pharmaceutical and medical practice in Europe. *British Medical Journal* 3: 749-52.

Fitzgerald, S. J. Kevin. 2008. Medical enhancement: A destination of technological not human betterment. In Gordijn and Chadwick, eds., 39-53.

Fukuyama, Francis. 2002. *Our Posthuman Future: Consequences of the Biotechnology Revolution*. New York: Picador.

Gillik, Muriel R. 2009. Medicine as ecoculture. *Annals of Internal Medicine* 151: 577-80.

Gordijn, Bert, and Ruth Chadwick, eds. 2008. *Medical Enhancement and Posthumanity*. Amsterdam: Springer. See "Introduction," 1-5.

Greely, Henry, Barbara Sahakian, John Harris, et al. 2008. Towards responsible use of cognitive-enhancing drugs by the healthy. *Nature* 456: 702-5.

Groopman, Jerome. 2008. *How Doctors Think*. New York: Houghton Mifflin.

Hart Research Associates. 2009. *Nanotechnology, Synthetic Biology and Public Opinion*. A report for the Project on Emerging Nanotechnologies, The Woodrow Wilson International Center for Scholars. Washington, DC: Hart Research Associates: http://www.nanotechproject.org/process/assets/files/8286/nano_synbio.pdf, accessed July 14, 2011.

Herlitz, Leal C., Glen S. Markowitz, Alton B. Farris, et al. 2010. Development of focal segmental glomerulosclerosis after anabolic steroid abuse. *Journal of the American Society of Nephrology* 21: 163-72.

Huxley, Aldous. 1932. *Brave New World*. London: Chatto and Windus.

International Narcotics Control Board. 2009. *Psychotropic Substances*. New York: United Nations.

Jung, John. 2001. *Psychology of Alcohol and Other Drugs: A Research Perspective*. Thousand Oaks, CA: Sage Publications, Inc.

Kamm, Frances M. 2005. Is there a problem with enhancement? *The American Journal of Bioethics* 5 (3): 5-14.

–. 2009. What is and is not wrong with enhancement? In *Human Enhancement*, ed. J. Savulescu and N. Bostrom, 91-130. Oxford: Oxford University Press.
Kass, Leon R. 2002. Preventing a brave new world. In Kristol and Cohen, eds., 219-41.
Kristol, William, and Eric Cohen, eds. 2002. *The Future Is Now: America Confronts the New Genetics*. Lanham, MD: Rowman and Littlefield. See "Introduction: The Future Is Now, xv–xix.
Kurzweil, Ray. 2005. *The Singularity Is Near: When Humans Transcend Biology*. New York: Viking Press.
Lewis, G. 1993. Some studies of social causes of and cultural response to disease. In *The Anthropology of Disease*, ed. C.G.N. Mascie-Taylor and G. Lewis, 73-124. Oxford: Oxford University Press.
Loustaunau, Martha O., and Elisa J. Sobo. 1997. *The Cultural Context of Health, Illness, and Medicine*. Westport, CT: Bergin & Garvey.
Luby, Joan L., Xuemei Si, Andy C. Belden, Mini Tandon, and Ed Spitznagel. 2009. Preschool depression: Homotypic continuity and course over 24 months. *Archives of General Psychiatry* 66 (8): 897-905.
Maher, Brendan. 2008. Poll results: Look who's doping. *Nature* 452: 674-75.
Mandelblatt, Jeanne S., Kathleen A. Cronin, Stephanie Bailey, et al. 2009. Effects of mammography screening under different screening schedules: Model estimates of potential benefits and harms. *Annals of Internal Medicine* 151: 738-47.
Marsh, G.N., R. B. Wallace, and J. B. Whewell. 1976. Anglo-American contrasts in general practice. *British Journal of Medicine* 1: 1321-25.
Marx, Patricia. 2010. Four eyes: Looking for glasses. *The New Yorker*, March 29, 46-50: http://www.newyorker.com/reporting/2010/03/29/100329fa_fact_marx, accessed July 14, 2011.
Mayes, Rick, and Allan B. Horwitz. 2005. DSM-III and the revolution in the classification of mental illness. *Journal of the History of the Behavioral Sciences* 41 (3): 249-67.
McCabe, Sean E., John R. Knight, Christian J. Teter, and Henry Wechsler. 2005. Non-medical use of prescription stimulants among U.S. college students: Prevalence and correlates from a national survey. *Addiction* 99: 96-106.
McKibben, Bill. 2003. *Enough: Staying Human in an Engineered Age*. New York: Henry Holt.
Mehlman, Max J. 2009. *The Price of Perfection: Individualism and Society in the Era of Biomedical Enhancement*. Baltimore, MD: The Johns Hopkins University Press.
Mossman, Kenneth L. 2006. *Radiation Risks in Perspective*. Boca Raton, FL: Taylor & Francis Publishing Group.

National Institute of Drug Abuse, National Institutes of Health. 2003. *Preventing Drug Abuse among Children and Adolescents*. 2d ed. NIH Publication No. 04-4212(A): http://drugabuse.gov/pdf/prevention/redbook.pdf, accessed July 14, 2011.

Nessim, Susan, and Dianne S. Smith. 2002. Survivorship: Obstacles and opportunities. In *Everyone's Guide to Cancer Therapy: How Cancer Is Diagnosed, Treated and Managed Day to Day*, ed. M. Dollinger, E. H. Rosenbaum, M. Temparo, and S. J. Mulvihill, 274-77. Kansas City, MO: Andrews McMeel Publishing.

Nolte, Ellen, and C. Martin McKee. 2008. Measuring the health of nations: Updating an earlier analysis. *Health Affairs* 27 (1): 58-71.

Payer, Lynn. 1996. *Medicine and Culture: Varieties of Treatment in the U.S., England, West Germany and France*. New York: Henry Holt.

President's Council on Bioethics. 2003. *Beyond Therapy: Biotechnology and the Pursuit of Happiness*. Washington, DC: Dana Press.

Sandel, Michael J. 2004. The case against perfection. *Atlantic Monthly* 293 (3): 51-62: http://www.theatlantic.com/magazine/archive/2004/04/the-case-against-perfection/2927/, accessed July 14, 2011.

–. 2009. The case against perfection: What's wrong with designer children, bionic athletes, and genetic engineering? In *Human Enhancement*, ed. J. Savulescu and N. Bostrom, 71-89. Oxford: Oxford University Press.

Schwartz, Peter H. 2005. Defending the distinction between treatment and enhancement. *The American Journal of Bioethics* 5 (3): 17-18.

Setlik, Jennifer, G. Randall Bond, and Mona Ho. 2009. Adolescent ADHD prescription medication abuse is rising along with prescriptions for these medications. *Pediatrics* 124 (3): 875-80.

Stock, Gregory. 2002. *Redesigning Humans: Our Inevitable Genetic Future*. New York: Houghton Mifflin.

Substance Abuse and Mental Health Services Administration, U.S. Department of Health and Human Services. 2006. *Results from the 2005 National Survey on Drug Use and Health: National Findings*. Rockville, MD: Office of Applied Studies.

Talbot, Margaret. 2009. Brain gain: The underground world of "neuroenhancing" drugs. *The New Yorker*, April 27: http://www.newyorker.com/reporting/2009/04/27/090427fa_fact_talbot, accessed July 14, 2011.

Van de Werf, Frans, Eric J. Topol, Kerry L. Lee, et al. 1995.Variations in patient management and outcomes for acute myocardial infarction in the U.S. and other countries: Results from the GUSTO trial. *Journal of the American Medical Association* 273: 1586-91.

The (In)Feasibility of Regulating Enhancement

Gary E. Marchant and Alexandra López

While transhumanism involves an often untidy matrix of technologies, processes, goals and beliefs, the central core of transhumanism is human enhancement. As defined by its advocates, transhumanism is "[t]he intellectual and cultural movement that affirms the possibility and desirability of fundamentally improving the human condition through applied reason, especially by developing and making widely available technologies to eliminate aging and to *greatly* enhance human intellectual, physical, and psychological capacities" (WTA 2003). The debate over transhumanism and its key corollary of human enhancement has largely focused, appropriately, on the feasibility and capabilities of various existing or future technologies to modify humans, the human and social impacts of any such enhancements, and the debate on whether such human enhancements should be favored or discouraged.

Less often discussed is the practical problem of whether we could stop human enhancement even if we wanted to do so. That question is the focus of this chapter. The answer is critical to much of the discourse on human enhancement and the larger project of transhumanism, for, if as argued herein, we likely lack the capability to stop human enhancement, then much of the debate and hand-wringing over whether we should try to stop it becomes an academic exercise. The issue becomes simply when, not whether, human enhancements occur once they have proven to be technologically feasible.

Any effective restrictions on human enhancement are likely to rely on the legal system to adopt and enforce such prohibitions. While nonlegal measures such as social norms, religious doctrines, or funding restrictions may also slow or hinder the development of human-enhancement technologies, these measures are unlikely to stop such development permanently in the absence of enforceable legal proscriptions. Accordingly, this chapter begins with an exploration of the effectiveness of law in restricting human behavior generally and the factors that may modulate the effectiveness of laws. This exploration focuses on some specific examples where law has sought to restrict certain behaviors that may be analogous to attempts to prohibit human enhancement. Next, data on public opinion on human enhancement are canvassed, since, as argued below, any significant beachhead of support for enhancement is likely to be destabilizing for any legal restrictions and will tend to push much of the population toward enhancement. This is followed by a discussion of some additional problems that will limit the effectiveness of any attempt to enforce legal restrictions on the process. Finally, the regulatory irony of trying to stop enhancement is presented – human-enhancement technologies will flourish to the extent they are shown to be safe and effective – yet safeguarding the safety and efficacy of enhancement technologies is the one function that regulatory oversight can, and should, aspire to achieve. Accordingly, the one form of useful regulation of human enhancement that the law can offer will have the overall effect of promoting the process.

Legal Attempts to Control Human Behavior

A primary function of law is to control and change human behavior. As one legal scholar has written, "[O]ne thing is irreducibly clear: at its most basic, every legal system exists to effect some change in human behavior. That is, law is a lever for moving human behavior" (Jones 1997, 167). Over time, our society has increasingly resorted to the law to modify, regulate, or channel human behavior, a trend sometimes referred to as "legalism," as the authority and power of other social institutions to control human behavior has diminished (Callahan 1996). Accordingly, any effective attempt to prohibit or restrict human enhancement will inevitably need to be based in the law. While ethical inducements, religious dictates, social norms, and individual self-restraint can play some role in resisting the temptation of enhancement, these forces are unlikely to stem human enhancement unless leveraged by enforceable legal proscriptions.

To be sure, the influence of law on modifying human behavior goes beyond simple command-and-enforcement models in which citizens comply with the law only because they fear being caught and punished for violation. The direct threat of enforcement and sanctions *does* compel at least some compliance with laws, as evidenced by the sudden slowing of drivers on a highway as they approach a police car or speed radar post along the highway. But it is also true that many people comply with laws when there is little or no chance they would be caught or sanctioned for noncompliance (e.g., littering and pooper-scooper laws). In these situations, it is the expressive and internalization functions of law that modify behavior, as government action to proscribe a particular action conveys a message to its citizens, which is often internalized, that such actions are socially unacceptable. This expressive and internalization function can operate both by internal individual responses based on feelings such as guilt and self-esteem and by the threat of second-order sanctions in the form of peer disapproval and public shaming (Scott 2000).

Not all types of human behavior are equally controllable by law, either by the direct threat of enforcement or the expressive and internalization functions of law. The dynamics, incentives, and pressures associated with human enhancement suggest that this will be a type of human behavior that will be particularly difficult for law to control. In particular, two aspects of human enhancement will make this activity especially intractable to control through law. First, the public is less likely to comply with laws that restrict behaviors that are perceived as ethically acceptable notwithstanding their illegality. Second, law is challenged to control actions that might give an individual a competitive advantage. These two factors are elaborated below.

Controlling Ethical Behaviors

Legal rules are most effective in modifying behavior when normative beliefs run parallel with the legal requirements (Ellickson 1987). Law will, therefore, often be least effective in controlling human behavior when it tries to restrict behaviors that are not perceived as unethical or otherwise normatively objectionable. In such contexts, the expressive and internalization functions of law will provide little or no leverage for compliance. Rather, compliance will be based solely on avoiding being caught and sanctioned, which then places a heavy burden on designing and implementing a credible and robust enforcement system that can detect and take action against a substantial proportion of violations. Of course, the interaction of law and norms is dynamic not static, and the publicity and expression of lawmaking can help create or modify norms over time (McAdams 1997). Examples include laws against littering and smoking in public, which have helped to shape social norms to conform to legal expectations. Yet the leverage of law to shift norms still depends on convincing individuals that an action is wrong. Passing a law that says an action is unlawful can help, particularly if a person's perceptions are neutral or weak. But if an individual feels strongly that an action is morally permissible, laws that seek to prohibit such actions tend to be ineffective in bringing about both changes in norms and behavior.

A paradigmatic case in point is the recent ineffectiveness of legal sanctions to control illegal downloading of music and other materials from the Internet in violation of copyright law. A large proportion of the population does not view such downloading as unethical, likely because downloading materials from the Internet does not impose any direct physical costs on the content provider, given that the marginal cost of an addition digital copy is zero. Of course, this view does not take into account the consequences of failing to pay content providers with regard to the costs and incentives to produce original content in the first place; rather, this perception somewhat unrealistically views the creation of content as a given and then considers only the marginal cost of making an addition copy of that content. Despite attempts by content providers to instill a more systemic understanding of the consequences of illegal downloading, public opinion has barely budged on this issue, and most people continue to believe that unauthorized downloading of copyrighted material is ethical (Freestone and Mitchell 2004).

In an attempt to deter copyright infringement, in 2003 the Recording Industry Association of America (RIAA) began filing thousands of lawsuits against individual file sharers. This aggressive legal campaign was aimed at educating music fans about the law and encouraging them to turn to legal music-downloading websites. Although the number of lawsuits filed to date is inexact, commentators believe that it swelled from 261 lawsuits in 2003 to around 30,000 by 2007 (EFF 2008). However, critics questioned this legal campaign's overall effectiveness, as the popularity of peer-to-peer (P2P) file-sharing networks seemed to continue to rise with time. Although surveys administered just after the campaign started show that it slightly discouraged people in downloading music illegally, more recent surveys demonstrate that such effect was only transitory (Bridy 2009). In fact, although the RIAA lawsuits may have motivated some consumers into using authorized music downloading Web sites – such as iTunes Music Store or Amazon.com – the reality is that the effort to eradicate illegal file trading through these lawsuits fell short and that the RIAA eventually discontinued its litigation campaign. One analysis summarized the results:

> [T]he number of downloads sold to date continues to pale when compared to the number of files swapped over P2P networks. The recording industry's own international industry group, the IFPI, estimated in 2008 that there were 20 unauthorized downloads for every legitimate download purchased – in other words, as of January 2008, 95% of all digital music downloads were from unauthorized sources. In short, all of the authorized music services together do not yet amount to a drop in the digital music downloading bucket. (EFF 2008)

If anything, these lawsuits have moved people to look continually for alternate means – the so-called darknet solutions – to circumvent copyright protections. For example, the use of new file-sharing software that protects the identity of uploaders, or even swapping iPods with friends, may prove to be convenient ways for music lovers to share their files in violation of copyright laws without the risk of being sued. Naturally, with the ready availability of means to circumvent copyright protections, any legal model focused on limiting people's rights over their music will probably prove unsuccessful. Such has been the experience in the U.S. Evidently, the law cannot effectively regulate music file sharing or downloading unless society, in general, starts viewing such behavior as morally unacceptable.

Competitive Advantage

Another signpost of behaviors that are difficult to control using the law is behaviors that provide a competitive or evolutionary advantage to the actor. It has been suggested that "[l]aw will encounter resistance that varies according to the strengths of evolved predispositions to those behaviors that law may attempt to regulate" (Jones 1997, 172). It is, therefore, important that laws not be "misforged at the outset by ignorance of human dispositions in thought and behavior. Effective law must be vigilant and attentive to what people do. What people do will be influenced by what they and their ancestors have done over thousands of years" (Rodgers 1993, 75). As Margaret Gruter has written, "The effectiveness of law will be proportional to the degree to which the function of a particular law complements the function of the behavior that the law intends to regulate" (1991, 21).

Evolved behaviors such as seeking competitive social (hence, indirectly reproductive) advantage and particularly the drive not to be left behind by other members of the community ("keeping up with the Jones") are one of the most entrenched and unbendable human instincts. Thus, attempts to restrict individual attempts to better oneself and one's immediate family members, especially with techniques that have been demonstrated to be safe and effective and are being used successfully by others, are likely to be ineffective.

An acute example of this dynamic is the type of hoarding, looting, and other antisocial behaviors that occur in times of crisis or emergency. Citizens who are otherwise law abiding are often observed to engage in illegal or proscribed activities in situations where they believe they may be severely disadvantaged or threatened by staying within the law (Gostin and Berkman 2007). This tendency toward lawbreaking is exacerbated by evidence that other citizens are engaging in the prohibited actions, igniting competitive tension that results in a cascade effect (Lang and Lang 1976).

From this brief discussion of factors influencing noncompliance with law, it is evident that a law that tries to prevent citizens from engaging in activities (e.g., such as human enhancement) that are perceived as ethical and that give adopters a competitive social advantage is likely to be very difficult to enforce. While implementing such an unenforceable law may have some benefit in pushing social mores toward the law's objective, this benefit does not come without social cost. Thus, while the legal prohibition on alcohol in the United States from 1920 to 1933 did reduce alcohol consumption, it had other corrosive effects: "It encouraged criminality and institutionalized hypocrisy. It deprived the government of revenue, stripped the gears of the political system and imposed profound limitations on individual rights" (Okrent 2010, 373). Similarly, while the recent legal strategies to crack down on illegal downloading of music has had some minor effect in deterring such actions, this legal heavy-handedness has also imposed significant social costs:

> [T]he single certain consequence from this battle has been one our government is strangely oblivious to: its rendering a generation criminal. A concerted campaign ... has convinced kids that their behavior violates the law. But that law breaking continues. We call our kids

> crooks; after a while, they believe it. … They get used to being criminal. This fact is deeply corrosive. As with prohibition, it is profoundly corrupting. And over time, it will only weaken our kids' respect for the law. (Lessig 2008)

Laws prohibiting human-enhancement actions that are otherwise safe and effective would seem to fit this dynamic – very hard if not impossible to enforce because enhancement technologies will be seen by many both as ethically acceptable and also as providing competitive advantages (including competitive disadvantages for those who do not partake). Accordingly, the experience and knowledge we have gained about why people obey laws suggest that antienforcement laws may have limited effectiveness but significant corrosive effects for respect for the law.

Public Demand for Enhancement

Public opinion and personal preferences are critical factors affecting the feasibility of controlling human behavior regarding enhancement. If even a minority of the population believes that enhancement is ethical and/or advantageous, some of those individuals will almost certainly pursue such enhancement. Should that enhancement prove to be safe and effective, other members of the population less inclined to pursue enhancement will be tempted to follow suit to avoid being left behind. In this sense, human-enhancement technologies are likely to be destabilizing, in that successful enhancement by some individuals in some countries is likely to spark a cascading demand for similar enhancement by competitors at either the individual or national level (Gardner 1995). Recent public-opinion polls suggest that a sufficient subset of the population will be inclined to engage in available enhancement, thereby setting in motion the cascade of enhancement.

For example, in 2004 the Genetics and Public Policy Center at Johns Hopkins University published the results of a comprehensive survey of the public's perceptions of reproductive genetic technologies – including those that could be used for purposes of enhancement, such as prenatal genetic diagnosis (PGD) (Genetics and Public Policy Center 2004). While there was strong public support for using prenatal genetic testing to screen out or prevent serious childhood diseases, there was much less support for the use of reproductive genetic technologies to select for "socially desirable traits such as intelligence, strength, or hair and eye color" (ibid. 16). Nevertheless, more than one-quarter of the respondents did favor using prenatal genetic testing to select for such traits, creating a wedge of the population that might be willing to experiment with enhancement technologies, which, if successful, would likely lead to much larger portions of the population to follow suit. In fact, three-quarters of the survey respondents agreed or strongly agreed with the statement "Technology will inevitably lead to genetic enhancement and designer babies" (ibid. 17).

A *Time*/CNN poll found that 25 percent of Americans supported the use of genetic engineering to improve a person's physical appearance, while 34 percent favored using this technology to improve a person's intelligence (Elmer-Dewitt 1994). A public-opinion survey by Virginia Commonwealth University in 2003 found that 37 percent of respondents were somewhat or very likely to use gene therapy to try to extend their lives. A survey by *Nature* found that 20 percent of respondents to an online survey took a cognitive-enhancing medication without a prescription and that one-third of respondents said that they would feel pressured to give these drugs to their children if other children were using them (Maher 2008). Further evidence of the latent demand for enhancement technologies can be seen by the use of off-label cognitive-enhancing drugs such as Provigil, Ritalin, and Adderall by college students, which appears to already occur in 5-15 percent of college students and seems to be increasing rapidly, apparently already exceeding 25 percent of students at some colleges (McCabe 2004; Schermer et al. 2009).

In summary, technologies to enhance characteristics that are not related to treatment of disease enjoy some degree of popular support, although not to the same extent as health-related enhancements. There will almost always be some initial volunteers who will, out of curiosity or ambition, try any available enhancement technology, regardless of how low the prospects of success (Baylis and Robert 2004). All it takes is a relatively small number of initial adopters to try the enhancement technology, and, if it succeeds, interest and support will quickly snowball. Indeed, taking a look at the different enhancements available today, one can perceive the increasing public acceptance that these technologies enjoy. Botox, cosmetic surgery, and dietary supplements, among many others, are all examples of common enhancement technologies that now enjoy a wide acceptance, even though not all of them are used for health-related purposes. That being so, it follows that future enhancement technologies will be favored with the same kind of public demand, especially if pertinent authorities found them to be safe and effective. As the *Economist* predicted in its "Genomics" column (2010), "Thirty years ago the qualms felt by some about in-vitro fertilization melted in the face of the first gurgling child born using the new technology. The same is likely to happen for the first 'enhanced' human, assuming the gurgling is happy."

Additional Challenges for Potential Legal Restrictions on Human Enhancement

In addition to the problems described above, a number of additional challenges would make prohibiting biomedical human enhancements remarkably difficult.

For example, most enhancement technologies will likely result from attempts to develop treatments for legitimate health problems, an undertaking that would be politically difficult, and perhaps ethically unacceptable, to try to stop. Second, how would the government monitor illegal biomedical enhancements? It is likely that an effective strategy for monitoring and enforcing compliance with restrictions on human enhancement would unduly intrude on and burden individual freedom. Third, any national attempt to restrict human enhancement could easily be circumvented by many citizens by going abroad for such enhancement. Finally, attempts to restrict human enhancement might run afoul of constitutional limitations on governmental powers, particularly in the U.S. These four additional challenges are elaborated below.

The Therapy/Enhancement Linkage

Human-enhancement technologies will emerge, at least initially, under the guise of unobjectionable attempts to address human suffering and loss due to legitimate health conditions (Mehlman 2009). Oft-cited examples include the development of neural implants to give quadriplegics the capacity to communicate that will also open the door to neural enhancements; the development, testing, and regulatory approval of cognitive-enhancing drugs to treat conditions such as Alzheimer's disease; and the perfection of human genetic manipulation to treat serious genetic diseases that can then be applied to genetically enhancing human attributes. It is likely to be politically and ethically infeasible on humanitarian grounds to stop the development of such dual-use technologies. Putting aside the difficulty of distinguishing therapy from enhancement, trying to ban enhancement applications while allowing legitimate therapeutic applications of the identical technology to proceed would likely represent an unacceptable governmental intrusion into the practice of medicine.

In the U.S., the Food and Drug Administration (FDA) has traditionally stated that it has no authority under the law to regulate the practice of medicine and that such regulation would contravene the legislative history and spirit of the Food, Drug and Cosmetic Act the agency administers (Adams et al. 1997). Off-label use of approved drugs – which refers to the prescription of pharmaceuticals for uses other than those approved by the FDA – falls within what constitutes the practice of medicine. As a result, it is not unlawful for medical practitioners to prescribe drugs for purposes other than those approved and stated on the label of the product. In implementing this policy, the FDA recognizes that, once a drug is approved, the discovery of new uses is conceivable and that those new uses are often useful or even necessary in healthcare delivery (Adams et al. 1997). Today, modern drugs approved for legitimate therapeutic purposes are being used off-label as a means of enhancement.

For example, the drug Provignil (modafinil) – approved by the FDA for the treatment of narcolepsy and excessive sleepiness caused by shift work or obstructive sleep apnea – is used by a growing number of healthy people allegedly to improve cognitive performance (Repantis et al. 2010; Schermer et al. 2009; Turner 2008; Turner et al. 2003). If future biomedical enhancements are derived from medical products or therapies approved for legitimate medical purposes, as is likely to occur, the FDA will lack authority to restrict their usage for enhancement purposes under current law (Markwood 2005; Schermer et al. 2009).

Enforcement and Monitoring

Effective enforcement of prohibitions or restrictions on human enhancement would be difficult if not impossible. Enforcement would likely focus, at least initially, on the supply side against the providers of enforcement technologies, whether they be genetic therapies, neurological implants, or cognition-enhancing drugs. Because many of these products would have legitimate health applications, they could not be banned outright but would need to have their use restricted. The limits and challenges of such an enforcement strategy are demonstrated today by the widespread availability of drugs such as Adderall and Ritalin to college students, whereby college students can and easily do obtain such restricted prescription drugs, approved by the FDA for prescription for attention deficit hyperactivity disorder (ADHD), over the Internet or from black-market sources (McCabe 2004; Schermer et al. 2009). Even for products that are banned outright, including drugs such as marijuana, cocaine, and heroin, the so-called war on drugs has been frustrated by noncompliance and the limited success (and some would argue outright failure) of supply-side enforcement.

Ultimately, effective enforcement of a ban on enhancement would likely require not only prohibitions, monitoring, and sanctions on the providers of enhancement technologies but also similar enforcement techniques against the consumers of enhancement – i.e., individual citizens. This issue of enforcement and monitoring is especially unsettling. Suppose for a moment that the government eventually has access to the necessary technology to detect illegal biomedical enhancements in people. This kind of detection will most likely pry into people's private lives and decision making (Mehlman and Rabe 2002). As has been persuasively argued, enhancement enforcement against individuals would invoke "big brother" concerns:

> We would have to endure testing whenever we competed – at school, at work, and ... at home. Moreover, because the positive effects of enhancements might persist after the use of enhancements ceases ... testing would have to take place on some schedule "outside of competition" – in other words, during our private lives. (Mehlman 2009, 152)

The need for vigorous governmental surveillance of biomedical enhancements is not at all farfetched. In fact, we may find an analogous example in current antidoping surveillance programs to which Olympic athletes are subjected (Mehlman 2009). In the U.S., for example, it is required for Olympic athletes to submit reports to authorities about their daily schedules and subject themselves to surprise antidoping tests at any time (ibid.). While these kinds of programs are premised on the principle of fair competition, to what extent will a ban on biomedical enhancements justify the government's intrusion into the general public's private life? Moreover, how likely would the public tolerate such intrusions?

International Complexities

Another problem becomes apparent when one takes into account the difficulty of enforcing a ban in an increasingly globalized world. If the U.S., in the long run, decided to ban human enhancement technologies, it would most likely promote the rise of black markets, as well as the development and use of enhancements abroad (Bostrom and Sandberg 2009). It would likely be infeasible to screen out enhancement products imported illegally into the U.S. or to stop people who decided to enhance themselves or their offspring in more permissive foreign jurisdictions from returning to the country. The cost of implementing such a prohibition, along with the possibility of foreign countries being willing to endorse or at least turn a blind eye toward enhancement practices within their jurisdiction, certainly reduces the chances or effectiveness of a ban on enhancement practices at the national level (Mehlman 2009). Of course, one alternative would be to try to implement an international prohibition, but such an undertaking would be extremely challenging if not infeasible, as the cooperation of all countries may be impossible to obtain (Baruch et al. 2005).

Constitutional Limits

Constitutional provisions, particularly in countries such as the U.S. with strong constitutional restrictions on government powers, may further impede any attempts to prohibit human enhancement (Glahn 2003). State and federal courts have widely recognized that the right of privacy is one of the major fundamental constitutional rights in the United States (Roe 1973). In particular, the protection of this right extends to the personal choices a person may make regarding life activities, such as marriage, procreation, and child rearing, among other intimate decisions (Glahn 2003; Loving 1967; Pierce 1925; Roe 1973; Skinner 1942).

Whenever government regulations threaten to hinder the exercise of fundamental rights, courts shall review such legislations under what has been termed the strict scrutiny test (*Attorney General* 1986). In essence, this requires the state to demonstrate two things, namely, that there is a compelling state interest and that the state is employing the least restrictive measure to further such interest (*Roe* 1973). Accordingly, the state must justify its intrusion into people's fundamental rights by showing that it furthers a countervailing interest and that there are no alternative mechanisms of lesser impact (ibid.).

A ban on biomedical enhancements would undoubtedly need to endure strict scrutiny, as it would arguably involve a governmental intrusion into people's fundamental rights. For instance, a law that prohibits the use of assisted reproductive technologies to enhance children genetically may in effect interfere with the parents' fundamental rights of privacy, reproductive freedom, and procreation (Mehlman 2009). As such, the government must have a compelling state interest to justify its intrusion on these rights and prohibit the birth of genetically enhanced children. This, of course, is open to question. On the one hand, courts may find that the government does have such a compelling state interest if there are concerns regarding the health and safety of enhanced children or if there is a strong showing that society is likely to suffer substantial harm (Markwood 2005). On the other hand, it can easily be argued that, even if these technologies were found to be somewhat risky, competent adults should be able to choose whether they wish to assume those risks, without governmental intervention. As one analysis recently concluded, "For the government to deny parents the right to provide their children with the best possible starting point and, instead, force them to rely upon random chance would be more than a bad policy choice – it would be an unconstitutional infringement of a fundamental right" (Glahn 2003).

Solutions?

The factors discussed above suggest that enforcement of any restrictions or prohibitions of human enhancement will necessarily be imperfect. Imperfect enforcement alone does not disqualify a legal intervention, as no law is completely enforceable and as even nonperfect compliance can result in beneficial reductions in the frequency of a disfavored behavior (Fukuyama 2002). For example, prohibiting the illicit sale and possession of heroin is generally (although not universally) considered a beneficial policy, even though it is obvious that some individuals will continue to sell, buy, and possess heroin illegally. Even the prohibition on alcohol in the U.S. in the 1920s, largely regarded as a failed and unenforceable policy, was partially successful in its intended purpose of reducing alcohol consumption (Okrent 2010).

Imperfect enforcement of human enhancement invokes a different dynamic, however, one that is unstable and will inevitably tumble toward widespread use of any safe and effective enhancement technology. At the individual level, successful enhancement by one's peers, competitors, or even neighbors will create a growing pressure to engage in similar enhancements to "keep up", even if one was initially disinclined to engage in such enhancement (Gardner 1995). The more people give in to this pressure, the stronger will grow the pressure on the remaining hold-outs. Even if some individuals resist to the end, a substantial proportion of the population will have undertaken the enhancement. The same phenomenon will occur at the international level between nations, as successful enhancement by some populations will create growing pressures on competing or adversarial nations to follow suit. This dynamic has been described as a "cascade slope," a stronger and more dramatic form of the slippery slope (Gardner 1995).

Banning biomedical enhancements based on the perceived perils that these technologies could pose to patients and society may, thus, be unwise and ill-founded. Such a legal strategy is bound to fail. Moreover, overinclusive regulations would certainly encroach on the autonomy of those who wish to be enhanced and have the capacity to consent and assume the risks of these procedures. Equally persuasive is the fact that paternalistic regulations intended to prohibit or limit human enhancements, based primarily on perceived unproven harms rather than strong scientific data, would certainly interfere with medical research and medical practices that could prove beneficial in the long run.

Rather than shielding the development and use of enhancements altogether and in order to protect those who wish to be enhanced, a wiser approach would be for the government to assure that these technologies are, in fact, safe, effective, and used ethically (Greely et al. 2008). In this way, the government would not only be respecting people's autonomy and freedom of choice, but it would also be fostering the use of safer enhancements. This could, in turn, reduce the motivation for black markets and the dangers of people getting enhanced in more permissive foreign countries.

In effect, government resources would be better spent – and societal costs reduced – by regulating, rather than prohibiting, enhancement technologies. Given that existing regulatory schemes may not be adequate to monitor human biomedical enhancements effectively and in view of the plausible risks they represent, a more sensible approach would be to tailor regulations to assure the safe and ethical development of these technologies (Mehlman 2009; Schermer et al. 2009). Of course, by ensuring that enhancement technologies are safe and effective, government regulation would have the net effect of encouraging human enhancement.

References

Adams, David G., et al. 1997. *Fundamentals of Law and Regulation: An In-Depth Look at Therapeutic Products*. Washington, DC: Food and Drug Law Institute.

Attorney General of New York v. Soto López, 476 U.S. 898. 1986.

Baruch, Susannah, et al. 2005. Human Germline Genetic Modification: Issues and Options for Policymakers: http://www.dnapolicy.org/images/reportpdfs/HumanGermlineGeneticMod.pdf, accessed July 14, 2011.

Baylis, Francois, and Jason S. Robert. 2004. The inevitability of genetic enhancement technologies. *Bioethics* 18: 1-26.

Bostrom, Nick, and Anders Sandberg. 2009. Cognitive enhancement: Methods, ethics, regulatory challenges. *Science and Engineering Ethics* 15: 311-41.

Bridy, Annemarie. 2009. Why pirates (still) won't behave: Regulating P2P in the decade after Napster. *Rutgers Law Journal* 40: 565-611.

Callahan, Daniel. 1996. Escaping from legalism: Is it possible? *The Hastings Center Report* 26: 34-35.

Electronic Frontier Foundation (EFF). 2008. RIAA v. the people: Five years later: http://www.eff.org/riaa-v-people, accessed July 15, 2011.

Ellickson, Robert C. 1987. A critique of economic and sociological theories of social control. *Journal of Legal Studies* 16: 67-99.

Elmer-Dewitt, Philip. 1994. The genetic revolution: New technology enables us to improve on nature. How far should we go? *Time Magazine*, January 17.

Freestone, Oliver, and Vincent-Wayne Mitchell. 2004. Generation Y attitudes towards E-ethics and Internet-related misbehaviours. *Journal of Business Ethics* 54: 121-28.

Fukuyama, Francis. 2002. How to regulate science. *The Public Interest* 146: 3-22: http://www.nationalaffairs.com/public_interest/detail/how-to-regulate-science, accessed July 15, 2011.

Gardner, William. 1995. Can human enhancement be prohibited? *The Journal of Medicine and Philosophy* 20: 65-84.

Genetics and Public Policy Center. 2004. Reproductive genetic testing: What America thinks: http://www.dnapolicy.org/images/reportpdfs/ReproGenTestAmericaThinks.pdf, accessed July 15, 2011.

Genomics [column]. 2010. No hiding place. *Economist*, June 19-25, S15-16.

Glahn, Jason C. 2003. I teach you the superman: Why Congress cannot constitutionally prohibit genetic modification. *Whittier Law Review* 25: 409-39.

Gostin, Lawrence O., and Benjamin E. Berkman. 2007. Pandemic influenza: Ethics, law, and the public's health. *Administrative Law Review* 59: 121-76.

Greely, Henry, et al. 2008. Towards responsible use of cognitive-enhancing drugs by the healthy. *Nature* 456: 702-5.

Gruter, Margaret. 1991. *Law and the Mind: Biological Origins of Human Behavior*. Newbury Park, CA: Sage Publications, Inc.

Jones, Owen D. 1997. Law and biology: Toward an integrated model of human behavior. *Journal of Contemporary Legal Issues* 8: 167-208.

Lang, Kurt, and Gladys E. Lang. 1976. Planning for emergency operations. *Mass Emergencies* 1: 107-17.

Lessig, Lawrence. 2008. Don't make kids online crooks. *U.S. News & World Report*, December 29: 15, http://www.allbusiness.com/crime-law/criminal-offenses-cybercrime/12210243-1.html, accessed July 15, 2011.

Loving v. Virginia, 388 U.S. 1. 1967.

Maher, Brendan. 2008. Poll results: Look who is doping. *Nature* 452: 674-75.

Markwood, Sarah M. 2005. Creating a perfect human is not so perfect: The case for restricting genetic enhancement research. *Pennsylvania State Law Review* 110: 473-92.

McAdams, Richard. 1997. The origin, development, and regulation of norms. *Michigan Law Review* 96: 338-433.

McCabe, Sean E. 2004. Non-medical use of prescription stimulants among U.S. college students: Prevalence and correlates from a national survey. *Addiction* 100: 96-106.

Mehlman, Maxwell J. 2009. *The Price of Perfection: Individualism and Society in the Era of Biomedical Enhancement*. Baltimore, MD: The Johns Hopkins University Press.

Mehlman, Maxwell J., and Kirsten M. Rabe. 2002. Any DNA to declare? Regulating offshore access to genetic enhancement. *American Journal of Law and Medicine* 28: 179-213.

Okrent, Daniel. 2010. *Last Call: The Rise and Fall of Prohibition*. New York: Scribner.

Pierce v. Society of Sisters, 268 U.S. 510. 1925.

Repantis, Dimitris, et al. 2010. Modafinil and methylphenidate for neuroenhancement in healthy individuals: A systemic review. *Pharmacological Research* 62: 187-206.

Rodgers, William H. 1993. Where environmental law and biology meet: Of pandas' thumbs, statutory sleepers, and effective law. *University of Colorado Law Review* 65: 25-75.

Roe v. Wade, 410 U.S. 113. 1973.

Schermer, Maartje, et al. 2009. The future of psychopharmacological enhancements: Expectations and policies. *Neuroethics* 2: 75-87.

Scott, Robert E. 2000. The limits of behavioral theories of law and social norms. *Virginia Law Review* 86: 1603-47.

Skinner v. Oklahoma, 316 U.S. 535. 1942.

Turner, Danielle. 2008. Cognitive enhancement in the pharmacy. *The Pharmaceutical Journal* 280: 691-93.
Turner, Danielle C., et al. 2003. Cognitive enhancing effects of Modafinil in healthy volunteers. *Psychopharmacology* 165: 260-69.
Virginia Commonwealth University (VCU). 2003. VCU life sciences survey: http://www.vcu.edu/lifesci/images2/survey2003.pdf, accessed July 15, 2011.
World Transhumanism Association (WTA) (now Humanity+). 2003. Transhumanism FAQ: What is Transhumanism: http://humanityplus.org/learn/trans humanist-faq/#answer_19, accessed July 15, 2011.

Part III:
Transhumanism and the Human Person

Transhumanist Materialism: A Critique from Immunoneuropsychology

Steven A. Hoffman

Transhumanism can be viewed as an ideology, a philosophic view, and a technological agenda. Transhumanism insists that we ought to go beyond our current human condition. Presumably, we ought to be prepared for the drastic evolution of the human to a species as far removed from us as we are from the great apes. Accordingly, we have a responsibility to assist in this evolution and we should use nanotechnology and biotechnology, including genetic engineering, artificial intelligence, and neurocognitive technologies to enhance the human, eventually leading to the posthuman phase. The agenda of transhumanism is to eliminate disease, improve our physical capacities, enhance intelligence, improve our emotional condition, create a happier society for all, and ultimately eliminate aging. In the words of one of the transhumanist Web sites,

> Transhumanism is a loosely defined movement that has developed gradually over the past two decades. It promotes an interdisciplinary approach to understanding and evaluating the opportunities for enhancing the human condition and the human organism opened up by the advancement of technology. Attention is given to both present technologies, like genetic engineering and information technology, and anticipated future ones, such as molecular nanotechnology and artificial intelligence. The enhancement options being discussed include radical extension of human health-span, eradication of disease, elimination of unnecessary suffering, and augmentation of human intellectual, physical, and emotional capacities. (Bostrom 2003)

By focusing on nanotechnology, biotechnology (including genetic engineering), neurocognitive technologies, and artificial intelligence to enhance human attributes, transhumanism seeks to generate a new phase of human development: the posthuman. Allegedly, the posthuman phase will constitute a utopian society (or "extropian", according to one strand within the transhumanist discourse).

I argue that we ought to be cautious about transhumanism when it is viewed as an ideology, be critical of its philosophical views, and watch it carefully as a technological agenda. The transhumanist approach is problematic because it is both materialistic and reductionistic, thereby failing to understand the complexity of being human. Transhumanism overemphasizes the materialistic sciences at the expense of values that the material sciences fail to explain, values that only the humanities express or grapple with. Moreover, the transhumanist agenda is based on a reductionist conception of science that privileges molecular and cellular techniques, employing technological tools to advance the human condition. This shortcoming makes the transhumanist vision inherently inadequate either as an analysis of the human condition or as a scenario to improve it.

One young field of scientific inquiry has the ability to go beyond such a reductionistic approach – immunoneuropsychology (INP). INP goes by many different names, including psychoneuroimmunology, neuroimmunomodulation, neuroimmunology, alternative or complementary medicine, and the like. It focuses on integrating immunology, psychology (including social and cultural dimensions), and neuroscience (including neuroendocrinology) for the purposes of basic scientific understanding and medical practice. Thus, INP is able to bridge between the molecular/cellular, reductionistic sciences and the humanistic approach.

This paper claims that INP is a useful vantage point from which to critique transhumanism, as well as overcome its limitations. It begins with a brief explanation of INP as a distinctive scientific subfield. With a better understanding of INP, the paper examines the concept of happiness that is so central to the transhumanist project. Even though most transhumanists do not devote much attention to the concept of happiness, it is fair to say that many take for granted that "technology has … a great capacity for making people happier" (Sotala 2007). The chapter presents INP as an alternative, more adequate understanding of human well-being than transhumanism. Since all reflections on happiness necessarily use the concept of the self, the chapter then proceeds to analyze this concept in transhumanist discourse, exposing its reductionist assumptions. In short, INP not only offers a critical vantage point from which to expose the inadequacies of transhumanism, but it also provides a better theoretical framework within which to integrate the natural sciences, the social sciences, and the humanities.

Transhumanism as Reductionistic Materialism

The transhumanist program for human enhancement is based on advances in bioengineering, nanotechnology, information technology, and neuroscience. Bioengineering and nanotechnology seek to engineer living systems; they do so mainly through manipulation of genes. Whether or not they intend to improve a given organ or system, these technologies, in fact, alter the organism to which they are applied. In humans, biotechnology and nanotechnologies are used for the purpose of eliminating a particular disease. For example, severe combined immunodeficiency, which is deadly, can be eliminated by altering a single gene. Of course, very few diseases have single-gene etiologies. Furthermore, biotechnology can also be used to improve the functioning of more complex characteristics, but this would require manipulating multiple genes and understanding their interactions with their environment, which is currently well beyond our abilities.

The leading transhumanist, Max More, makes it clear that this is indeed the intent of transhumanism. On his Extropy Institute Web site, he says, "Extropy entails strongly affirming the value of science and technology. It means using practical methods to advance the goals of expanded intelligence, superior physical abilities, psychological refinement, social advance, and indefinite life spans. It means preferring science to mysticism, and technology to prayer. Science and technology are indispensable means to the achievement of our most noble values, ideals, and visions and to humanity's further evolution" (More 2003).

The morality, social soundness, and efficacy of More's agenda, particularly in the area of enhancing complex characteristics, has been thoroughly debated (Fukuyama 2002; Garreau 2005; Stock 2003), but I do not wish to focus on these much-discussed issues. Instead, I wish to expose the reductionistic and materialistic underpinning of transhumanism, precisely because it solely endorses biotechnology. I argue that transhumanism posits a reductionistic and materialistic conception of being human and that this view is philosophically untenable and scientifically unfounded. By "reductionistic" is meant here the view that everything, including psychological and social phenomena, can be explained in terms of more fundamental concepts and entities, eventually down to the level of chemistry and physics. This goes along with a materialism that says there is really nothing else in the world except these fundamental particles, energies, and entities of chemistry and (ultimately) physics. That is, all entities (including emotions and all mental and social phenomena) are made up of these fundamental constructs. This is the view behind the sciences and technology advocated by the transhumanists. I do not mean to say that transhumanists do not deal with ethical and societal issues. The recently published volume by Savulescu and Bostrom (2009) indicates that transhumanists are fully aware of such criticisms but that they are unable to address these critiques adequately. Precisely because transhumanists understand the human being as a bundle of molecular and cellular complexes, they welcome biotechnologies. There is nothing else to enhance, according to this view, other than the molecular/cellular and technological aspects of the human. All the problems of humankind can be addressed by mere technological advances, to the exclusion of social and cultural dimensions. Biotechnology accomplishes many good things and can bring about good results. Yet transhumanism is misguided in its approach to the development of human beings and the future of humanity because there is more to the human than molecules and cells. Advocates of transhumanism fail to see this simple but crucial point.

When we focus on making humans smarter by increasing the release of specific neurotransmitters, like dopamine, so that they can stimulate specific pathways in the brain, we are focusing on the molecular level. Most current cognitive enhancers work by increasing attention span and focus on task, rather than increasing "intellectual" abilities. We are trying to improve learning or memory or attention by manipulating the molecular interactions in a physiologic system, as if there were nothing to human intelligence besides these molecular and cellular processes. This brings us back to the age-old philosophic problem of trying to understand the relation between mind and body (Bunge 1980; Carruthers 2004; Chalmers 1996; P. M. Churchland 1984; P. S. Churchland 1986; Clayton 2004; Damasio 1994; Descartes 1641; Feigl 1958; Flanagan 1984; Schwartz and Begley 2002; Smart 1963). The attitude is equivalent to saying that human minds are nothing over and above neurophysiological processes or, more abstractly, information-processing systems (independent of the actual material substrate). This attitude is fundamentally materialistic (i.e., there is nothing over and above the material) and reductionistic (i.e., intelligence, wisdom, happiness, etc., can be reduced to neurophysiologic processes or, ultimately, physical and chemical processes).

Let's take the case of human happiness. Bostrom and Sandberg (2009, 395) say that "evolution has not optimized us for happiness." Rather, it has led to mechanisms that contribute to psychological distress and frustration. Bostrom and Sandberg argue that this may have been adaptive at one point in our evolutionary history but now leads only to human suffering and reduces our well-being. They say that "an intervention that caused an upward shift in hedonic set-point, or that down-regulated some of these negative emotions" could be beneficial in our current times (396). Bostrom and Sandberg's statement, however, makes sense only against a very specific understanding of happiness (and suffering), which they do not disclose. This view can be easily identified as a form of hedonism. So, what exactly is happiness? Is it simply a matter of shifting some set-points by manipulating some cellular and molecular interactions in the brain? This is assumed to be the case, based on a mechanistic view of the human and happiness, but this is unlikely to be the best view of happiness. Below we will point out the materialistic and reductionist underpinnings of transhumanism, reducing happiness to a set of molecular and cellular reactions in the brain.

Another transhumanist goal is immortality or approximating it as much as possible either biologically through radical life extension or cybernetically through the uploading of human consciousness into supercomputers. Radical life extension could presumably be attained if we bioengineer ourselves so as to eliminate disease (which by itself would only increase lifespan by a few years) and eliminate the molecular mechanisms of aging. Cyber immortality could be achieved through downloading our minds into powerful computers. As in the case of happiness, the transhumanist goal of immortality attests a mechanistic, materialistic understanding of the human that fails to grasp the complexity of the human organism. By the same token, transhumanism takes a reductionistic and materialistic approach to human cognition because it identifies the mind with brain processes. The advocates of cyber immortality do not explain how the mind can be downloaded into a computer, and it is very unlikely that this is doable. But whether this is doable or not, we first need to inquire if this is in principle desirable. Does this program offer us an adequate conceptualization of the human self? I reject the transhumanist program because it fails to grasp the complexity of the human self and the interplay between physiological and nonphysiological factors.

We shall now show how psychoneuroimmunology avoids the reductionistic materialism of transhumanism by offering us a much more sophisticated understanding of the human self. By juxtaposing transhumanism and psychoneuroimmunology, we will be more aware of the inadequacies of transhumanism, on the one hand, and offer a richer and scientifically more accurate notion of the human "self" and of human happiness.

INP – Beyond Materialistic Reductionism

Immunoneuropsychology is the relatively young scientific discipline that integrates immunology, neuroscience (including neuroendocrinology) and psychology (Ader et al. 1991, 2006; Fabris et al. 1994; Schedlowski and Tewes 1999; Siegel and Zalcman 2009). It goes by other names, including psychoneuroimmunology, psychoneuroendocrinimmunology, neuroimmunomodulation, and the like. The new discipline is related to neuroimmunology, but the latter is a more traditional medical discipline, focusing on neuroimmunologic diseases like multiple sclerosis and myasthenia gravis (Raine 1988). Both INP and neuroimmunology, however, deal with understanding the interactions between the nervous and immune systems, so there is a good amount of overlap.

Like traditional neuroimmunology, INP is interested in how the immune system can alter normal nervous-system functioning. Whereas in neuroimmunology the focus is on pathology and how these interactions can lead to mental or neurologic diseases, in INP the focus is on normal physiologic functioning and how the nervous and immune systems communicate with and modulate one another. There is also a focus on pathology in INP. For example, how does stress impact the immune system and health? It is now well known that chronic stress can have detrimental effects on the immune system and one's health (Kemeny and Schedlowski 2007). Some of the molecular and cellular mechanisms that underlie this have also been elucidated (N. Cohen 2006; Irwin 2008; Zalcman and Siegel 2006).

In addition, the focus in INP is not just on neuro-mmune interactions but on the interaction between the nervous (endocrine) and immune systems in relation to psychosocial factors. That is, the psychological, social, and cultural side of the equation is brought into play. Immunoneuropsychologists address questions like

(1) How do psychosocial factors impact the immune system and health? (2) How does our immune system influence our mental functioning? (3) What are the molecular and cellular mechanisms by which the nervous and immune systems interact with one another (both pathologically and physiologically)? These, of course, generate other subquestions. For example, under (1) we might consider the following questions: (a) How do the negative emotions, moods or states, like stress, depression, and anxiety, affect the immune system? (b) Do the different negative emotions affect the immune system in the same way? (c) Do positive emotions have an impact on the immune system, independent of their ameliorating effects on the negative emotions?

There is certainly a healthy materialist and reductionistic foundation to INP. As question (3) above shows, there is a good deal of interest in the molecular and cellular mechanisms underlying INP. This is the difference between INP and similar but older fields of study such as psychosomatic medicine. The research questions here get into identifying the mechanisms by which the nervous system and the brain in particular can modulate the immune response. If these interactions are physiologic, then the nervous system must "know" what it is doing, that is, the immune system must signal the brain as to its current state. Thus, a good deal of research must be devoted to the immunological signaling mechanisms.

Since INP studies the relation between mind, brain, and immunity, it would seem obvious that there would be some philosophical discussions with regard to the relation between mind and body. Unfortunately, there has not been a lot of discussion on the philosophical foundations of INP. Philosophically it is possible to identify several positions as the foundation of INP. A large number of these INP researchers would probably categorize themselves with those thinkers who view mind as materialists and reductionists, saying that the mind is nothing more than brain or its computational functions (P. M. Churchland 1984; P. S. Churchland 1986; Damasio 1994; Dawkins 2006; Dennett 1978, 1991; Monod 1972; Pinker 1997; Sagan 1977; Smart 1963). As long as we can understand the molecular and cellular interactions between the nervous and immune systems, that is all we can establish with respect to how mind, brain, and immune system are related. Other INP researchers would argue that this leaves out the psychological underpinnings of the field, not to mention the social and cultural milieu within which psychological processes take place, that the psychological, social, and cultural ingredients are equally important as the molecular and cellular interactions. In fact, it would seem that a purely reductionist attitude would eliminate the "psychology" in INP and eliminate a lot of the questions outlined above.

The uniqueness of INP is the integration of the mechanistic, molecular, and cellular underpinnings of science with an equal focus on the human being, within a sociocultural milieu. The trick will be in how best to understand this integration philosophically. A pure materialistic identity theory, which says that mental events are nothing over and above brain processes (P. M. Churchland 1984; P. S. Churchland 1986; Place 1956; Smart 1963), or epiphenomenalism, which says that mental events arise from brain processes but cannot have an effect on anything (Huxley 1874), would both seem to be inadequate. They say either that there are no psychological states or that they are inefficacious and that psychological states play an important causal role in INP. Those positions that would seem to be consistent with INP include the following:

- neutral identity theory (or dual aspect theory), which argues that mind and brain are identical (they are two aspects of the same thing) but identify each with some third entity (Broad 1925; Spinoza 1677) rather than one side of the identity or the other, i.e., brain (as in materialism) or mind (as in idealism)
- interactionistic dualism (Chalmers 1996; Descartes 1641; Popper and Eccles 1977) which says that mind and brain both exist and causally interact with one another.
- some form of complementarity, which says that neurophysiological and psychological interpretations of human phenomena are mutually exclusive, depending on the experimental conditions for trying to understand that phenomena but that both are necessary for a complete understanding of our world (Bohr 1943, 1958; Hoffman 1975)
- emergentism, which states that consciousness arises out of more fundamental processes, viz., neurophysiological yet can also affect those more fundamental processes (Broad 1925; Clayton 2004; Schrodinger 1967)
- a functionalist account (Flanagan 1984), which says that mind is a functional concept, either causing or being caused by something (consistent with INP as long as it doesn't eliminate the mental)

Which of these views is best as a foundation for INP is, however, open to debate.

Not only do we have to understand the molecular and cellular interactions between the immune and nervous systems, but we also have to understand the influence of psychosocial factors. Stress can impact the immune system and health. For example, one study found that a delayed type hypersensitivity (DTH) response was reduced in distressed subjects (Smith et al. 2004). This is the simple skin test used in allergy testing which is known to be a consequence of cell-mediated immunity. In another interesting study, subjects in a tandem parachute jump (first-time jumpers) showed effects on their natural killer cells (Schedlowski et al. 1993). In this particular case, the stressor is considered something positive (eustress), although still stressful. How do we want to understand these examples? We can use a materialistic identity theory, where we would say that "distress" is simply certain brain processes, which, in turn, caused the cellular phenomena associated with the reduced DTH. Of course, this leaves out distress and its role in human life. That is, the subjective experience of distress, or eustress, is irrelevant here. This seems to miss the point of INP research.

In INP research, we ask (among other things), "What impact does stress have on the immune system and health?" Additionally, stress is a human phenomenon where factors other than corticosterone and norepinephrine release come into play. Stress is also dependent on the individual. What is stressful for one person may not be stressful for another. In addition, the context of the situation is important, as well as the cultural milieu. What is stressful in one society may not be stressful in another. How we treat stress in one society may be inadequate in another. This is where the human dimension becomes important, and this dimension is necessarily culturally and socially embedded. No reduction to molecular and cellular interactions can possibly explain stress or deal with its consequences.

For example, studies show that disclosure, i.e., writing or talking about one's traumatic experiences, can be beneficial to health and boosts the immune system (Petrie et al. 1995). One study (Esterling et al. 1994) showed that Epstein-Barr virus viral capsid antigen (EBV-VCA) antibody titers significantly decreased following a verbal or written disclosure session, while subjects talking about trivial events showed no changes. The most effective immune response to a viral infection is usually a cell-mediated response (as opposed to a humoral, antibody, response). Thus, when antibodies to a virus increase, this is generally viewed as detrimental, indicating a less effective antibody response or reactivation of the virus. The decrease in EBV-VCA antibody titers following the disclosure intervention suggests a beneficial response of the immune system. A similar intervention was shown to have a beneficial effect on human immunodeficiency virus and T cell response (Petrie et al. 2004). It would seem that such an intervention is culture-dependent. That is, in a well Westernized society, the disclosure of one's innermost thoughts and feelings might be beneficial. What, however, would occur in another society, perhaps one in which talking about ones' inner thoughts and feelings was taboo, or potentially dangerous, because black magic could be used against the individual if such things were known. Talking or writing about one's life traumas might be traumatic in itself, and the impact on the immune system might be opposite of what Esterling and colleagues found in their study. The impact of culture on psychosocial interventions and the immune response has to be better developed (Wilce 2003). When we are talking about the social and cultural dynamics that affect this situation, we are going beyond a simple discussion of molecular and cellular interactions.

In addition to exploring how psychosocial factors influence the immune system and health, we should note that the reverse is also taking place. That is, we have to examine how our health, via the immune system, impacts our mental life. It is well known that immunologic dysfunction can affect the brain, leading to neurologic and psychiatric disorders, as in diseases like multiple sclerosis, myasthenia gravis, and systemic lupus erythematosus (Hoffman and Sakic 2009). In addition, there are many studies showing how the immune system communicates with the brain (Siegel and Zalcman 2009). Thus, the immune system may affect mental functioning to a greater extent than what is normally believed. We must keep in mind that stress and negative emotions may not only impact the immune system and health but that our immune status may make individuals more or less susceptible to these same negative emotions and stress. Stress may contribute to the genesis, or exacerbation, of a disease like lupus or rheumatoid arthritis, but the immunologic events going on (independent of the fact that an individual has a chronic condition) in these autoimmune states may also contribute to his or her emotional status (Miller 2010). There is even research showing that we may be able to vaccinate against depression (Lewitus et al. 2009). Not only has it been shown that the immune system can affect our emotional states, but it can also affect our cognitive functioning (Brynskikh et al. 2008; Hoffman et al. 1998; Palumbo et al. 2010; Shatz 2009)!

INP must also go beyond the negative emotions and stress and ask the question of how a variety of emotions interact with the immune system. For example, do positive emotions impact the immune system and do they do it independently of the negative emotions. Positive events may affect the immune system and health by simply counteracting the negative impact of the negative emotions. There is evidence, however, that positive emotions have their own impact. The effect of the positive emotions or states is not clear cut. For example, the influence of optimism is a complex one. Some research has shown it has a positive effect on the immune system, while other research does not (Segerstrom 2005). More recent research suggests the effects of optimism depend on the situation (Brydon et al. 2009). Positive affect has also been shown to depend on the situation. Normally, positive affect is thought to play a protective role in health, by suppressing an inflammatory response, and preventing its deleterious effects (Prather et al. 2007). During cancer therapy, however, positive affect was found to correlate with markers of inflammation (Sepah et al. 2009). This may be because, during cancer, an enhanced inflammatory and cell-mediated immune response may be important for combating the disease, as well as eliminating the dead and dying tissue that is a consequence of the therapy.

The current happiness research featured in the *Journal of Happiness Studies* has done a lot to explore the influence of positive emotions on health (Cohen and Pressman 2006; Steptoe et al. 2009). INP research goes beyond this by looking at the impact on the immune system, as well as the underlying molecular and cellular mechanisms (Brydon et al. 2009; Marsland et al. 2006; Prather et al. 2007;

Segerstrom 2005; Sepah and Bower 2009; Von Ah et al. 2007). Indeed, to make progress in this area, we have to understand what exactly "happiness" is and how we wish to define and study it. When talking about studying the influence of happiness, we must also consider the possibility of studying the virtues and whether they have an impact on health via the immune system. Let me explore these issues in some detail.

Transhumanists focus on the sciences and technology in improving humanity, but their focus on genetic engineering, nanotechnology, and neuroscience fails to deal with the complexity of being human. I argue that only if we have a broader understanding of the human, as offered by the discipline of INP, can we reach the proper perspective on the molecular and cellular functions of the human organism. There may be other research disciplines that can offer a similar integration of humanistic perspectives and mechanistic science, but there is probably not a lot. In order to have a complete view of the human, and adequately understand how the human can be enhanced, we must go beyond the transhumanist goal of simply using the reductive, materialistic sciences and integrate this with more humanist perspectives. This is something INP can do. Let me illustrate this point in regard to the concept of happiness, one of the main goals of transhumanism.

Happiness: Beyond Hedonism

Attaining happiness is a major goal of the transhumanist project. Yet the transhumanist discourse does not provide us with a sufficiently deep analysis of its understanding of happiness. What does it mean for a human being to be happy? How will posthumans be happy in a way that humans are not? What will happiness mean in a posthuman society, and does the concept at all apply to an environment that will be radically different from ours? To date, transhumanist thinkers have promised happiness, but they have not offered an analysis of their conception of that state. They have not answered the question "Why should we pursue transhumanism if our future will not be a happier one?"

For transhumanism, technological enhancement of the human is the path toward happiness. Since transhumanists equate happiness with feeling good, it is no surprise that their happiness is secured through the use of chemical substances: "A cornucopia of drugs will soon be on sale to improve everything from our memories to trust in others" (Edmonds 2009). This extensive use of drugs to control moods leads Max More (2003) to promote Extropy as "practical optimism": "Extropy entails espousing a positive, dynamic, empowering attitude. It means seeking to realize our ideals in this world, today and tomorrow." Going further, More states, "Living vigorously, effectively, and joyfully, requires prevailing over gloom, defeatism, and negativism." Furthermore,

> [p]ractical optimists question limits others take for granted. Observing accelerating scientific and technical learning, ascending standards of living, and evolving social and moral practices, we can project and encourage continuing progress. Today there are more researchers studying aging, medicine, computers, biotechnology, nanotechnology, and other enabling disciplines than in all of history. Technological and social development continue to accelerate. Practical optimists strive to maintain the pace of progress by encouraging support for crucial research, and pioneering the implementation of its results. (More 2003)

In "Transhumanist Values", Nick Bostrom (2001) explores this point further:

> In contrast to many other ethical outlooks, which in practice often reflect a reactionary attitude to new technologies, the transhumanist view is guided by an evolving vision to take a more proactive approach to technology policy. This vision, in broad strokes, is to create the opportunity to live much longer and healthier lives, to enhance our memory and other intellectual faculties, to refine our emotional experiences and increase our subjective sense of well-being, and generally to achieve a greater degree of control over our own lives.

Eliminating or reducing diseases is certainly a worthy goal and would seem to make for a happier future for humanity. Improving replacement limbs or body parts would also seem to be beneficial. Improving memory, intelligence and cognitive functioning would also seem to be worthwhile … or would it? Can we simply manipulate neural wiring or brain functions to "increase our subjective sense of well-being" – i.e., create a happier person? This is where we start getting into a morass of complexity and confusion. When we start manipulating mental function, it is not that straightforward as to what must be done or what the consequences may be. We do not have a clear idea of what intelligence is or, specifically, how to improve it. There are currently "smart drugs" that assist in enhancing cognitive performance, including focusing attention, improving memory, and enhancing creativity (Stix 2009). These drugs are, however, far from perfect, not always doing what they are supposed to do. They may also come with unforeseen consequences, as has been seen with memory enhancement in mice (Tang et al. 1999; Lehrer 2009), such as an increase in pain sensitivity. Nonetheless, the genetic manipulation to wire the brain for enhanced performance is a long way off.

Perhaps we can simply make people happier, or "increase our subjective sense of well-being," through the use of the appropriate drugs; certainly, we can combat depression by using antidepressants. If we can better understand the neurochemistry of pleasure and happiness, then we could use genetic engineering techniques to rewire the brain, allowing individuals to have a propensity toward happiness. There are many arguments for and against such drug-induced forms of happiness or genetically engineered rewiring of the brain. For example, Arthur Caplan believes that the arguments against enhancement of our brains to allow for happiness or satisfaction are ill conceived: "We do not have to 'earn' our happiness to be really and truly happy" (2009, 207). The trouble with most of these arguments, both pro and con, is that we haven't examined the concepts involved. What kind of sense does it make to say that we can make individuals happier through the use of drugs or genetic enhancement? The only sense for a materialistic view, as described above, is a hedonic one, which is the basis of the transhumanist view of happiness. These views have been previously critiqued (Tirosh-Samuelson 2007).

Clearly, part of the problem in this debate is conceptual and pertains to the definition of terms. It is not my purpose here to engage the actual definitions of *happiness*, since that would take another full paper (or several) and has been partially done by others (e.g., see Haybron 2000, 2007a, 2007b); rather, my purpose is simply to point out this deficiency and discuss some of the questions involved. For example, what is happiness, and how will we know if we are achieving it? Will increasing our subjective sense of well-being be consistent with happiness? There are currently studies underway to investigate happiness and its impact on one's health and well-being (Allmark 2005; Barak 2006; Chida and Steptoe 2008; Ryff et al. 2004). What exactly are these happiness researchers studying? When you look at the literature, you can see there are different definitions and ways of measuring happiness. The debate about transhumanism must have a better understanding of happiness, or well-being, to be able to quantify it in some reasonable way. So far, scientists and philosophers have not collaborated sufficiently close in happiness research. When they do begin to collaborate, it will become clear that there is no consensus on definitions of happiness and that quantifying them to measure human happiness is quite difficult. Most of the research utilizes hedonic views of happiness, although one or two discuss utilizing eudaemonic definitions. Ryff et al. 2004 compared eudaemonic with hedonic definitions and found that the former more closely associated with biological and immunological markers of improved health. Nonetheless, definitions of hedonic, or eudaemonic, well-being, or happiness, differ from study to study and should be analyzed critically. We could go farther in discussing the philosophic underpinnings of existing research, but this would again take us far beyond the purpose of this paper. Suffice it to say that this should be done and that philosophers should be helping these researchers come up with clearer and more appropriate definitions of happiness. Conversely, happiness researchers should be testing the various definitions to give some feedback to the philosophers concerning the best definitions in terms of human behavior and health. Most philosophers would insist that empirical findings would be useless in conceptualizing happiness and trying to figure out what it is. This may be the case, but it would seem that knowing which definitions (after being operationalized) are best at contributing to health and well-being would be important in deciding which theories of happiness are best. There are some philosophers who feel that an interchange between philosophers and scientists would be beneficial. Nancy Snow (2008) has argued that empirical findings can contribute to a better understanding of happiness. Philosophers could give more rigor to the definitions of *happiness* being used, while the researchers could compare those different views based on their relation to immunological markers and health.

We have said that happiness researchers should pay attention to what philosophers are saying with respect to happiness. This is, of course, easier said than done, since there are many different philosophical views about happiness. Two of the major positions derive from hedonism and eudaemonism. Modern-day forms of hedonism originate largely with Jeremy Bentham (1789) and John Stuart Mill (1863), emphasizing pleasure. It is probably the predominant ethical view of modern times. As an ethics, it focuses on the ends achieved. That is, what is right should be based on the results of an action. It utilizes the principle of utility (utilitarianism), which says act so as to maximize the resulting good. The "good" is defined in terms of pleasure, although there are many variants on what is pleasure, from physical pleasures to mental ones. Happiness is maximizing our pleasure, or subjective well-being. In contrast to the utilitarian approach to happiness, Aristotle (d. 344 BCE) articulated what is known as the eudaemonian conception of happiness. Here, happiness is not defined simply in terms of pleasure but rather in terms of self-actualization of the inherent human function to reason. Reason defines the distinctive mark of humans and actualizing that capacity through the study of philosophy enables humans to attain their end (*telos*). The end of human life could be attained only if one acquires and cultivates the virtues, namely, the character traits that enable one to perform "just right": to act in the right manner, for the right reason, not too much and not too little. Aristotle distinguished between moral and intellectual virtues and the relationship between these sets of virtue is complex; but in the eudaemonian approach to happiness, pleasure does not constitute human well-being. Rather, it is the contemplation of God, the Unmoved Mover, which is the ultimate end of human life. A person cannot be happy without being virtuous (although one can be virtuous without being happy).

As Snow emphasizes, according to the eudaemonist thesis, "there is a kind of deep and enduring happiness that is impossible without virtue" (2008, 225). She points out that this thesis can be viewed as either a conceptual or empirical one. As a conceptual thesis, if counterexamples to the connection between virtue and happiness can be convincingly made, then the thesis is disproved. Alternatively, as an empirical claim, it is about whether an individual's happiness is dependent on virtue. For example, the impact of a virtuous life on one's biomarkers and health can be studied. Snow argues that the thesis is, to a large extent, an empirical one and that there are psychological studies that confirm the importance of the eudaemonist interpretation of happiness.

I do not wish to debate the merits of hedonism versus eudaemonism but rather to note that there are several disputed conceptions of happiness. Transhumanism proposes to create a better and happier human being (although this may not be the end-stage of the posthuman) without examining what the concept of happiness means. With its focus on genetics, nanobiology, artificial intelligence, and neuroscience, there is a gaping hole where happiness could be examined. If transhumanism included in its scientific agenda INP, then perhaps it could avoid this deficiency.

Transhumanist vision, however, could help advance INP. The field should include in its research an exploration of happiness and the virtues and the relationship between human health and well-being. This is being done to some extent with respect to happiness, but only serendipitously with respect to the virtues. Remember that INP studies how psychosocial factors can influence the immune system and health, as well as how the immune system can influence psychosocial dynamics. Most of the former research has focused on the negative emotions, particularly stress. Recent research has realized the deficiency and has started focusing on the positive emotions, including happiness (Marsland et al. 2006; Segerstrom 2005; Von Ah et al. 2007; Ryff et al. 2004). As we discussed above, there is some research that has shown that positive emotions, or events, can have an independent impact on the immune system and our health (Chida and Steptoe 2008; Steptoe et al. 2009). There are also some researchers who are investigating the impact of happiness and are also thinking about what is happiness and how to measure it (Ryff et al. 2004). There should, however, be more interaction between philosophers and these researchers.

Daniel Haybron (2007a) illustrates how philosophy can enrich the field of happiness studies. He has shown the inadequacy of the concept of "life satisfaction" in happiness research by arguing that philosophers can help inform scientific psychological research by evaluating the constructs and instruments they use for quantifying concepts like happiness. Haybron (2000) has closely examined the concept of happiness and its relation to empirical research, focusing on how psychological research uses the construct of happiness in comparison to philosophical notions, as well as offering his ideas on what that notion of happiness should be for this kind of research. This interaction between philosophical analysis and scientific research is a direction that should be further pursued. He has also argued against an objective, Aristotelian virtue, or perfectionist account of well-being (Haybron 2007b), opting for a subjective component, although not against the importance of the perfectionist view in the bigger scheme of things of the good life. In any case, a consensus of two or three definitions of *happiness* should be developed by humanists and scientists, for the purposes of utilizing and testing the definitions. Immunoneuropsychologists and psychologists should then operationalize these definitions, so that instruments measuring these senses of happiness can be developed. After a period of empirical testing, for the purposes of seeing how happiness influences the immune system and health, the adequacy of the definitions should be evaluated. In addition, the different views of happiness behind these definitions should be compared based on the empirical findings. There should be at least a comparison of eudaemonic and hedonic theories of happiness (based on the appropriate definitions). Which of these has the greatest impact on the immune system and health? If a hedonic view has the greatest impact, then this may be telling us that this view is superior to the eudaemonist view. The opposite may be true, or there may be features of both views that impact our health and well-being. In this last case, it may be important to generate a hybrid of the two. For example, it has been suggested that purpose in life is important in health and well-being (McKnight and Kashdan 2009). In any case, in this way science may contribute to the conceptualization of happiness. It should not go unattended that, during this entire process, humanists should be analyzing the validity of the constructs being used by scientists. Thus, the process should be a continual movement, or dialectic, back and forth between the humanities and the material sciences.

When the concept of happiness is incorporated into INP research, it brings to the fore the concept of virtue, since they are closely tied to theories of happiness. In INP research, the key question is not just how negative and positive emotions can influence the immune system and health but all psychosocial influences. Eudaemonism argues that the virtues are important to the well-being of individuals. If true this would imply that the virtues should have an impact on the immune system and health. This can (and should) be tested. So far, only one INP study (Gouin et al. 2008) has addressed the notion of the virtues. Its purpose was not to test the impact of the virtues on the immune response but rather to study stress. Inadvertently, the authors studied one virtue – or rather one vice, namely, anger – and found that the ability to regulate the expression of an individual's anger had an impact on the rate of wound healing. In addition, as reported, this effect was independent of negative emotions, social support, and health behaviors. Individuals with lower anger control were slower wound healers. This ability to control one's anger can be considered a virtue. Thus, we are seeing an example of how the virtues could be studied in INP.

So far, we have emphasized the fact that determining the happiness of an individual is not an easy task, both from a conceptual and empirical perspective. I argue that when transhumanists discuss enhancing the subjective well-being of an individual, they should seek greater precision in their understanding of happiness. The simplistic, materialist/reductionist notion of happiness that underscores the transhumanist discourse is simply inadequate. How does one determine what happiness is purely from the interactions of molecules and cells? Only if we consult the rich traditions preserved by the humanities, can we begin to address this question. Conversely, the humanities alone are unable to fathom the meaning of human happiness, without proper attention to the natural sciences that study how the human body actually functions. This essay argues, therefore, that only if we combine the humanities and the natural sciences can we begin to fathom the meaning and depth of human happiness. The new discipline of INP offers us such integration.

The Self: Beyond Mind

Transhumanism argues that the human species as it currently exists will have to be transformed and even transcended by the posthumans. But what is the posthuman? The word *post* implies that that the posthuman will simply be a more evolved being that will overcome the limitations of the human. But it is not clear in what way such a species will be human. Does the posthuman being constitute a different species? If so how could the human and posthuman be compared? Will the posthuman really be an improvement on the human, and if so, in what ways? There is no way to answer these questions without some understanding of what it means to be human, but to do so, it is necessary to examine the concept of the "self." What is it that characterizes the essence of being human? We generally refer to this as the self, or, more broadly, the person. The self refers to those essential characteristics of a person that make that person unique (Braude 2005; Harle 2007; Olson 2007; P. F. Strawson 1959; G. Strawson 1997; Teichert 2004). Will the posthuman be a person – will it have a self? This question is especially pertinent since transhumanism envisions a machine-human interface as part of the posthuman future. Does that interface fit into our understanding of self or person? Western philosophers have debated the meaning of *self* (Perry 1975): some have identified it with the mind (Descartes 1641), others with the brain (Ramachandran and Hirstein 1997; Ramachandran 2003), and still others with the body (Shoemaker 2008). Others have characterized the self by denying its existence or importance (Hume 1739).

The dominant position has been to identify the self with the mind. Galen Strawson (1997) says that the Self is a subject of experience, a mental thing. Two of the current major views of personal identity are animalism and neo-Lockeanism, respectively, the views that persons are human animals or are identified by psychological continuity (Olson 2007; Shoemaker 2008). The animalism view is basically a bodily view of self, while neo-Lockeanism is a mental view. Both are consistent with materialism, particularly (in the case of neo-Lockeanism) if we maintain that psychological continuity is realized in the brain. The transhumanists tend to advocate such a view:

> A more radical kind of upgrade might be possible if we suppose a computational view of the mind. It may then be possible to upload a human mind to a computer, by replicating *in silico* the detailed computational processes that would normally take place in a particular human brain. Being an upload would have many potential advantages, such as the ability to make back-up copies of oneself (favorably impacting on one's life-expectancy) and the ability to transmit oneself as information at the speed of light. Uploads might live either in virtual reality or directly in physical reality by controlling a robot proxy. (Bostrom 2011)

This views the self as mind, which is really just the brain or the information processing going on within the substrate of brain. We can upload ourselves to a computer because the self is simply mind. Is the view that self is mind (or the brain) an adequate view? Many seem to think so (Ramachandran and Hirstein 1997; Ramachandran 2003; Shoemaker 2008; G. Strawson 1997).

The science of immunology also investigates the self: in order for an effective immune response to take place, the immune system must distinguish between self and nonself. If the immune system cannot do this, then a pathologic autoimmune reaction takes place, and the immune system starts destroying the very organism it is designed to protect. It has been argued by some immunologists and philosophers (Silverstein and Rose 1997; Matzinger 1998; Pradeu and Carosella 2006) that the self paradigm in immunology is misleading. They feel that there is no immunological self: there are only danger signals, which determine whether an immune response will be made. The concept of danger signals is a useful one in immunology, but it should be asked, "What is the danger in reference to?" The danger has to be with respect to someone or something. In other words, there is danger only because a self can be exposed to that danger. Thus, danger signals only make sense within the context of a self.

It would seem that an immunological concept of self would be a substance-oriented one, i.e., a thing or object, within the confines of materialism. But analysis of the immunological self reveals that it is not a substance-based view. In immunology, one of the first views of self is that the major histocompatibility complex (MHC) constitutes self (Tauber 1994). The MHC is a set of genes that codes for immunologically important proteins. There is so much diversity within this gene complex that virtually every person has a different MHC type. Identical twins, of course, will have identical MHC. These genes determine whether a transplant will be accepted or rejected. If the transplant (e.g., skin, heart, etc.) comes from a person who is genetically identical at the MHC gene loci to the recipient, then the transplant will be accepted. If the MHC genes are different between the donor and recipient, then the graft will be rejected, plus, the closer the match, the better the chances of graft acceptance. In addition, there is a phenomenon within immunology known as "MHC restriction." Simply put, this is the idea that, in order to generate an immune response, the immune system has to recognize antigen (foreign molecules) within the context of self MHC! Without the foreign molecules being presented by (cells bearing) self MHC, no immune response is generated. This is a form of tolerance or nonresponsiveness to an antigen.

The above can lead some to identify (immunological) self with MHC. One problem, of course, is that MHC cannot uniquely individuate persons. As mentioned, identical twins have identical MHC, but they are different persons. Plus, their immune systems develop differently, based on their respective environments and experiences. The most important problem is that MHC does not fully explain the phenomenon of an immune response and tolerance to self. There are receptors on cells of the innate immune system, which include phagocytic and antigen presenting cells such as macrophages, which recognize conserved molecular configurations on pathogens (i.e., nonself), such as bacteria and viruses. These receptors help to activate the innate immune system, forming a first line of defense, contributing to the maintenance of the integrity of the individual. These receptors bind to nonself (pathogens) and eliminate these microorganisms. This is one, very primitive, view of self (Medzhitov and Janeway 1997), based on a strict substance view. There is no knowledge of self, only of other. This is an extension of the MHC view, but is itself still incomplete.

In order to generate an appropriate immune response, without a pathologic autoimmune reaction, we need a variety of other signals, such as cytokines and costimulatory receptors, within the context of the appropriate cellular interactions. The point is that it is not simply recognition of some simple substances that determines whether an immune response will be generated but rather a complex set of interactions within an environmental context. For example, the MHC molecule is never seen by itself but is always seen (by the T cell and its receptor) as a complex of MHC plus antigen (as peptide). The T cell (receptor) will then either recognize this complex and bind to it or not. If it binds, then a signal will be sent into the T cell, but this is still not enough to activate the T cell (and the immune response). Activation is also dependent on costimulatory signals, delivered by other receptors. The process we are describing can now be seen to be a complex, dynamic one, involving learning what self is by the system, for whether the T cell will recognize the antigen is dependent on a maturation process immunologists call "positive/negative selection." This is the process whereby T cells are selected so that they can recognize self MHC, in order to be able to generate an immune response, without recognizing self antigens that would generate a pathologic response to self. This is basically a learning-and-weeding out process for the T cells. In positive selection, thymocytes (maturing T cells) learn to recognize self MHC. If they cannot recognize self MHC, then they are eliminated since they would not be able to generate an immune response and are useless. In negative selection, thymocytes that react against antigens (molecules) that are found in the body are destroyed since these would mature to become T cells that would react against self and generate an autoimmune disease. There are exceptions, it is currently thought that some self-reactive thymocytes are allowed to mature and become regulatory T cells, which are involved in regulating an immune response, some of which prevent autoimmune disease. Thus, there are actually self-reactive cells of the immune system whose role is to protect against destruction of self by the immune system.

Notice that the above is a dynamic process of learning, as well as defining, what is self. It is not just a static concept of self, based on certain substances of the body, like MHC, or self antigens, because the self is always changing. Plus, the concept of self is not just defined within these central mechanisms of positive/negative selection (in the thymus or bone marrow for B cells), by eliminating auto-reactive lymphocytes. There are also important mechanisms outside these central organs, in the periphery (e.g., lymph nodes, spleen, mucosal tissue) that help to prevent a destructive autoimmune response, such as the regulatory T cells (which themselves are autoreactive). These peripheral mechanisms are equally important in defining the immunologic self. The key concept is that the immune system is dynamic and integrative. The distinction between self and nonself is not a clear one. The immune system must recognize self (viz., MHC) in order to generate a response to nonself, and it can only recognize self (antigen) by recognizing other. That is, the immune system does not really see self (except for MHC, or in the case of regulatory T cells), since the self reactive lymphocytes are (for the most part) eliminated, but *in not seeing self, it knows self.* In order to know nonself (other), the immune system must know self (foreign antigens must be presented by self MHC) and, paradoxically, in order to know self, the immune system must be able to recognize other (the immune system only responds to other). The distinction between self and nonself becomes even more blurred when we consider another concept of immunology.

For the most part, the above theories view autoreactivity as pathologic. That is, there ought to be no response made to self, and the immune system goes through elaborate processes to prevent such a response. As we have seen, however, this is not totally correct: there are autoreactive cells that are physiologic and help maintain a healthy balance in the immune response. One example is the regulatory T cell. There are also current theories about the beneficial effects of some autoreactivities. These are the theories that focus on natural autoantibodies, arguing that autoreactive cells and antibodies are a natural component of the immune system, which plays an important role in regulating normal functioning (I. Cohen 1991; Poletaev and Osipenko 2003), as opposed to the classical views that autoreactivity is a threat to the survival of the organism. These theories originate from network theory (Jerne 1974), which talks about a network of autoreactive interactions within the immune system that are regulatory. One of the key concepts from this is that of idiotypic interactions. That is, the generation of an antibody response will result in an antibody response against the original antibody. These are called anti-idiotypic interactions, which are known to exist. According to network theory, these kinds of antiself interactions will eventually result in equilibrium, bringing the system to a new steady state. What is debated is the significance of these interactions and whether they are regulatory. One of the theoretical consequences of these idiotypic interactions is that of "internal image." This says that, for every antigen in the external universe (i.e., outside an individual), there is a corresponding internal image within the person. What this implies is that, for everything in the external world, there is something in the internal system that looks the same. This means that autoreactivity is the rule, rather than the exception! It also means that, immunologically speaking, *there is little or no distinction between self and nonself (at least from a substance view)!*

Initially, it might be thought that this view eliminates the distinction between self and nonself. What has actually happened, however, is that it has transposed the view of self from a substance-oriented one to a dynamic one. Self must no longer be viewed in terms of antigens (molecules) and what they look like, but rather in terms of a dynamic equilibrium. Self must be defined in terms of the network of interactions and the ever-changing states of equilibrium in which the system finds itself. This is not only a consequence of network theoretic and natural autoantibodies views but of the immunologic views that have been developing since MHC as self.

This information implies that a substance view of self is inadequate. What is suggested here is that the *self* not only refers to the psychological concept of Self, viz., the "I" of introspection, but to the immunological locus of self as well. Both the psychological and the immunological concepts of self are equally important. The psychological concept of Self only identifies one aspect of the self. It focuses on the thoughts, feelings, and plans of the individual. Another way to identify an individual is via the immune system. It does it in a way which is different from simply pointing to a person's body, as might have been thought to be the case when thinking about immunology. It views the self as dynamic and complex. If the immune self, which is apparently bodily, cannot be adequately accounted for by a wholly substance view, then it is unlikely that the psychological Self can be. We cannot simply identify self with body, or for that matter, with brain or brain processes. For the same reasons, we cannot identify Self with some incorporeal, spiritual entity. The psychological and immunological are two necessary aspects of the self (there are likely others). The implications for the transhumanist views are obvious.

The above is not as farfetched as it might at first seem. There is good evidence from INP that the psychological and immunological are mutually interdependent (Hoffman and Sakic 2009; Siegel and Zalcman 2009). As already discussed in the first section, psychosocial processes (e.g., stress, anxiety, mood) can affect immune-system functioning and one's health. Conversely, a change in one's immunological functioning can affect one's psychological functioning. This state of affairs points to an inextricable interweaving of the immunological, neurophysiological, endocrinological, psychological, and social. We can no longer view the immune system as a strictly material system, disconnected from the psychological and cultural, but must view them all as integrated.

The self is not a substance, whether material or immaterial. This also means that the self is not primarily identified with the mental. The predominant transhumanist view that the human is primarily identified with reasoning and, since it is a materialist philosophy, with the brain, or computational processes, can no longer be viewed as adequate. We cannot download the brain into a computer and assume the Self is continuing since it's only part of the original self. We may be able to download the contents of the brain into a computer, although Barry Ritchie in this volume has given us good reasons to doubt that this will occur in the near future, if ever; but whatever the results it would be very different from the original self and the human.

I am more than just my mind. I am also my athletic ability, my musical and artistic talents, and my immune system integrated into a complex physiological system that interacts with its external environment to create a unique individual. What does this imply for the human? It implies that the essence of the human is more than just rationality. The human is also an athletic creature, capable of participating in sports and competitions; it is also a game-playing creature, a musical creature, an artistic creature, an emotional creature. The essence of the human is an antiessence, i.e., it is the diversity of that which is unique in the creature known as "human." The posthuman might be homo-exquisitus, or beyond that cyber-immortalus – of course, what this means remains to be seen – but will that creature have some of what makes humans unique? Certainly, posthumans will have rationality, since that is a focus of transhumanists, but this in itself is not the human.

Beyond the implications of the above for the self and the human, it should also be kept in mind that the immune system combats disease and is one of the major factors in influencing our life spans. Insofar as a major goal of transhumanism is life extension, it will have to take into account the progress of immunology. It will be the ability of immunologists to understand and manipulate the immune system, so that it can better combat infectious diseases and tumors and eliminate immunologic disorders (like autoimmunity and immunodeficiency), which will play a major role in extending our life span, as well as improving our quality of life. As can be seen in the above, to a good extent, this will entail being able to manipulate individual immune systems, since each one is unique, just like the self.

Conclusion

The transhumanist commitment to the betterment of humanity is laudable to the extent that it seeks to alleviate pain and suffering. We must not quench the desire to improve the human condition through biotechnology, as transhumanism calls on us to do, but we must not believe naïvely that the material sciences, and by extension technology, can accomplish the betterment of humanity. Rather, we must turn to the humanities (especially the disciplines of philosophy and history) and the social sciences (especially the discipline of psychology) to forge a richer and deeper understanding of being human. This paper has shown how the new discipline of INP provides a good model for integrating the reductionistic, natural sciences and the humanities. First, the reductionistic nature of transhumanism was emphasized and how this makes it one-dimensional with respect to a propaedeutic for the future of humanity (and beyond humanity). Next, the nature of a relatively new scientific discipline, INP, was elucidated, with the intention of showing how this science can be both materialistic and humanistic. More of a focus on the future of disciplines such as this could help transhumanism move away from its reductionistic underpinnings. Leading transhumanists such as Bostrom and Sandberg (2009) indicate that they understand the point because they discuss immunology, stress, and the placebo effect and how the latter might be used for enhancing the human. The placebo effect is in the domain of INP research (Kemeny et al. 2007). A better understanding and elucidation of INP in the transhumanist agenda might allow for a better appreciation of the necessity for humanistic perspectives in charting out a course for the future.

The problems of an adequate conceptualization of happiness and the self were the next two topics to be explored with respect to INP and transhumanism. The reductionistic attitudes of the latter, and the sciences they emphasize, are inadequate to deal with these two important elements of a human (or posthuman) future. Immunology and INP, if developed properly, are designed to handle these ideas. We cannot simply tweak the neural circuitry of an individual to make them happier. We cannot make an individual happier until we truly understand what happiness is, and this is not simply a matter of neurotransmitters and neural circuitry. This is where philosophy and the humanities can help. It is also where INP can help philosophers, or more accurately, where the two together can help one another. We can develop an outlook for a happier future by not only developing the brain sciences but also by developing our understanding of what happiness is through the humanities working with the sciences.

Likewise, if we are talking about enhancing the human, and possibly creating the posthuman, then we have to understand what the human is and those characteristics that are essential to the human. We have to understand what the self is. Who am I? What is the self we are trying to enhance, and does it make sense to download the self into cyberspace? Will the same individual be retained after such a download? What will be changed, and how essential is it to the self? Will we alter the self, by genetically reworking the brain? This is where an interaction between science and the humanities can again be beneficial. More specifically, immunologists can contribute something to the philosophers' reflections on the self, personhood, and human nature, just as philosophers can contribute to our better understanding of these for the scientist and transhumanist. In sum, current forms of transhumanism are too reductionistic and materialistic because of their emphasis on specific sciences and technologies to the exclusion of the humanities. Immunoneuropsychology is a discipline that can show the way toward a better integration of the humanities and the hard-core sciences.

References

Ader, Robert, Robert Dantzer, Ronald Glazer, et al., eds. 2006. *Psychoneuroimmunology*. 4th ed. New York: Academic Press.

Ader, Robert, David L. Felten, and Nicholas Cohen, eds. 1991. *Psychoneuroimmunology*. 2d ed. New York: Academic Press.

Allmark, Peter. 2005. Health, happiness and health promotion. *Journal of Applied Philosophy* 22: 1-15.

Aristotle. 1941. *Ethica Nicomachea.* In *The Basic Works of Aristotle.* Edited by Richard McKeon. New York: Random House.

Barak, Yoram. 2006. The immune system and happiness. *Autoimmunity Reviews* 5: 523-27.

Bentham, Jeremy. 1789. *An Introduction to the Principles of Morals and Legislation.* Oxford and London: Clarendon Press.

Bohr, Niels. 1943. *Atomic Theory and the Description of Nature.* New York: MacMillan Company.

–. 1958. *Atomic Physics and Human Knowledge*. New York: Wiley.

Bostrom, Nick. 2001. Transhumanist values: http://www.nickbostrom.com/tra/values.html, accessed July 15, 2011.

–. 2003. Human genetic enhancements: A transhumanist perspective: http://www.nickbostrom.com/ethics/genetic.html, accessed July 15, 2011.

Bostrom, Nick, and Anders Sandberg. 2009. The wisdom of nature. In Savulescu and Bostrom, eds., 375-416.

Braude, Stephen E. 2005. Personal identity and postmortem survival. *Social Philosophy and Policy Foundation* 22: 226-49.

Broad, C. D. 1925. *The Mind and Its Place in Nature.* London: Kegan Paul.

Brydon, Lena, Cicely Walker, Andrew J. Wawrzyniak, et al. 2009. Dispositional optimism and stress-induced changes in immunity and negative mood. *Brain, Behavior and Immunity* 23: 810-16.

Brynskikh, Anna, Ted Warren, Julia Zhu, and Jonathan Kipnis. 2008. Adaptive immunity affects learning in mice. *Brain, Behavior and Immunity* 22: 861-69.

Bunge, Mario. 1980. *The Mind-Body Problem: A Psychobiological Approach.* New York and Oxford: Pergammon Press.

Caplan, Arthur L. 2009. Good, better or best. In Savulescu and Bostrom, eds., 199-209.

Carruthers, Peter. 2004. *The Nature of Mind: An Introduction*. New York and London: Routledge.

Chalmers, David J. 1996. *The Conscious Mind: In Search of a Fundamental Theory*. Oxford and New York: Oxford University Press.

Chida, Yoichi, and Andrew Steptoe. 2008. Positive psychological well-being and mortality: A quantitative review of prospective observational studies. *Psychosomatic Medicine* 70: 741-56.

Churchland, Patricia Smith. 1986. *Neurophilosophy: Toward a Unified Science of the Mind-Brain*. Cambridge, MA: MIT Press.

Churchland, Paul M. 1984. *Matter and Consciousness.* Cambridge, MA: MIT Press.

Clayton, Philip. 2004. *Mind and Emergence: From Quantum to Consciousness.* Oxford: Oxford University Press.

Cohen, Irun R. 1991. The self, the world and autoimmunity. In *Immunology: Recognition and Response*, edited by William E. Paul, 98-108. New York: W.H. Freeman and Co.

Cohen, Nicholas. 2006. The uses and abuses of psychoneuroimmunology: A global overview. *Brain, Behavior and Immunity* 20: 99-112.

Cohen, Sheldon, and Sarah D. Pressman. 2006. Positive affect and health. *Current Directions in Psychological Science* 15: 122-25.

Damasio, Antonio R. 1994. *Descartes' Error*. New York: G. P. Putnam.

Dawkins, Richard. 2006. *The God Delusion.* Boston and New York: Mariner Books.

Dennett, Daniel C. 1978. *Brainstorms: Philosophical Essays on Mind and Psychology*. Boston: The MIT Press.

–. 1991. *Consciousness Explained.* New York and London: Little, Brown and Company.

Descartes, René. 1641. *Meditations on First Philosophy*. In *The Philosophical Works of Descartes*. 1969. Translated by E. S. Haldane and G.R.T. Ross. Cambridge: Cambridge University Press.

Edmonds, David. 2009. The age of enhancement. *Prospect* 162, September 3: http://www.prospectmagazine.co.uk/2009/09/the-age-of-enhancement/, accessed July 15, 2011.

Esterling, Brian A., M. H. Antoni, M. A. Fletcher, Scott Margulies, and Neil Schneiderman. 1994. Emotional disclosure through writing or speaking modulates latent Epstein-Barr virus antibody titers. *Journal of Counseling and Clinical Psychology* 62: 130-40.

Fabris, Nicola, Branislav M. Markovic, and N. Herbert Spector. 1994. *Neuroimmunomodulation: The State of the Art*. New York: New York Academy of Sciences.

Feigl, Herbert. 1958. *The "Mental" and the "Physical"*. Minneapolis: University of Minnesota Press.

Flanagan, Owen J. 1984. *The Science of the Mind*. Cambridge, MA: MIT Press.

Fukuyama, Francis. 2002. *Our Posthuman Future*. New York: Picador.

Garreau, Joel. 2005. *Radical Evolution*. New York: Broadway Books.

Gouin, Jean-Philippe, J. K. Kiecolt-Glaser, W. B. Malarkey and Ronald Glaser. 2008. The influence of anger expression on wound healing. *Brain, Behavior and Immunity* 22: 699-708.

Harle, Rob. 2007. Disembodied consciousness and the transcendence of the limitations of the biological body. *Janus Head* 9: 589-603.

Haybron, Daniel. 2000. Two philosophical problems in the study of happiness. *Journal of Happiness Studies* 1: 207-25.

–. 2007a. Life satisfaction, ethical reflection and the science of happiness. *Journal of Happiness Studies* 8: 99-138.

–. 2007b. Well-being and virtue. *Journal of Ethics and Social Philosophy* 2: 1-24.

Hoffman, Steven A. 1975. Conscious States, Neurophysiological Processes and the Principle of Complementarity, PhD. diss. Ann Arbor: University Microfilms (reprints: http://disexpress.umi.com/dxweb), accessed July 15, 2011.

Hoffman, Steven A., Ronald J. Harbeck, and David William Shucard. 1998. The immune system can affect learning: Chronic immune complex disease in a rat model. *Journal of Neuroimmunology* 86: 163-70.

Hoffman, Steven A., and Boris Sakic. 2009. Autoimmunity and brain dysfunction. In *The Neuroimmunological Basis of Behavior and Mental Disorders*, edited by Allan Siegel and Steven S. Zalcman. New York: Springer Science.

Humanity+. n.d.: http://humanityplus.org/learn/philosophy, accessed July 15, 2011.

Hume, David. 1739. *A Treatise of Human Nature.* Edited by A. Selby-Bigge. Oxford: Clarendon Press.

Huxley, Thomas H. 1874. On the hypothesis that animals are automata, and its history. *The Fortnightly Review*, 16: 555-80. Reprinted in *Method and Results: Essays by Thomas H. Huxley*. New York: D. Appleton and Company, 1898.

Irwin, Michael R. 2008. Human psychoneuroimmunology: 20 Years of discovery. *Brain, Behavior and Immunity* 22: 129-39.

Jerne, Niels K. 1974. Towards a network theory of the immune system. *Annals of Immunology* (Paris) 125C: 373-89.

Kemeny, Margaret E., L. J. Rosenwasser, R. A. Panettieri, R. M. Rose, et al. 2007. Placebo response in asthma: A robust and objective phenomenon. *Journal of Allergy and Clinical Immunology* 119: 1375-81.

Kemeny, Margaret E., and Manfred Schedlowski. 2007. Understanding the interaction between psychosocial stress and immune-related diseases: A stepwise progression. *Brain Behavior and Immunity* 21: 1009-18.

Lehrer, Jonah. 2009. Neuroscience: Small, furry … and smart. *Nature* 461: 862-64.

Lewitus, Gil M., Adi Wilf-Yarkoni, Yaniv Ziv, Maytal Shabat-Simon, et al. 2009. Vaccination as a novel approach for treating depressive behavior. *Biological Psychiatry* 65: 283-88.

Marsland, Anna L., S. Cohen, B. S. Rabin, S. B. Manuck. 2006. Trait positive affect and antibody response to hepatitis B vaccination. *Brain, Behavior and Immunity* 20: 261-69.

Matzinger, Polly. 1998. An innate sense of danger. *Seminars in Immunology* 10: 399-415.

McKnight, Patrick E., and Todd B. Kashdan. 2009. Purpose in life as a system that creates and sustains health and well-being: An integrative, testable theory. *Review of General Psychology* 13: 242-51.

Medzhitov, Ruslan, and Charles A. Janeway. 1997. Reply to Silverstein and Rose "On the mystique of the immunological self". *Immunological Reviews* 159: 208-10.

Mill, John Stuart. 1863. *Utilitarianism*. Rept. Seattle: Pacific Publishing Studio (2010).

Miller, Andrew H. 2010. Depression and immunity: A role for T cells? *Brain, Behavior and Immunity* 24: 1-8.

Monod, Jacques. 1972. *Chance and Necessity: An Essay on the Natural Philosophy of Modern Biology*. New York: Vintage Books.

More, Max. 2003. *Principles of extropy*. Version 3.11, Extropy Institute Web site: http://www.extropy.org/principles.htm, accessed July 15, 2011.

Olson, Eric T. 2007. What are we? *Journal of Consciousness Studies* 14: 37-55.

Palumbo, M.L., M.C. Canzobre, C.G. Pascuan, H. Ríos, et al. 2010. Stress induced cognitive deficit is differentially modulated in BALB/c and C57Bl/6 mice: Correlation with Th1/Th2 balance after stress exposure. *Journal of Neuroimmunology* 218: 12-20.

Perry, John, ed. 1975. *Personal Identity*. Berkeley: University of California Press.

Petrie, Keith J., R. J. Booth, J. W. Pennebaker, K. P. Davison, and M. G. Thomas. 1995. Disclosure of trauma and immune response to a Hepatitis B vaccination program. *Journal of Consulting and Clinical Psychology* 63: 787-92.

Petrie, Keith J., I. Fontanilla, M. G. Thomas, R. J. Booth, and J. W. Pennebaker. 2004. Effect of written emotional expression on immune function in patients with human immunodeficiency virus infection: A randomized trial. *Psychosomatic Medicine* 66: 272-75.

Pinker, Steven. 1997. *How the Mind Works*. New York: W. W. Norton and Company.

Place, U. T. 1956. Is consciousness a brain process? *British Journal of Psychology* 47: 44-50.

Poletaev, Alexander, and Leeza Osipenko. 2003. General network of natural autoantibodies as immunological homunculus (Immunculus). *Autoimmunity Reviews* 2: 264-71.

Popper, Karl R., and John C. Eccles. 1977. *The Self and Its Brain: An Argument for Interactionism*. New York: Springer International.

Pradeu, Thomas, and Edgardo D. Carosella. 2006. The self model and the conception of biological identity in immunology. *Biology and Philosophy* 21: 235-52.

Prather, Aric A., Anna L. Marsland, M. F. Muldoon and S. B. Manuck. 2007. Positive affective style covaries with stimulated IL-6 and IL-10 production in a middle-aged community sample. *Brain, Behavior and Immunity* 21:1033-37.

Raine, Cedric, ed. 1988. *Advances in Neuroimmunology*. New York: New York Academy of Sciences.

Ramachandran, V. S. 2003. The emerging mind. BBCs Reith Lectures: http://www.bbc.co.uk/radio4/reith2003/lectures.shtml, accessed July 15, 2011.

Ramachandran, V. S., and W. Hirstein. 1997. Three laws of qualia: What neurology tells us about the biological functions of consciousness. *Journal of Consciousness Studies* 4: 429-57.

Ryff, Carol D., Burton H. Singer, and Gayle Dienberg Love. 2004. Positive health: Connecting well-being with biology. *Philosophical Transactions of the Royal Society of London* 359: 1383-94.

Sagan, Carl. 1977. *The Dragons of Eden: Speculations on the Evolution of Human Intelligence*. New York: Ballantine Books.

Savulescu, Julian, and Nick Bostrom, eds. 2009. *Human Enhancement*. Oxford: Oxford University Press.

Schedlowski, Manfred, R. Jacobs, G. Stratmann, S. Richter, et al. 1993. Changes of natural-killer-cells during acute psychological stress. *Journal of Clinical Immunology* 13: 119-26.

Schedlowski, Manfred, and Uwe Tewes, eds. 1999. *Psychoneuroimmunology: An Interdisciplinary Introduction*. Dordrecht: Kluwer Academic and New York: Plenum Publishers.

Schrodinger, Erwin. 1967. *What is Life? Mind and Matter*. Cambridge: Cambridge University Press.

Schwartz, Jeffrey M., and Sharon Begley. 2002. *The Mind and the Brain*. New York: Harper.

Segerstrom, Suzanne C. 2005. Optimism and immunity: Do positive thoughts always lead to positive effects? *Brain, Behavior and Immunity* 19: 195-200.

Sepah, Saviz C., and Julienne E. Bower. 2009. Positive affect and inflammation during radiation treatment for breast and prostate cancer. *Brain, Behavior and Immunity* 23: 1068-72.

Shatz, Carla. 2009. MHC class I: an unexpected role in neuronal plasticity. *Neuron* 64: 40-45.

Shoemaker, Sydney. 2008. Persons, animals, and identity. *Synthese* 162: 313-24.

Siegel, Allan, and Steven S. Zalcman, eds. 2009. *The Neuroimmunological Basis of Behavior and Mental Disorders*. New York: Springer Science.

Silverstein, Arthur M., and Noel R. Rose. 1997. On the mystique of the immunological self. *Immunological Reviews* 159: 197-206.

Smart, J.J.C. 1963. *Philosophy and Scientific Realism*. London: Routledge and Kegan Paul.

Smith, Alison, Ute Vollmer-Conna, Barbara Bennett, Denis Wakefield, et al. 2004. The relationship between distress and the development of a primary immune response to a novel antigen. *Brain, Behavior and Immunity* 18: 65-75.

Snow, Nancy. 2008. Virtue and flourishing. *Journal of Social Philosophy* 39 (2): 225-45.

Sotala, Kaj "Xuenay." 2007. Transhumanism: Happiness, equality, choice. Live journal: http://www.xuenay.net/transhumanism.html, accessed July 15, 2011.

Spinoza, Benedict de. 1677. *Ethica Ordine Geometrico Demonstrata*. Produced by Tom Sharpe in the Kindle Version (Amazon.Com). Translated R.H.M. Elwes: http://www.semantikon.com/philosophy/spinozaEthics.pdf, accessed July 15, 2011.

Steptoe, Andrew, Samantha Dockray, and Jane Wardle. 2009. Positive affect and psychobiological processes relevant to health. *Journal of Personality* 77: 1747-76.

Stix, Gary. 2009. Turbocharging the brain. *Scientific American* 301 (4): 46-55.

Stock, Gregory. 2003. *Redesigning Humans*. New York: Mariner Books.

Strawson, Galen. 1997. The self. *Journal of Consciousness Studies* 4: 405-28.

Strawson, P. F. 1959. *Individuals: An Essay in Descriptive Metaphysics*. New York: Anchor Books.

Tang, Ya-Ping, Eiji Shimizu, Gilles R. Dube, Claire Rampon, et al. 1999. Genetic enhancement of learning and memory in mice. *Nature* 401: 63-69.

Tauber, Alfred I. 1994. The immune self: Theory or metaphor? *Immunology Today* 15: 134-36.

Teichert, Dieter. 2004. Narrative, identity and the self. *Journal of Consciousness Studies* 11: 175-91.

Tirosh-Samuelson, Hava. 2007. Facing the challenges of transhumanism: Philosophical, religious, and ethical considerations. *The Global Spiral*: http://www.metanexus.net/Magazine/Default.aspx?TabId=68andid=10169and SkinSrc=[G]Skins%2f_default%2fNo+SkinandContainerSrc=[G]Containers%2f_default%2fNo+Container, accessed July 15, 2011.

Von Ah, Diane, Duck-Hee Kang, Janet S. Carpenter. 2007. Stress, optimism, and social support: Impact on immune responses in breast cancer. *Research in Nursing and Health* 30: 72-82.

Wilce, James. 2003. *Social and Cultural Lives of Immune Systems (Theory and Practice in Medical Anthropology*). London: Taylor and Francis.

Zalcman, Steven S., and Allan Siegel. 2006. The neurobiology of aggression and rage: Role of cytokines. *Brain, Behavior and Immunity* 20: 507-14.

Being Human versus Being Transhuman: The Mind–Body Problem and Lived Experience

Craig T. Nagoshi and Julie L. Nagoshi

Transhumanism offers diverse visions of "enhanced" humanity that range from modest extrapolations of current medical and pharmaceutical technologies designed for modifying human physiological functioning to attain greater physical and cognitive abilities to farfetched scenarios of discarding the physical human body entirely and uploading human consciousness unto artificially intelligent "immortal" machines. These visions implicitly assume a mind-body dualism, in which the human body is perceived as merely an imperfect, burdensome machine to be tinkered with by a separate, rational, free-willed consciousness. This consciousness includes the experience of personhood, about being self-aware and being able to will the mental products deriving from self-awareness onto the physical world. For many, that consciousness and free will are the essence of "being human" that supposedly separates our species from the "lower animals." While the physical substrate may change, the human mind will presumably maintain its essential properties in the transhuman.

In this essay, we consider the nature of personhood and the related concept of identity. We argue that the experiences of personhood and identity are inextricably linked with the experiences of the body on its journey through life. Most proponents of transhumanism, basing their ideas on Western rationalist traditions, treat consciousness as merely knowledge and knowledge as objective information (*logos*) that exists separate from the knower and the knower's body. Such knowledge is readily analogized as computer programs and data that can, with sufficient technology, be recorded and transported to more indestructible and efficient media. We counter that our understanding of ourselves and others as sentient beings is derived from knowledge as *mythos*, namely, lived experiences self-understood and shared through inherently subjective, personally meaningful, bodily based narratives of such experiences. We explore these issues by considering the meaning of suffering in the context of medical treatment and then segue into issues of the use of medical procedures for various aspects of treating or enhancing gender-related behaviors, appearance, and identity. We conclude by arguing that understanding how new technologies are changing what it means to be "human" requires not just recognizing the changes in ideas about the nature of humanity but also requires recognition of the more subtle ways that our physical being, personal and social functioning, and personal narratives of our existences are also simultaneously evolving alongside these technologies.

The Questions of Personhood and Transhumanism

According to Julian Savulescu (2009, 211-14) likely future enhancements of human beings include the use of trans-species and human genetic engineering, as well as new pharmaceuticals, all for the sake of eliminating aging and increasing memory, cognitive functioning, social bonding, and athletic ability. Since these predictions are based on extrapolating from existing medical technologies, it is reasonable to assume that these forms of human enhancements will come to pass. A less proven technology, but still not outside our current understanding of how the body works, is the proposal that nanotechnology would be used to reconstruct and enhance the parts and functions of the human body, for example, by creating "artificial blood cells with greater life, durability, and oxygen carrying capacity" (ibid., 214). Savulescu, however, ends this section with the famously outlandish proposal associated with transhumanism (e.g., Hughes 2004) that it will eventually be possible to upload human minds into immortal artificially intelligent machines. This scenario, however, is most problematic: not only would the machine-based "mind" not be recognizably "human," but the scenario also manifests a very narrow and superficial meaning of "personhood." At the foundation of the transhumanism project, then, there is a flawed understanding of the human.

At first blush, transhumanist ideas seem to be based on a naïve materialism that takes for granted that all aspects of human nature, including personhood, consciousness, and free will, are based in the physical workings of the human body. Hughes proposes that, "since computers powerful enough to model human brains should be common in thirty years, those computer models may then be able to run software simulations of our brains and bodies. Presumably these backups of our minds, if switched on, would be self-aware and have an independent existence" (2004, 41). Such beliefs overlook the tricky metaphysical and epistemological problems of figuring out where this "mind stuff" comes from (e.g., where in the brain can conscious experience be located?) and how it works (e.g., how does one's experience of being a self-aware entity, seemingly able to "will" sensations, thoughts, and emotions in an imaginary mental space, emerge from neural processes?). The proposal of uploading minds into machines, however, reveals that transhumanists are really implicit Cartesian dualists, who believe that their personhoods, their sense of Self, exist in an immaculate reality separate from their bodies. Tinkering with the body to make it more durable, neurally efficient, and physically stronger just allows for that personhood to have a longer, more physically comfortable existence, before technologies become available to dispense with the corruptible, mortal thing for good. Hayles (1999), in fact, argues that the theme that characterizes the "posthuman" future that already manifests itself in our information-based, virtual-reality existences is disembodiment. Taken to its logical extreme, personhood in an immortal, powerful machine with access to all the knowledge of the world would then be as close to godhood as one could imagine.

The typical questions raised about transhumanism center on whether technologies can fundamentally alter what it means to be human and on the ethics of allowing such technologies to proceed (e.g., Daniels 2009). Such questions cannot be answered without an understanding of what it means to be "human," which, in turn, centers on the issue of what defines a "person." We now consider personhood and identity in the context of the use of medical technologies to alleviate suffering.

The Person in Treatment and the Meaning of Suffering

As Sandel (2009) points out, medical treatment and medical enhancement both have the goals of fulfilling human desires and easing overall human suffering. However, since treatment has the goal of alleviating suffering by restoring the person to some "normal" state of functioning, the benefits versus the costs of such treatment are more easily defined. Thus, treatment supposedly has far fewer ethical issues associated with it than enhancement. Sandel, in fact, argues that enhancement is ultimately about mastering nature, which is in itself ethically questionable, and also fosters collateral damages, such as the erosion of the ethical sensitivities that come from accepting the "giftedness" of life and children (78-80). It turns out, however, that the ethics of using medical treatments to alleviate suffering are not so cut and dried, once one considers the issue of defining personhood.

Suffering is a seemingly inescapable part of the human condition, and it doesn't take much observation of life to realize the horrendous levels of suffering that can befall any of us at any time. Providing people with the means to cope with suffering is one of the flashpoints in the conflict of ideas between science and religion, with the former promising ever more effective technologies for physically eliminating suffering, while the latter promises beliefs that provide meanings for enduring suffering and perhaps a final supernatural release from all suffering. One basic problem here, however, is that suffering, separate from physical pain, is always relative to the perceptions of the person who experiences a possibly suffering-inducing event. Brock thus notes that deafness, which would cause suffering for many in the hearing community, is perceived as merely a difference and even an advantage for many in the deaf community, where "deaf culture and sign language represent reasonable alternatives to the language and culture of hearing persons" (2009, 273).

Cassell (2004) addresses the issue of suffering and personhood from the point of view of medicine, while Hauerwas (1990) addresses the issue from the point of view of Christian theology. Each, in his own way, bases his criticisms on first attacking Cartesian dualism/interactionism, which assumes a separation of a nonphysical, rational/mental, conscious, free-willed, spiritual realm from the physical, bodily, nonconscious, determined, material realm. As noted above, such a dualism seems necessary since suffering is not synonymous with "physical" pain. In many cases, it is the "meaninglessness" of some event, for example, the death of one's young child that is focused on by both Cassell and Hauerwas, which creates great suffering in someone who has not otherwise been directly physically harmed.

Cassell describes how the increasing incorporation of seemingly objective scientific and technological advances into medicine, particularly in the last fifty years, banished the "subjective and anecdotal" from the discipline and "demote[d] the individuality of the physician to the level of a contaminant" (2004, 18). These historical developments facilitated the promulgation and widespread acceptance of a conceptualization of Western medicine that explicitly separated subjective suffering from objective pain by relegating suffering to the realm of the mind, while arguing that the objective doctor should only be concerned about eliminating the pain emanating from the body. Against this view, Cassell argues that suffering and its counterpart, meaning, are expressions of the entire person. Personhood is not just the "mind," not just a sense of self-awareness and identity, but includes individual and socially collective mental and physical/bodily manifestations, some unconscious, that emerge through the dynamic, interactive developmental trajectory of the person, as he/she moves through the space/time of his/her life. In this view, mental and physical experiences are intimately intertwined and inseparable, with suffering and the choice of appropriate medical treatment only understandable within this more holistic conception of personhood.

For Hauerwas (1990), modern theology, ironically influenced by Western rational philosophy and the achievements of science, separates God and spirituality from bodily existence, such that believers are taught to choose to believe in a spiritual meaning to justify and overcome their suffering. Hauerwas sees medicine operating from the same principle that it is from the mental realm, in this case, through human intellect and technology, that physical suffering can be overcome. He proposes that suffering comes from desire, which is a choice that people can make about their existence. The highest desire one can choose is to believe in God, which creates the greatest suffering, because it creates the desire for meaning for all that happens in what may be an essentially meaningless physical existence. Nevertheless, the gift of God was to give humans this capacity not only to experience but to choose desires, which is the highest essence of being alive. It can be implied here that knowing God and, hence, having a meaning in life and in suffering are about simultaneously experiencing the process of life as intertwined physical hardship and spiritual transcendence. Here again, understanding suffering, in order to choose appropriate medical and perhaps spiritual treatments, requires a holistic understanding of the person, in this case as a free-willed, meaning seeking being in continuous, dynamic interaction with and against the limits of their physical body and the physical world.

Going back to Sandel's (2009) distinction between treatment and enhancement, one can see the conundrums generated by the above more inclusive and dynamic definitions of personhood and suffering. How do physicians, medical technologists, and medical ethicists define the "normal" state of a person's being that medical treatment is supposed to restore the person to? How do we know the basis of any person's suffering, so that we can predict whether some medical treatment will actually alleviate that person's suffering in the present and future? If one of the most "human" of desires is to achieve self-perfection, based on some consciously chosen ideal of perfection derived from the narrative of a person's life experiences, then is it not the most "human" to use medical-enhancement technologies to alleviate the suffering caused by "naturally" falling short of perfection? Kass (2003) raises similar arguments in criticizing the supposed distinction between treatment and enhancement and in providing a moral argument against the unbridled use of medical enhancement technologies. It turns out that these abstract questions have, in fact, been debated in the realm of gender identity and gender-related body modification.

Transgenderism: Untenable Distinction between "Treatment" and "Enhancement"

We want to examine the case of gender identity as a way to problematize the distinction between "treatment" and "enhancement." In particular, we want to pay attention to the phenomenon of transgenderism as a useful vantage point from which to explore the links between personhood, narrative, and suffering. It is only when this link is fully understood that the limitations of the transhumanist project become clear.

Gender is undoubtedly the first socially imposed identity category that humans incorporate into their sense of personhood. For the vast majority of heteronormative, "straight" individuals, gender is so fundamental a part of their overall identity that their gender identity, their self-perceived membership in the category "male" versus "female," is taken for granted. The given idea is that one is born biologically male or female, which is determined by the child's genitalia at birth. The official determination is made by a doctor, who is required to assign a biological sex on the birth certificate, in spite of the sometimes ambiguous genitalia that are presented (Preves, 2003). Of course, with the common use of ultrasound scans before birth, by the time of birth, parents and their larger society have already imposed this identity category on the fetus.

This assigning of a sex then has profound consequences on the individual, as it sets in motion a trajectory of events, where the anatomy of the individual is linked to actually socially constructed expectations, that somehow the biological "essence" of gender determines innate physiological differences between the male and female body that, in turn, determine innate sex differences in psychological functioning. Gender roles are then prescribed in order to stay in line with these expected biological differences. Men are expected to behave in a "masculine" manner centered on instrumental problem solving, with much leeway for competitiveness and aggression, because of the naturally strong and stoic male body. Women are expected to behave in a "feminine" manner centered on emotional responses and maintaining social relationships. As many feminists would point out, however, this leads to the social expectation that it is "natural" for women to take a passive, more subordinate role in society, based on the supposedly weaker, more fragile female body that is primarily designed for childbearing and childrearing. Opposite-sex sexual orientation and its supposedly inevitable development into a "straight" sexual identity are also taken for granted by many as a natural consequence of the essential nature of gender identity.

The rub with this supposedly natural system is that it is not natural at all. Gender is a social construct based on mentally derived ideals for rationalizing and subjugating the actually messier sex-related manifestations that arise in real human bodies. As pointed out by Butler (1990), the social environment essentializes gender identity by forcing individuals to conform to the expectations of gender-identity categories, and the repeated performances of individuals in conformity with these expectations also act as an essentializing force. The phenomenon of transgenderism and the experiences of transgenders, however, vivify the problems that arise from Western societies' implicit mind-body dualism with regard to gender.

Transgenders are individuals who defy socially defined gender roles and gender identity and/or go across the boundaries of one gender to another gender (Green 2004). One subgroup of transgenders are intersex individuals, those born with ambiguous genitalia at birth due to chromosomal (e.g., Turner's syndrome, where apparently female infants are actually missing an X chromosome) or physiological reasons (e.g., congenital adrenal hyperplasia, where the body's endocrine system produces excess androgens, thus masculinizing an otherwise female fetus; or androgen insensitivity syndrome, where the lack of key androgen receptors prevents the masculinization of an otherwise male fetus). As many as two in one thousand births feature ambiguous external genitalia, and as Preves (2003) documents, up until recently nearly all intersex infants were immediately diagnosed with a medical disorder. The parents of these infants were informed by physicians that medical treatments involving surgeries to "normalize" the child's genitalia (e.g., by shortening enlarged clitorises or by constructing penises or vaginas) were required, even though, in the vast majority of cases, there was no danger to the physical health of the child and even though the surgeries themselves carried risks in terms of the later physiological and sexual functioning of the child/adult. The reason given for these highly invasive medical treatments was that such treatments would prevent the *future* suffering of a child/adult who did not otherwise fit within one of the gender-identity categories required for "normal" human development.

Gender-reassignment surgery for intersex children would seem to be an obvious example of the use of science to superimpose a more perfect nature onto the child, in essence acting as God. Such surgery raises very similar ethical issues as raised by Sandel (2009) with regard to parents using medical-enhancement technologies to preempt the future suffering that would be caused by their child's being less able to compete against other children, particularly those who had been enhanced by their parents. Preves's (2003) interviews with intersex individuals revealed that nearly all felt that the surgeries, hormonal treatments, and medicalized lifestyle they experienced growing up were traumatic and unnecessary. Ironically, for many interviewed intersex individuals, being a medical curiosity became an important part of their identity and personhood, as much so as their gender identity. Also ironically, but perhaps not surprisingly, for many their gender identity came to be seen as much more fluid and socially and self-constructed, with several individuals changing their gender identity in the course of their lives and even having surgery to reverse what was done to them in childhood.

Another important subset of transgenders is transsexuals, transgenders who undergo psychological, hormonal, and surgical interventions to become the opposite sex of what they were chromosomally born as. This would seem to be a compelling example for the ideas of transhumanism, since this is a fundamental alteration of the body, with profound implications for the definition of personhood and personal identity.

In the U.S., self-requested gender-reassignment surgery is only allowed if the individual requesting it has a diagnosis of Gender Identity Disorder from the Diagnostic and Statistics Manual of the American Psychiatric Association, i.e., has a "disease" in need of "treatment." There is, however, much controversy over whether those who feel psychological distress because they are in the "wrong-gender body" actually have a disorder. Many argue that transsexuals are otherwise healthy individuals suffering from the prejudice and oppression of a society that rigidly socializes everyone into a biologically based binary gender-identity system that determines physical appearance, behaviors, thoughts, emotions, and sexual preferences (Ault and Brzuzy 2009). If those who seek sex-reassignment surgery do not have a disorder, then such surgery would be an enhancement, much like the cosmetic surgery and body modification (Nagoshi and Nagoshi 2008) discussed below.

Many transgender and transsexual individuals are searching for a physical embodiment that conforms to their personal sense of Self. Yet, many transsexuals are not comfortable identifying as simply "male" or "female" before or after the surgery, and neither are they aspiring to meet the stereotypical ideals of being a male or female in their postoperative life (Nagoshi 2008). Having sex-reassignment surgery does help facilitate being perceived by others as a man or woman, thereby allowing individuals to fit better into society (Green 2004). In general, society requires people to fit into the male or female gender box throughout one's daily functioning, including one's driver's license, work histories, birth certificates, school transcripts, parents' wills, and what public restroom to use (Green, 2004). The difficulty of needing to conform to society's binary-gender arrangements often becomes a secondary motivation for transsexuals to have the surgery.

Scholars and activists debate what rights transsexuals and transgenders should have regarding sex-reassignment surgery. Feinberg (1996) argues that it is the right of the individual to be able to modify his or her body through surgery. Feinberg points out that women already get hormone-replacement therapy for menopause and fertility assistance, and many have cosmetic surgery, such as breast implants, breast reductions, face lifts, or belly tucks. In contrast to cosmetic surgery, as noted above, sex-reassignment surgery patients must be diagnosed as having Gender Identity Disorder and must undergo extensive evaluations. To get around these institutional barriers, some transsexuals buy hormones on the street, get prescriptions from underground doctors, or travel to other countries for the surgery, placing them at further health risks (ibid.).

As discussed in Nagoshi and Brzuzy (forthcoming), the phenomenon of transgenderism and the social oppression of transgenders posed fundamental challenges to both feminist and queer-theory conceptions of gender and sexual identity. Feminism challenged the social oppression of women by arguing that gender roles, particularly those in service to a male-dominated social order, are social constructs and, hence, subject to questioning and self-determined change. Feminist theorists, however, were ambivalent about whether the identity categories of gender itself could be deconstructed versus being "essential" (Hesse-Biber, Gilmartin, and Lydenberg 1999). If women's personal and social power derive from their essential identity as women, then transgenders either become the oppressor or the oppressed, depending on which gender identity they choose to be (Heyes 2003).

Queer theory (e.g., Sedgwick 1998) addressed the intersections of gender and sexual identity and oppression by arguing that, in fact, both gender and sexual identity are social constructs that could be challenged by the individual. Here is where transgenderism would seem to meet transhumanism, where the gendered body is merely the vehicle carrying the person whose identity is otherwise capable of being freely chosen and constructed. One could suppose that, without the gendered body, the uploaded minds of transhumans would no longer have gender as a component of identity and personhood.

The problem with queer theory conceptualizations of transgenderism, however, was that such conceptualizations often did not correspond to the actual experiences of gender and sexual identity/personhood described by many transgenders and transsexuals. In addition to asserting the need for their gendered bodies to match their gender identities, many transgenders and transsexuals also reported that, even after sex-reassignment surgery, they continually negotiated their gender, sexual, and overall personal identity. A "transgender" theory, thus, developed as a critique of queer theory. Roen (2001) asserted that transgenderism had to include more than just an "either/or" conceptualization that accepted the fluidity of gender identity but still retained the gender binary. Roen argued that transgenderism also included a "both/neither" conceptualization of a gender identity outside the gender binary. Monro (2000), in turn, argued for the need for understanding the lived experiences of transgenders, as well as the limitations on the fluidity of gender imposed by the body and biology. She pointed out that postmodernist models of gender failed to account for the embodied aspects of one's sense of self or the impact of social structures on the fluidity and plurality of gender expression.

Transgender theory, thus, reasserted the importance of the body in gender and sexual identity, but body identity was not a fixed, essentially physically defined base upon which a Self and socially constructed, mental, social identity superstructure were overlaid. Building on the ideas of Shotwell and Sangrey (2009), Nagoshi and Brzuzy (forthcoming) propose a transgender theory of identity within a social categorization as a continually dynamic interaction among (1) a social environment that essentializes, defines, and enforces social-identity categories and individuals' performances of appropriate appearances and behaviors within those categories (Butler 1990); (2) the bodily experiences of being forced to conform to or internally resisting social pressures to conform to an identity category; and (3) a subjective consciousness that freely wills the construction of aspects of self-identity. These three components of self/personhood can only be integrated and understood by the self and others through the narratives of the lived experiences and actions of the person that embodied and minded these interactions in the course of existence (Nagoshi and Brzuzy, forthcoming). This is consistent with Alcoff's idea that "a more plausible account of the self ... would hold that neither public identity nor lived subjectivity are separable entities, fundamentally distinct, or entirely independent of the other" (2006, 93). This is also consistent with Cassell's (2004) holistic, dynamic definition of personhood.

The Person in Enhancement and Gender-related Body Modification

In a transhumanist world, seeking perfection by enhancing the body is viewed as merely trying to obtain the mentally defined ideal of what the person can be. This can already be seen today in the large number of easily available procedures for permanently modifying the external appearance of the body to approach some ideal for gendered appearance and sexual appeal. These procedures range from semipermanent liposuction and botox and collagen injections to minimally invasive but permanent tattoos, permanent makeup, and body piercings to the outpatient surgery required for face and body tightening and face, breast, and buttock implants to the major surgery required for gender reassignment. What is revealing here is the fact that such procedures are largely undertaken by women, rather than men and how the physical features and motivations for these enhancements contrast with the kinds of physical enhancements of athletic and cognitive abilities touted by transhumanist (mostly male) proponents. As Nagoshi and Nagoshi (2008) have discussed, debates concerning women's choice to have these procedures done revolve around whether this choice is an expression of a woman's freedom for self-enhancement or a socially coerced self-mutilation by women feeling the need to conform to societal stereotypes of the ideal physical form for women.

Jeffreys's (2005) historical overview describes how feminist theorists of the1970s criticized "beauty" practices that caused women to diet and makeup to conform to masculine aesthetic standards, making women feel that their bodies were somehow inadequate in their natural state. By the 1980s and 1990s, however, this critique itself came under attack by feminist theorists who argued that feminism had given women the choice to use makeup and body-modification technologies to feel good about themselves, not just to conform to the standards of a male-dominated society. Postmodernist feminists, basing their ideas on queer theory and rejecting essentialist ideas that tied gender roles to physical gender differences, also argued that the body was merely a "text" that could be modifiable at will. Much like the arguments of many proponents of transhumanism, extreme modifications of the body through extensive tattoos and piercings and through surgery were idealized by some feminist theorists as a form of creative self-expression (Jeffreys 2005).

Eric Gans (2000) describes weight lifters and exercise practitioners as body modifiers who nevertheless retain those bodies as works of nature and contrasts these body modifiers with those who modify their bodies through tattoos, piercings, and surgery. Gans argues that these latter body modifiers turn their bodies into created exhibits of "the arbitrary and painful meaningfulness of the inscribed sign" (160). In this view, body modification becomes a narrative, where each succeeding modification creates both significance and a historical record for the person's life, with such modifications being particularly attractive for a youth culture rebelling against conventional social norms and exalting its freedom and mastery to achieve "the gratuitous and unproductive extremes of physical and spiritual experience" (165). A provocative aspect of this is that, while erotic needs are clearly a major motivation for body modifiers, the self-description of many body modifiers as "modern primitives" reflects a desire to "humiliate the flesh," a harkening back to ancient self-sacrificial, self-flagellating practices in the name of spiritual enlightenment. One can perhaps hear echoes here of transhumanist proponents' seeming desire to dispense ultimately with the corruptible body in order to achieve a more perfect state of mental personhood.

Pitts's (2003) interviews with body modifiers confirm many of the emotional and political motivations and fulfillments described by Gans (2000), but she is uncomfortable with the postmodern feminist idea of the body as a purely created object. Women expressed mixed messages in the meanings they ascribed to their body modifications, and Pitts wonders about the extent to which such ascribed meanings are merely reactions to conventional social norms. She is concerned that important distinctions of race, gender, sexual orientation, social class, etc., are glossed over by an emphasis on the created body. Finally, she questions how an emphasis on individual control of the body fits in with a feminist perspective on social reality that emphasizes the relationships and interconnections between people.

Jeffreys (2005) firmly comes down on the side that argues that beauty practices in Western societies, ranging from the use of cosmetics to cosmetic plastic surgery, are "harmful cultural practices," where the culture of Western male dominance causes socially accepted practices that harm women to occur with frequency. International human-rights organizations already recognize the idea of harmful cultural practice with regard to the brutal body modification practiced in several African, Middle Eastern, and Asian countries of female genital mutilation, which involves cutting off the clitoris to reduce sexual pleasure and ostensibly ensure marital fidelity. One can note the echoes here of the American medicine practice described above of shortening the enlarged clitorises of intersex girls to conform to societal expectations of "normal" female appearance. Jeffreys notes how, in Western societies, women have in the past been willing to put toxic chemicals on their faces and force restrictive diets on themselves to conform to male conceptions of the ideal physical form for women. Now women are demonstrating an increased willingness to have their bodies cut into, with body parts removed or implants inserted, as a response to this societal coercion. Jeffreys argues that, in such a coercive society that continues to objectify women in so many ways (pornography, prostitution, fashion, advertising, etc.), the idea that women have the ability to "consent" to the self-mutilation inherent in body modification procedures is dubious at best.

Logos versus *Mythos*: The Limits of Mind–Body Dualism

What is apparent from the above discussion is that the meaning and ethics of body modification/enhancement can only be understood in terms of the life narratives of the individuals undertaking the enhancement within the social context that oppresses or empowers those individuals. While transhumanism and enhancing humans are really about enhancing persons, the nature of persons does not fit the naïve materialist nor implicit Cartesian dualist mind-body orientations that most transhumanist proponents operate under. Ironically, given transhumanism's emphasis on the biological sciences, many neuroscientists reject such materialist and dualist conceptions of human nature. Rose (2005), for example, discusses how modern science has historically operated from a positivistic Western rationalist framework that assumes that the separate rational mind can objectively make sense of the physical world, in order to understand, predict, and control it. In contrast, his description of what the biological and psychological sciences have determined about the evolution of life, the evolution of the human nervous system, and the development of human cognitive/emotional function (as well as the development of science) argues that all of it can be understood as a dynamic, interactive developmental trajectory, where changes in the organism can only be understood in terms of the context of changes in other parts of the organism and the environment in which the organism is developing. Changes in the organism, in turn, not only produce changes in the contexts in which development occurs but also change the ways the organism will respond to future changes in the developmental context. He argues that the goal of all neural processing is meaning, which is driven by "feelings" in the context of the entire existence of the organism, not just information, and that human consciousness and free will are emergent properties of an entire organism that has evolved a certain kind of neural physiology in a particular evolutionary context. Thus, a purely biological/physiological approach that does not take into account the meaning-making capacities of the human body is tunnel-visioned in its efforts to enhance humans.

Foerst (2004) observed the interactions of engineers designing, building, and working with robots and noted how the humans came to attribute human attributes approaching personhood to their machine creations. She makes the important distinction between two kinds of knowledge, *logos*, factual statements that are subject to justification, calculation, and reason, because such knowledge is about truths that exist independently of the knower, and *mythos*, stories/narratives that are bound by the subjective realities of the knower/storyteller and the audience for the story (48-49). All the *ologies* in our society demonstrate the privileged place that *logos* holds as the basis for truth, while the low regard held for *mythos* is shown in the pejorative connotations associated with some item of knowledge being a myth. It is, therefore, not surprising to find that proponents of transhumanism understand being human and personhood from a purely *logos* perspective. The point Foerst makes, however, is that we can only understand being human, particularly those aspects of consciousness and free will that are essential for personhood, through *mythos*, through interactions and relationships with other sentient and seemingly sentient beings.

Cassell (2004) and Hauerwas (1990) explicitly extol the virtues of the narrative as a source of truth. The rational didactic approach assumes that there is a reasonably objective truth that exists separate from the truth-giver and that is then passed on from the truth-giver to the learner through logic and empirical support. In contrast, when a story conveys truth, it can only do so because of the relationship between the storyteller and the audience. That truth, in a lot of ways, exists only in that relationship. Thus, in dealing with the issue of suffering, Cassell argues that a doctor needs to understand his patient, while his patient needs to understand medicine. It is only in their enfolding relationship with each other that an understanding of the patient's suffering and how best to treat it will be found. Hauerwas, in turn, implicitly argues that theologians and Christians need to understand suffering in this way, with the implication that God should be understood as the ground within which the story of one's existence as a living being proceeds. Transgender theory (Nagoshi and Brzuzy, forthcoming) asserts that the narrative of one's lived experiences is what holds together the ever-changing relationships among the embodied and constructed aspects of one's identity, while "transcendant narratives" about transforming the narrative of one's life can empower one to overcome oppression (Ekins and King 2006). One can go out on a limb here about how perhaps the proponents of science and those of religion can be brought together by the realization that understanding nature (Rose 2005) and understanding God are both about truths that exist in narratives of dynamic, motivated relationships, not in absolute objects or ideas.

In terms of the question of whether human-enhancement technologies will lead to transhumans who are no longer recognizably "human," the extreme idea of uploading minds into artificial intelligent machines disregards most of what we know about how minds exist in biological substrates. On the other hand, the notions of embodiment and narrative truth discussed here imply that humans as a species are already increasing the pace at which our "human nature" is being changed, perhaps at some fundamental level. With each succeeding generation, the technologies we've been immersed in change us in terms of our psychology, our physiology, and the narratives we construct of our existences and the meaning of those existences. For example, epidemiological research suggests that widespread long-term exposure of infants and young children to television produces deficits in language, cognition, and attentional capacity (Christakis 2009). Given what is known about neural development in infancy and childhood, it is likely that such psychological effects reflect differences in neuronal growth and proliferation, compared to that of previous generations, that undoubtedly fundamentally alter how these children will process information in their environments throughout their lives. It should not be surprising that writers like Clark (2003) propose that the increasing integration of technologies with human functioning already makes us transhuman.

Recognizing the more general impact of technology on how we live as humans needs to come first, before we debate whether various specific technologies for human enhancement alter human nature in unethical ways. Technology works in subtle, complex, and reflexive ways (see the chapter by Braden Allenby in the present volume), like the dynamic natural systems Rose (2005) describes, such that most of us are likely not aware of how technology has already steadily and fundamentally changed how we live and how we perceive and morally evaluate our existences. Noble (1999) decries the destructiveness and insatiability of the "religion of technology" that promises a transcendence of the imperfections of the body and mortal existence, while Borgmann condemns the "device paradigm, a life where we pay our dues to the machinery of the device through labor and where in our leisure time we surrender to the diversions of commodities" (2003, 123), as "deeply inhospitable to grace and sacrament" (126). Noble (1999) quotes Cockburn (1985) in arguing that the response to the moral ravages of technology involves "bring(ing) men back down to earth" (1999, 208). Borgmann (2003), in turn, urges the countering of the device paradigm through communal celebrations and the associated narratives of religion, sports, arts, music, etc. We would explicitly argue that what Noble and Borgmann propose is a mythic, relational undertaking that must include the intertwined embodied and mental experiences of the participants.

The challenge is that, as several authors cited here have in one way or another pointed out, the advance of scientific and technological development has accelerated the already persistent privileging of *logos* over *mythos* in Western society. The promises and perils of transhumanism are in many ways merely another reflection of this. The privileging of *logos* over *mythos* and the triumph of the device paradigm are also reflected in the decline of the humanities in academe over the past two decades (Clayton 2009). This derision of the humanities, however, hamstrings our ability to evaluate ethically the impact of human-enhancement technologies. It can be argued that what particularly makes us human and what particularly needs to be included in the discussion of the ethics of human enhancement are the cultural, religious, historical, and literary/artistic narratives that connect humans to each other and provide temporal, spatial, and emotional context for our existences. In terms of understanding human and transhuman nature, the ones who can tell us where we're going are the keepers of the stories that tell us where we've been and of the lives we lived to get there.

References

Alcoff, Linda M. 2006. *Visible Identities: Race, Gender, and the Self.* New York: Oxford University Press.

Ault, Amber, and Stephan/ie Brzuzy. 2009. Removing gender identity disorder (GID) from the Diagnostic and Statistical Manual of Mental Disorders Fifth Edition: A call for action. *Social Work* 54 (2): 187-89.

Borgmann, Albert. 2003. *Power Failure: Christianity in the Culture of Technology.* Grand Rapids, MI: Brazos Press.

Brock, Dan W. 2009. Is selection of children wrong? In Savalescu and Bostrom, eds., 251-76.

Butler, Judith. 1990. *Gender Trouble: Feminism and the Subversion of Identity.* New York: Routledge.

Cassell, Eric J. 2004. *The Nature of Suffering and the Goals of Medicine.* 2d ed. New York: Oxford University Press.

Christakis, Dimitri A. 2009. The effects of infant media usage: What do we know and what should we learn? *Acta Paediatrica* 98 (1): 8-16.

Clark, Andy. 2003. *Natural-Born Cyborgs: Minds, Technologies, and the Future of Human Intelligence.* Oxford: Oxford University Press.

Clayton, Philip. 2009. The crisis of the humanities in America: An analysis and concrete proposal for action. Templeton Research Lecture given at Arizona State University, School of Historical, Philosophical and Religious Studies, October 26: http://www.scribd.com/doc/17922700/Transdisciplinarity-in-Science-and-Religion-No-4-2008, accessed July 14, 2011.

Cockburn, Cynthia. 1985. *Machinery of Dominance.* London: Pluto Press.

Daniels, Norman. 2009. Can anyone really be talking about ethically modifying human nature? In Savulescu and Bostrom, eds., 25-42.

Ekins, Richard, and Dave King. 2006. *The Transgender Phenomenon.* London: SAGE Publications.

Feinberg, Leslie. 1996. *Transgender Warriors*. Boston: Beacon Press.

Foerst, Anne. 2004. *God in the Machine: What Robots Teach Us about Humanity and God.* New York: Dutton.

Gans, Eric. 2000. The body sacrificial. In *The Body Aesthetic: From Fine Art to Body Modification*, edited by Tobin Siebers, 159-78. Ann Arbor: University of Michigan Press.

Green, Jamison. 2004. *Becoming a Visible Man.* Nashville, TN: Vanderbilt University Press.

Hauerwas, Stanley. 1990. *God, Medicine, and Suffering*. Grand Rapids, MI: William B. Eerdmans Publishing Co.

Hayles, N. Katherine. 1999. *How We Became Posthuman.* Chicago: University of Chicago Press.

Hesse-Biber, Sharlene, Carol Gilmartin, and Robyn Lydenberg, eds. 1999. *Feminist Approaches to Theory and Methodology: An Interdisciplinary Reader.* New York: Oxford University Press.

Heyes, Cressida J. 2003. Feminist solidarity after queer theory: The case of transgender. *Signs: Journal of Women in Culture and Society* 28 (4):1093-1120.

Hughes, James. 2004. *Citizen Cyborg: Why Democratic Societies Must Respond to the Redesigned Human of the Future*. Cambridge, MA: Westview Press.

Jeffreys, Sheila. 2005. *Beauty and Misogyny: Harmful Cultural Practices in the West*. London: Routledge.

Kass, Leon R. 2003. Ageless bodies, happy souls: Biotechnology and the pursuit of perfection. *The New Atlantis* 1: 9-28.

Lind, Amy, and Stephan/ie Brzuzy, eds. *Battleground: Women, Gender, and Sexuality*. Westport, CT: Greenwood Publishing Group.

Monro, Surya. 2000. Theorizing transgender diversity: Towards a social model of health. *Sexual and Relationship Therapy* 15 (1): 33-45.

Nagoshi, Julie. 2008. Transgenderism and transexuality – Sex-reassignment surgery. In Lind and Brzuzy, eds., 527-30.

Nagoshi, Julie L., and Stephan/ie Brzuzy. Forthcoming. Transgender theory: Embodying research and practice. *Affilia*.

Nagoshi, Julie, and Craig Nagoshi. 2008. Plastic surgery, tattooing, and piercing. In Lind and Brzuzy, eds., 389-95.

Noble, David F. 1999. *The Religion of Technology: The Divinity of Man and the Spirit of Invention*. New York: Penguin.

Pitts, Victoria L. 2003. *In the Flesh: The Cultural Politics of Body Modification.* New York: Palgrave Macmillan.

Preves, Sharon E. 2003. *Intersex and Identity: The Contested Self.* New Brunswick, NJ: Rutgers University Press.

Roen, Katrina. 2001. "Either/or" and "both/neither": Discourse tensions in transgender politics. *Signs: Journal of Women in Culture and Society* 27 (2): 501-22.
Rose, Steven. 2005. *The Future of the Brain: The Promise and Perils of Tomorrow's Neuroscience*. New York: Oxford University Press.
Sandel, Michael J. 2009. The case against perfection: What's wrong with designer children, bionic athletes, and genetic engineering. In Savulescu and Bostrom, eds., 71-89.
Savulescu, Julian. 2009. The human prejudice and the moral status of enhanced beings: What do we owe the gods? In Savulescu and Bostrom, eds., 211-47.
Savulescu, Julian, and Nick Bostrom, eds. 2009. *Human Enhancement*. New York: Oxford University Press.
Sedgwick, Eve. 1998. What's queer? *Gender Inequality: Feminist Theories and Politics*, edited by Judith Lorber, 205-9. Los Angeles: Roxbury Publishing Co.
Shotwell, Alexis, and Trevor Sangrey. 2009. Resisting definition: Gendering through interaction and relational selfhood. *Hypatia* 24 (3): 56-76.

Prenatal Human Enhancement and Issues of Responsibility

Michael J. White

In what ways might human enhancement impinge on the freedom of persons and the responsibility of those persons for their actions?[1] This obviously is a question that is large, vague, and speculative. I, therefore, begin by attempting to limit the question in ways that are controversial but that, in my judgment, are necessary to make the discussion more tractable. First, I shall not really be concerned with issues of human *freedom* except insofar as such an issue is relevant to the *responsibility* of adult persons for their actions. Second, I shall regard issues of responsibility as essentially social and cultural. In other words, I shall not be concerned with more traditional metaphysical or theological questions of the "ultimate" or "deep" moral responsibility of persons for their actions. Rather, insofar as there are "facts" about the responsibility that persons bear with respect to their various actions, I shall be concerned only about the "facts" of the existence of social-cultural norms of responsibility-attribution – norms that vary culturally and temporally but that also seem to exhibit some cross-cultural and cross-temporal constancy. I also certainly do not rule out the possibility that there are different *kinds* of responsibility that may, in different social contexts within a given culture or society, be attributed to persons; and perhaps some of these varieties should be denominated as distinctively "moral" and others not. However, little if anything in the following discussion depends on this issue.

In this chapter, I make two principal claims that I regard as rather modest. The first is that our conception(s) of human persons' responsibility depends on assumptions of *normalcy* with respect to human nature. Were enhancements to provide sufficient grounds for substantial alteration of certain of these assumptions about what is and what is not normal, then it is likely that our current norms of responsibility-attribution would simply fail to apply to persons whose natures thus "diverge from the norm." It is reasonable to assume that, under such conditions, our criteria of responsibility-attribution would be somehow modified for the class of relevantly altered agents. The second claim is that it seems likely that there will arise novel *legal* issues of responsibility – as in tort law, for example – in connection with prenatal enhancements that turn out to be unwanted by those who receive them.

---

1 My thanks to my colleague Jeffrie G. Murphy and to members of the Arizona State University faculty seminar on transhumanism for comments on and criticism of an earlier draft of this chapter. And I especially thank Hava Tirosh-Samuelson for her editorial suggestions.

Here I emphasize a point in a way that I hope does not belabor the obvious. My two claims deal with two very *different* "issues of responsibility." The first pertains to changes in criteria of responsibility-attribution that might result from certain concrete kinds of prenatal interventions, interventions that change our concept of human normalcy in certain ways. The second claim, which does not seem to me to be related closely to the first, pertains to potential changes in legal responsibility on the part of those that effect (what turn out to be unwanted) prenatal interventions in human germ cells.

Before I turn to direct discussion of these two claims, I briefly address two other preliminary matters. The first pertains to the relevance of my two principal claims to transhumanism. The second is an invocation of Aristotle's seminal but nonetheless highly suggestive account of human responsibility as particularly apposite to my discussion of these issues.

Transhumanism and Human Responsibility

A common criticism of many transhumanist programs is that the sort of genetic intervention they envision amounts to "playing God [or Nature]" with respect to the modification of future generations. One version of this criticism "concentrates upon the potential invasion of autonomy that genetic intervention can bring about" (Coady 2009, 174). In other words, "genetically programmed persons might no longer regard themselves as the sole authors of their own life history; and second, they might no longer regard themselves as unconditionally equal-born persons in relation to previous generations" (Habermas 2003, 79). The idea appears to be that substantial genetic intervention *ipso facto* yields a less "autonomous" or "free" person than the person whose genotype has been produced by God or Nature (or even nature with a small *n* – that is, natural selection, genetic mutation, and whatever other mechanisms prove to be relevant).

This idea seems to me to be mistaken. The classical metaphysical "problem of freedom of the will" has been formulated in terms of the consistency – or lack thereof – between universal causal determinism and the possession of "freedom" (or autonomy, or moral responsibility) by individual human agents. If the "external" causal determination of an agent's "nature" is thought to be relevant to the autonomy or freedom of the agent possessing that nature, it would hardly seem to matter whether that external determination is derived from God, nature, or prenatal genetic intervention. Concrete, real-world questions of an agent's moral responsibility typically arise within a context in which the agent's possession of a given "nature" (genetic endowment, character, etc.) is *assumed.* However, if the external causal determination of that nature is thought to be relevant to the agent's responsibility for some action, the source or nature of that external causal influence would not seem to be relevant.

So, with respect to a common version of the classical metaphysical problem of freedom of the will – according to which the issue of the causal determination of an agent's nature *is* relevant – genetic intervention would not seem, in the abstract, to raise any more or less a threat to an agent's autonomy than any other external causal factors relevant to an agent's possessing the nature he or she in fact possesses. In my view, intentional human genetic manipulation of (potential or future) agents' natures does indeed raise a host of serious and fundamental moral problems. However, these are not problems of particular relevance to the metaphysical problem of freedom of the will.

Where genetic intervention *would* peculiarly impinge on issues of responsibility, I shall suggest, is in cases where a given intervention would tend to affect our attributions of responsibility to altered agents relative to those not receiving such an alteration. Aristotle's relatively commonsensical and nonmetaphysical account of human responsibility proves to be a useful framework for discussing the implications of such interventions with respect to human agents' responsibility for their actions. In particular, Aristotle focuses on the conditions relevant to *responsibility-attribution* as a social practice. This focus nicely brings out the relativity of assessments of responsibility, in concrete cases, to accepted "norms of human nature" in terms of our judgments concerning an agent's capacity to withstand (or not) various kinds of external causal influences on his or her behavior. In other words, attributions of (degrees of) responsibility depend on current social conceptions of what is and what is not "normal" with respect to human agents' capacities to conform their behavior to moral expectations in the face of external causal factors opposing such morally approved behavior.

Aristotle on Responsibility

In what might be termed the Western canon, the history of philosophical reflection on the relation between the responsibility for their actions that we typically attribute to humans, on the one hand, and the various external influences – causal and otherwise – to which human actions are subject, on the other hand, extends back at least to Aristotle. Aristotle begins his discussion of this issue in what seems to me to be the correct way: he implicitly acknowledges that social practices that involve bestowing praise and blame, approbation and disapprobation, punishment and reward on the "passions and actions" of human agents presuppose that there is a fundamental sense in which these agents are responsible for those actions and passions. In other words, the "default" assumption is that adult human agents are, generally and in most contexts, responsible for their behavior. Aristotle proceeds to designate two kinds of responsibility-defeating or -diminishing factor: compulsion and ignorance.[2] "That is compulsory," he says, of which the moving principle is outside, being a principle in which nothing is contributed by the person who acts or is acted upon, e.g., if he were to be carried somewhere by the wind, or by men who had him in their power" (Aristotle 1984, vol. 2, *Nicomachean Ethics* [*EN*] 1110a1-3). With respect to the sort of ignorance that is relevant to responsibility, he says,

> Now every wicked man is ignorant of what he ought to do and what he ought to abstain from, and error of this kind makes men unjust and in general bad; but the term "involuntary" tends to be used not if a man is ignorant of what is to his advantage – for it is not ignorance in choice that makes action involuntary (it makes men wicked), nor ignorance of the universal (for *that* men are *blamed*), but ignorance of particular circumstances of the action and the objects with which it is concerned. For it is on these that both pity and forgiveness depend, since the person who is ignorant of any of these acts involuntarily. (*EN* 1110b28-1111a2)

Ignorance of the fact of what one takes to be a toy pistol but that, in fact, is a loaded, real pistol, may defeat one's responsibility for murdering one's fellow actor during the rehearsal of a play. If fact, the absence of what lawyers term *mens rea* in such a case means that no murder was committed, although a physical act of killing (which, in *other* circumstances, might have constituted murder) occurred.[3]

The "clear cases" of responsibility-defeating compulsion are cases of what might be termed physical *force majeure*. Aristotle makes clear that not *every* "external" influence on an agent should be conceptualized as compulsion: "But if one were to say that pleasant and noble objects have a compelling power, forcing us from without, all acts would be [for the agent] compulsory; for it is for these objects that all men do everything they do" (*EN* 1110b9-11). But he does allow that some actions done, say, "from fear of greater evils" have an ambiguous character: "e.g., if a tyrant were to order one to do something base, having one's parents and children in his power, and if one did the action they were to be saved, but otherwise put to death" (*EN* 1110a5-7). Aristotle says that, like jettisoning valuable cargo, such a base action might be judged involuntary "in the abstract", for "one would never choose any such act in itself" (*EN* 1110a19). But, in concrete circumstances (as to save one's children or parents or to save one's life in a storm at sea), such an act might be the result of conscious and even rational choice and, hence, voluntary.

In the somewhat more elaborate discussion of responsibility in the *Eudemian Ethics*, Aristotle's fundamental principle is that a person is generally responsible for

2 Aristotle's doctrine concerning this "default assumption" is at home in many of the more sophisticated contemporary compatibilist accounts of responsibility. See, for example, Glannon 2002, 41: "[L]ike Aristotle, I assume from the outset that the agent is responsible for what he does barring evidence of ignorance, coercion, or compulsion."

3 Not surprisingly, there is an immense amount of legal scholarship on this topic. See, in particular, Turner 1936 and Hart 2008. For a clear, text-book account of *mens rea*, see Dressler 2006.

that behavior which is expression of that person's "internal tendency" (Aristotle 1984, vol. 2, *Eudemian Ethics* [*EE*] 1124a22); consequently, "it is only when something external moves a thing, or brings it to rest against its own internal tendency, that we say that this happens by force" (*EE* 1224b6-8). Aristotle proceeds, in effect, to argue that, since humans are motivated by factors that sometimes are in conflict, such as fear, desire, and thought, the terminology of faculty psychology might suggest that, in some human behavior, one mental *faculty* acts with compulsion or "force" on another. In general, he is loath to ascribe diminished responsibility to the *person* on the basis of such an "internal" struggle:

> Now of the parts of the soul this may be said; but the soul as whole, whether in the continent or the incontinent, acts voluntarily, and neither acts on compulsion. (*EE* 1224b26-28)

Nonetheless, he is not entirely unsympathetic to the idea that a person's responsibility for an action may sometimes be eliminated or mitigated by the force of external stimuli that at are odds with what the agent in the circumstances judges that he or she *ought* to do. The element of his discussion that I wish particularly to emphasize is his appeal to a notion of normalcy – what the "normal person" could either withstand or not withstand – in his attempt to provide at least a rough-and-ready delimitation of when responsibility is eliminated or diminished:

> Again perhaps one might say that some such acts [viz., those due to external stimuli but which, we might say, the agent did unwillingly] were voluntary and some not. For of those acts that a man does without wishing them some he has the power to do or abstain from doing; these he always does voluntarily and not by force; but those in which he has not this power, he does by force in a sense (but not absolutely), because he does not choose the very thing he does, but the purpose of which it is done, since there is difference, too, in this. For if a man were to murder another so as not to be caught in blind man's buff he would be laughed at if he were to say that he acted by force, and on compulsion; there ought to be some greater and more painful evil that he would suffer if he did not commit the murder. For then he will act on compulsion and by force, or at least not by nature. … Hence, many regard love, anger in some cases, and natural conditions as involuntary, as being too strong for nature; we pardon them as things capable of overpowering nature. A man would more seem to act from force and involuntarily if he acted to escape violent pain [as in torture] than if to escape gentle pain, and generally if to escape pain than if to get pleasure. For that which depends on him – and all turns on this – is what nature is able to bear; what it is not, what is not under control of his natural desire or reason, that does not depend on him. Therefore those who are inspired and prophesy, though their act is one of thought, we still say have it not in their power either to say or not say what they said, or to do what they did. (*EE* 1225a8-30)[4]

4 Cf. *EN* 1110a23-25: "On some actions praise indeed is not bestowed, but forgiveness is, when one does what he ought not under pressure which overstrains human nature and which no one could withstand." See also (Aquinas 1948, *ST* I^{a} II^{ae} q. 96, a. 2: "now human law is framed for a number of human beings, the majority of whom are not perfect in virtue. Wherefore human laws do not forbid all vices, from which the virtuous abstain, but only the more grievous vices, from which it is possible for the majority to abstain."

The two principal morals that I take away from this discussion are the following. First, that in assigning (degrees of) responsibility, we often explicitly or tacitly appeal to the idea of what the "normal person" could or could not withstand in what we might term "psychological pressure" in considering pleas of eliminated or mitigated responsibility for an action.[5] Thus, for example, we might wish to attribute diminished responsibility to a soldier who reveals secret information under torture; however, we (in our "Western" culture) would probably be less likely to make a similar attribution because the soldier reveals the secrets under the threat of having his face painted black and being made to walk around naked. Of course, in different cultures (e.g., ones in which modesty is much more highly valued), having one's face painted black and being made to walk around naked might be so psychologically painful that this judgment would be radically different.

Second, while there is an empirical, "statistical" dimension to the idea of what is *normal* in this context – the sorts of psychological pressure that the "normal person" could or could not withstand – there is also an evaluative dimension (a "normative" dimension, so to speak) as well. This dimension is nicely illustrated by Aristotle's concluding remarks about the (lack of) responsibility of persons for utterances and actions performed by persons under divine inspiration. Clearly, Aristotle and most of the Greeks of his time were willing to countenance such behavior as rather obvious cases of mitigated responsibility on the part of the human "conduits." Most contemporary Westerners would probably not be so inclined – particularly if fraud were suspected. They might be willing to attribute diminished responsibility, however, if they suspected insanity or severe mental illness – but clearly on different grounds from Aristotle's. Conversely, many of us now would be prepared to recognize varieties of "addiction" (pharmacological and, perhaps, behavioral – as in "sexual addiction") as to some degree responsibility-mitigating, while such phenomena would not have been so conceptualized several generations ago.

Responsibility ("In General") and Enhancement

But what has all this to do with human enhancement? The general answer, I believe, is that the preceding discussion suggests that certain kinds of change in what we

5 For a more contemporary account of the role of normalcy in issues of responsibility, see de Tarde (1912) and Murphy (1992). In the words of Murphy (commenting on de Tarde), "what we really want to know about a man in judging his responsibility is (1) if he is sufficiently like his fellows in certain relevant respects and (2) if he has a sufficiently continuous conscious history to count as a person" (211); "de Tarde is inclined to let his theory rest upon an institutional fact – namely, that for all out talk about free will, it is really the notion of social similarity which operates in our actual practical judgments of excuse" (212).

consider "normal" with respect to human motivation and practical reasoning might affect our standards of responsibility-attribution with respect to altered human agents; that is, such changes might well affect our judgments concerning the circumstances when an altered agent is fully responsible for, is not responsible at all for, or bears some diminished responsibility for particular behavior.

Much "transhumanist" and "posthumanist" discussion of prenatal enhancement (genetic and otherwise) of humans has assumed both an individualist and market-driven perspective. In other words, the following assumptions frequently have been made: (1) that individual parents would be able to exercise considerable choice with respect to the selection of enhancements for their (potential) offspring; (2) that those choices would be made on the basis of what the parents deem to be safe and desirable enhancements for themselves and for those "near and dear" to them; and (3) that their enhanced offspring would tend to endorse those choices made on their behalf. This is the new "liberal eugenics" described by Michael J. Sandel (who is himself not a proponent of it): "Government may not tell parents what sort of children to design, and parents may engineer in their children only those traits that improve their capacities without biasing their choice of life plans" (Sandel 2009, 85). From such assumptions, it is perhaps natural to conclude that the only enhancements that are likely to survive and to evolve are those that will make people "better" (more intelligent, healthier, better looking, more athletic, more capable of sustained concentration, etc.) *without* affecting what we now take to be the "normal" structure of human preferences – the "normal" human desires and aversions, the "normal" human capacities for human reasoning in the face of conflicting rationally chosen ends, and the "normal" way that human emotions, fears, and so forth interact with our practical and theoretical reasoning. If this "natural conclusion" is true, there would seem to be little reason to think that enhancements would have *any* substantial effect on our social practices of responsibility-attribution. That is, there would be no obvious reason to believe that smarter, healthier, stronger, more persistent "enhanced humans" would significantly differ from us "unenhanced humans" with respect to judgments concerning what they/we are and are not responsible for.

But perhaps we should be a bit cautious about these assumptions. One relevant consideration is that, in applied science and engineering (including human engineering), there is always a possibility of unintended consequences.[6] With

6 Of course, many proponents of germinal choice technology (GCT) recognize such perils. Gregory Stock proposes to minimize unexpected consequences by the use of artificial chromosomes, as opposed to modifying the genes on one of our present forty-six chromosomes: "not only could geneticists add much larger amounts of genetic material, which would mean far better gene regulation, they could more easily test to ensure that the genes were properly placed and functioning correctly (2002, 66). My thanks to my colleague Joel Garreau for directing my attention to Stock's work.

respect to prenatal enhancement, it is not difficult to imagine such scenarios. Thoughtful prospective parents might well find attractive a prenatal intervention, genetic or otherwise, that produces a heightened ability to concentrate on the task at hand. After all, as we have all been told by parents and mentors, "application makes for success." Bostrom and Sandberg conjecture that "we may have evolved attention systems with a tendency to be too easily distracted in a modern setting," a form of response-readiness "that was more adaptive in past environments" (2009, 390). A prenatal "corrective" might be sold as a permanent and superior replacement for pharmaceutical treatment with products such as Ritalin or Adderall.

But suppose that an unintended consequence of this enhancement was that it worked so well that persons thus enhanced were *so* immediate-task oriented that they tended to discount the significance of competing stimuli (such as the yells for help of a drowning child). If such an enhancement were widely used and did indeed prove to have this consequence, would we be inclined to apply the same standards of responsibility to the class of persons thus enhanced as we do to the unenhanced population? I do not know. But I should expect that many persons would judge it *unfair* to apply to a person "enhanced" in the way I am imagining the exactly same moral (or even legal) standards of responsibility that we now customarily apply for, say, giving aid to passersby in dangerous situations.

Other enhancements might result in our applying more stringent criteria of responsibility. If an agent's capacity for practical reasoning were sufficiently enhanced beyond the norm, we might be less inclined to soften our judgments of moral responsibility for reasons of the agent's inadvertency, inattentiveness, or other defects of practical rationality that often mitigate the rigor of our attributions of moral responsibility to fallible human agents.

The particular plausibility of scenarios is less significant, it seems to me, than the general principle that they suggest: we simply have no idea how various sorts of enhancements might alter our mores of responsibility-attribution. But it seems at least possible that some enhancements might have the sort of consequences that would bring about such alterations – likely in ways that would result in applying different standards of responsibility to different classes of persons.

Thus far, I have been assuming that enhancements would be chosen by prospective parents for their offspring in accord with the parents' considered judgment about what, on balance, is in their offsprings' "best interest." This assumption seems to me to ignore two important facts. The first is that what we might desire for our offspring or others "near and dear" to us can diverge from what we judge to be of general social utility. The other fact is that moral and technological changes of the twentieth century have tended to diversify the kinds of relations, proprietary and otherwise, in which adult human persons stand to foetuses, embryos, zygotes, and gametes. To put the point more plainly, there was a time not so long ago when the "elements" of sexual reproduction were not really separated from what used to be called "the marital act" and the process of having children – that is, not separated from our roles as spouses and as parents. Nowadays, of course, it is quite possible for adult humans to separate their social roles of parenthood from their relations to gametes and zygotes (even their *own* gametes and zygotes). The potential upshot would seem to be the possibility of amassing "stockpiles" of gametes and zygotes toward which everyone stands in a much less "personal" relation than that of (potential) parent.

To consider but one scenario, a case can be made for the social usefulness of a class of citizens who are very good at taking orders. That is, their respect for authority leads them to value what they understand to be in the public interest over potentially competing considerations such as personal wealth, comfort, and safety; personal political and religious beliefs; and so forth. Indeed, in Plato's *Republic* 375a, such "guardians" are characterized as "philosophical" watchdogs. While Plato envisions the production of such a class by a combination of eugenics and education, let us consider the scenario in which a socially useful compliancy of character could be produced by prenatal engineering. While perhaps most parents would not choose such a character for *their* children, citizens might be much less reluctant to countenance the production of such socially useful citizens from a "public" stockpile of genetic material. And, again, if the tendency of persons thus enhanced "automatically" to obey authoritative commands were substantially greater than that of unenhanced persons, it might seem that different standards of responsibility-attribution should be applied to the two groups.

I do not fault the reader who fears that I have here ventured rather too far into speculation (utopian or dystopian?) more appropriate to the realm of science fiction. In fact, my "futurist" aspirations are quite limited: my aim has been to illustrate a general point that I have already made. There are many varieties of responsibility-attribution to be found in contemporary society. And depending on the form of such responsibility-attribution (e.g., a technical legal matter versus some issue of etiquette), the standards or criteria that are taken to be appropriate may vary. However, it seems to me that virtually all sorts of responsibility-attribution begin with some assumptions of what is "normal" with respect to the motivations of human persons and the ability of such persons to prioritize and exercise control over those motivations. Were prenatal enhancements, genetic or otherwise, to produce results that obviously undermine such assumptions of normalcy, there is reason to think that standards of responsibility-attribution might change. In particular, an enhancement-relative *multiplication* of standards of responsibility-attribution seems to be one possibility.

Legal Responsibility for Prenatal Enhancements

The second and final general claim that I wish to explore in this chapter is, to quote my initial characterization, the possibility that there will arise novel *legal* issues of responsibility – as in tort law, for example – in connection with prenatal enhancements that turn out to be unwanted by their recipients. This issue seems to me to involve somewhat less speculative than my earlier scenarios. In fact, it was the topic of a recent symposium featuring the scholarship of Kirsten Rabe Smolensky and others, which was published in the *Hastings Law Journal*. See Smolensky 2008a and 2008b, Cohen 2008, King 2008, Ouelette 2008.

The legal issues begin with the recognition that the "mechanization" of human reproduction and the widespread legalization of abortion have resulted in novel ways in which both parents and third parties can affect the lives of their offspring by what might be termed prenatal interventions, where "interventions" might be broadly construed to include both actions and certain kinds of inaction. Included among such potential interventions are prenatal "enhancements." As the number and variety of potential interventions increase, there will undoubtedly arise disagreements about whether some such interventions really are "enhancements" – or whether they should rather be understood to be "diminishments." In fact, such issues have *already* arisen in fertility clinics with respect to deaf parents who wish their children to be deaf, parents with achondroplasia (dwarfism) who wish their children to have the same characteristics – and in at least one reported case of parents wishing to conceive a child with Down's syndrome so that their Down's affected child would have a similar sibling (Smolensky 2008a, 404 ff.). At present, such choices involve the use of preimplantation genetic diagnosis (PGD) on embryos: only those exhibiting the desired traits are implanted; the others are discarded (to speak euphemistically) or stockpiled. But it does not seem fanciful to envision the increasing potential for direct genetic intervention with respect to embryos (or pre-embryonic material). It also does not seem excessively fanciful to imagine some humans who are the products of such actions becoming sufficiently dissatisfied with their lot that they attempt to hold either their parents or third parties legally responsible for their condition. A question that has received considerable attention is whether, under current law, tort actions of this sort might succeed – although, as far as I know, no such actions have been attempted as of this date.

In terms of the current status of fertility medicine, this legal issue has been connected to so-called wrongful-life tort actions, which have indeed been attempted. These are actions for the claimed injury of having been born (usually with certain disabilities). In most jurisdictions, these attempts have been unsuccessful.[7] There are a number of reasons for this lack of success. But one line of reasoning, pertinent to possible "diminishment-based" tort actions, goes as follows. The alternative to the actual condition of a person making such a claim is not some "better condition of existence" of *that* very person – but, rather, the nonexistence of that very person.

At this point in the argument, two threads have been conflated that perhaps should be conceptually distinguished. One is that, absent the claimant's experiencing "a life not worth living" in his or her current state, that state (although perhaps a seriously disabled one) is better than the alternative of nonexistence. Hence, the actions of that person's parents (or of third persons) in bringing about his or her life (with the actual conditions, including the perceived disabilities, of that life) should not be a legally cognizable harm to the person. The preceding argument obviously involves a normative assumption concerning the relative positive value of life (human existence) – even what we would regard as a non-trivially diminished existence – versus nonexistence. However, a closely related argument is purely conceptual. The crucial assumption is that a necessary condition for the truth of the claim that a person *P* has been harmed is that some worse state *B* of *P* has been brought about to the exclusion of some possible alternative better state *A* of *that same person P*. In the case where the alternative to the bringing about of the "worse" state *B* of *P* entails the nonexistence of *P*, this condition is not satisfied. Hence, one could not, as a logical-conceptual matter, truly claim that *P* has been harmed, irrespective of any normative claims about the value of various forms of impaired or diminished human existence relative to the nonexistence of the person in question. In other words, if the contemplated alternative to *P*'s existence in some diminished/impaired condition entails the nonexistence of *P*, one cannot coherently maintain that it is *P* who has suffered a harm from whatever or whoever produced this condition of *P* – although one might well admit that it was wrong to bring about the state of affairs of *P*'s-existing-in-the-diminished-condition.

What do these considerations have to do with tort liability for "enhancements" that come to be regarded by those on whom they have been wrought as diminishments? Smolensky (2008a, 301) conflates the two arguments I have just rehearsed under what she terms "Parfit's Non-Identity Problem" (Parfit 1987) to conclude that if, say, deaf parents brought about the deafness of one of their

7 See Shiffren 1999, 118n 4: "Only three states currently recognize the cause of action. Within these jurisdictions, the occasions of liability and the scope of damages have been significantly restricted. California originally approved suits even against parents who knew their child would be severely disabled, Curlender v. Bio-Science Labs, 106 Cal. App. 3d 811, 829 (1980), but the legislature subsequently precluded suits against parents. Cal. Civ. Code §43.6."

children as a result of the use of PGD to select for implantation an embryo with a trait for congenital deafness, there would be no legally cognizable harm that could serve as the basis of a tort action by the deaf son or daughter *P* against either parents or a third party. For the alternative to the existence of the deaf offspring *P* would *not* be the existence of *that* (identical) person *P* with normal hearing but the nonexistence of that person *P* (which, of course, might involve the existence of some *other* person *P'* who possesses normal hearing). However, Smolensky argues that, if the deafness of a child were produced by direct manipulation of embryonic DNA (which cannot yet, in fact, be done), then there might be a legally cognizable harm in tort law.

Smolensky's arguments have produced extended discussion; and some of that, as one might imagine, has regarded this consequence as a virtual *reductio* of her position. I. Glenn Cohen, for example, has considered various maneuvers for separating tort liability for intentional diminishment from Parfit's Non-Identity Problem. He has also considered the possibility of criminal responsibility rather than tort responsibility for prenatal interventions that are deemed to be diminishments or "negative enhancements" (Cohen 2008).

Although I personally find the details of this discussion fascinating, they probably are of most interest to philosophers and legal scholars. Thus, I shall not pursue these issues further in this chapter. Rather, I shall draw some general conclusions concerning enhancement and legal responsibility. (A) The "moral intuitions" of most persons suggest that cases can arise where legal responsibility (whether at tort or criminal law or through violation of some form of governmental regulation) *should* be attributed to agents for certain kinds of prenatal interventions. (B) There may well develop increased numbers of "gray areas" where there is dispute whether a particular (kind of) intervention is positive (an enhancement) or negative (a diminishment). (C) For legal and regulatory purposes, it would certainly seem to be useful to have some "objective" standards to decide whether a prenatal intervention is positive or negative; but any such proposed standards will almost certainly lead to moral controversy, especially controversy about the nature of personhood and what constitutes human flourishing or "happiness," in one (Aristotelian) sense of the term. (D) Should – as most post- and transhumanists believe – the development of more dramatic and "deep" prenatal interventions become a reality and the use of those interventions become widespread, there would be less and less of an empirical/statistical conception of human normalcy to ground a normative or evaluative conception of human normalcy that could be used as a "baseline" to make legal decisions concerning the question of whether given prenatal interventions are enhancements or diminishments. For example, if certain sorts of prenatal interventions that effectively produce cognitive capacities that most persons regard as "enhanced" become sufficiently widespread, could parents who refused to condone such interventions for their children be subject to legal action on the grounds that their refusal constitutes a "diminishment" of (opportunities for) their children?

Conclusion

As indicated at the beginning of this chapter, my aim has been limited and modest. I have argued that increased use of what might be conceived of as prenatal enhancement on the scale envisioned by many trans- and posthumanists has the potential for altering our conception of human normalcy to such an extent that our present conceptions of human responsibility would not remain unaltered. Although I think that it is impossible to predict particulars, the first section of this paper considered some scenarios that might affect what might be termed our "general assumptions" about human responsibility. In the latter part of the chapter, I considered the issue of legal responsibility for prenatal interventions, suggesting that our legal and governmental regulatory systems will almost certainly have to come to terms with the increase in such interventions should that increase occur, as it seems likely that it will. Here, too, I think it difficult to predict exactly how the legal system would respond. Such predictions are particularly difficult for me to make since I am not a lawyer or legal scholar. But the general moral that I draw is cautionary. A future of increased prenatal intervention will almost certainly be a future in which we encounter altered conceptions of responsibility. It is difficult to imagine the occurrence of such changes without heightened moral and legal disagreements.

References

Aquinas, Thomas. 1948. *St. Thomas Aquinas: Summa Theologica.* Translated by Fathers of the English Dominican Province. New York: Benziger Brothers, Inc.

Aristotle. 1984. *The Complete Works of Aristotle: The Revised Oxford Translation.* Edited by Jonathan Barnes. 2 vols. Princeton, NJ: Princeton University Press.

Bostrom, Nick, and Anders Sandberg. 2009. The wisdom of nature: An evolutionary heuristic for human enhancement. In Savulescu and Bostrom, eds., 375-416.

Coady, C.A.J. 2009. Playing God. In Savulescu and Bostrom, eds., 151-176.

Cohen, I. Glenn. 2008. Intentional diminishment, the non-identity problem, and legal liability. *Hastings Law Journal* 60 (2): 347-76.

Dressler, Joshua. 2006. *Understanding Criminal Law.* 4th Ed. Newark, NJ; San Francisco; and Charlottesville, VA: LexisNexis.

Glannon, Walter. 2002. *The Mental Basis of Responsibility*. Aldershot, UK: Ashgate.
Habermas, Jürgen. 2003. *The Future of Human Nature*. Maldon, MA: Polity.
Hart, Herbert L. A. 2008. *Punishment and Responsibility: Essays in the Philosophy of Law*. 2d Ed. Oxford: Oxford University Press.
King, Jaime. 2008. Duty to the unborn: A response to Smolensky. *Hastings Law Journal* 60 (2): 377-96.
Murphy, Jeffrie G. 1992. Moral death: A Kantian essay on psychopathy. In *Ethics and Personality: Essays in Moral Psychology*, edited by John Deigh. Chicago: University of Chicago Press. Originally in *Ethics* 89 (4) (1972): 284-98.
Ouelette, Alicia R. 2008. Insult to injury: A disability-sensitive response to Smolensky's call for parental tort liability for preimplantation genetic interventions. *Hastings Law Journal* 60 (2): 397-410.
Parfit, Derek. 1987. *Reasons and Persons*. Oxford: Oxford University Press.
Plato. 1997. *Plato: Complete Works*. Edited by John M. Cooper. Indianapolis, In: Hackett Publishing Company.
Sandel, Michael J. 2009. The case against perfection: What's wrong with designer children, bionic athletes, and genetic engineering. In Savulescu and Bostrom, eds.
Savulescu, Julian, and Nick Bostrom, eds. 2009. *Human Enhancements*. Oxford: Oxford University Press.
Shiffrin, Seana Valentine. 1999. Wrongful life, procreative responsibility, and the significance of harm. *Legal Theory* 5: 117-48.
Smolensky, Kirsten Rabe. 2008a. Creating children with disabilities: Parental tort liability for preimplantation genetic interventions. *Hastings Law Journal* 60 (2): 299-346.
–. 2008b. Parental tort liability for preimplantation genetic interventions: Technological harms, the social model of disability, and questions of identity. *Hastings Law Journal* 60 (2): 411-30.
Stock, Gregory. 2002. *Redesigning Humans: Our Inevitable Genetic Future*. Boston and New York: Houghton Mifflin Company.
Tarde, Gabriel (Jean-Gabriel) de. 1912. *Penal Philosophy*. Translated by Rapelje Howell. Boston: Little, Brown, and Company.
Turner, J.W.C. 1936. The mental element in crimes at common law. *Cambridge Law Journal* 6 (1): 31-66.

Neuroscience's Threat to Free Will

Walter Glannon

Cognitive and affective neuroscience has yielded important insights into the neurobiological underpinning of our capacity for practical and moral reasoning. Experiments involving human subjects undergoing functional magnetic resonance imaging (fMRI) while engaging in cognitive tasks have established correlations between brain states and the mental states that figure in our deliberation and decision making. This has resulted in a better understanding of the brain-mind relation. Neuroimaging has shown that the desires, beliefs, emotions, and intentions that issue in actions are mediated by interacting cortical and subcortical networks in the brain.

Some cognitive neuroscientists and psychologists claim that our understanding of the relation between the brain and behavior implies that mental functions can be completely explained in terms of unconscious mechanical processes in the brain. This suggests that the source of our actions is not within our conscious control and that our mental states have no causal role in the actions we perform. Free will consists in the capacity to initiate and execute plans of action. This involves the capacity to choose and act in accord with one's desires, beliefs, and intentions. It also implies that our actions have an impact on events in the world. But if we are not the source of our actions and our mental states are causally inert, then our idea of conscious free will is an illusion. Further, if free will is an illusion, then no one can be responsible for his or her actions or omissions. The practice of holding people responsible rests on the assumption that we have free will.

I argue that neuroscience does not undermine free will because it does not show that deterministic or mechanistic processes in the brain completely explain human behavior. Any plausible conception of free will is consistent with the idea that some mental states can causally influence actions while having physical causes in the brain. Because the brain generates and sustains the mind and the mind, in turn, can influence the brain, any satisfactory account of human agency must include both unconscious physical and conscious mental states and events as the causes of our actions. My aim is not to argue on practical grounds that, even if our belief in free will were an illusion, we would still praise, blame, and hold people responsible for their behavior. Rather, my aim is to show that the argument from illusion is misguided and flawed on theoretical grounds. Neuroscience does not threaten free will because nothing about normal brain function suggests that we lack the capacity to choose and act freely.

Human-machine interfaces and psychotropic drugs can substantially alter many of our physical and psychological properties. They may radically change the way we choose and act. In this respect, transhumanism poses a threat to free will. Yet because we can plausibly retain our commitment to free will in the face of neuroscience and because the capacity for free will is one of the properties that make us human, neuroscientific arguments against free will fail to support the claim that we are evolving from a human to a transhuman world.

Free Will as an Illusion

Psychologists Joshua Greene and Jonathan Cohen claim that neuroscientific evidence will show that "every decision is a thoroughly mechanical process, the outcome of which is completely determined by the results of prior mechanical processes". From this claim, they conclude that "new neuroscience will undermine people's common sense, libertarian conception of free will" (2004, 1781). Among other things, they hold that this conclusion should move us to reject our retributive model of punishment and replace it with a consequentialist one. Although Greene and Cohen mainly discuss the implications of neuroscience for the criminal law, their claims challenge common assumptions about free will. From a slightly different perspective, cognitive neuroscientist Martha Farah states that "all behavior is 100% determined by brain function, which is in turn determined by the interplay of genes and experience" (2005, 38). Expressing a third perspective, psychologist Daniel Wegner maintains that "the real causal mechanisms underlying behavior are never present in consciousness" (2002, 97). The most confident assertion of this third position is made by psychologist Henry Roediger and colleagues: "Clearly conscious intentions cannot cause an action if a neural event that precedes and correlates with the action comes before conscious intentions" (2008, 208).

These claims present three distinct worries from neuroscience about free and effective action. One worry concerns determinism. If the brain is a deterministic system, then we cannot be free because free will and free action are incompatible with determinism. A second worry concerns mechanism. If the brain is just a mechanism, then we cannot be free because free will and free action are incompatible with the idea that all natural phenomena can be explained by natural causes and mechanical principles. A third worry concerns epiphenomenalism. If our conscious mental states and events have no causal force, then none of our actions results from these states and events. Although these are distinct arguments, together they appear to threaten free will in two respects: (1) that we are the authors of our actions and (2) that, as conscious agents, we have a causal impact on events in the world. Determinism and mechanism appear to undermine (1), while epiphenomenalism appears to undermine (2). If these cognitive psychologists and neuroscientists are correct about the implications of neuroscience, then our idea of conscious free will is an illusion. Determinism, mechanism, and epiphenomenalism together form the argument from illusion.

The first neuroscientist to question the idea of conscious will and the presumed efficacy of our conscious mental states on the basis of empirical evidence was neuroscientist Benjamin Libet. In a series of experiments he conducted in the 1980s involving subjects who were asked to flex their wrist or finger, Libet (1985, 2001, 2004, 2010) noted that unconscious-brain events preceded the conscious intention to flex by 300-500 milliseconds. These events are readiness potentials measuring activity in the motor cortex that precedes voluntary muscle movement. The activity is recorded by electrodes placed on the scalp as part of an electroencephalogram (EEG). The brain formed the state associated with the intention before the subjects became aware of it. From his experiments, Libet concluded that "the discovery that the brain unconsciously initiates the volitional process well before the person becomes aware of an intention or wish to act voluntarily … clearly has a profound impact on how we view the nature of free will" (2004, 201). For most neuroscientists, the impact is negative. For example, on the basis of the data from Libet's experiments, neuropsychologist Patrick Haggard claims that because "conscious intention occurs after the onset of preparatory brain activity," it "cannot … cause our actions" (2005, 291). Contrary to what many of us believe, the processes preceding action appear to take place entirely at the unconscious level. If our actions are the result of unconscious deterministic or mechanistic processes in the brain, then we do not have free will and cannot be responsible for what we do.

To assess the argument from illusion, it will be helpful to place it within the historical philosophical debate on free will. For philosophers, the main threat to the control necessary for free will has come from causal determinism. This says that natural laws and events in the past jointly determine a unique future. More precisely, causal determinism says that a complete description of the state of the world at a particular time, in conjunction with a complete formulation of the natural laws, entails the truth about the physical state of the world at later times. This means that any action one performs at a particular time is the only action one could have performed at that time. Causal determinism rules out alternative possibilities (APs) to do otherwise than what one actually does. Incompatibilists hold that APs are necessary for free will and that causal determinism is incompatible with APs. Hard incompatibilists believe that causal determinism is true and that we do not have free will. Libertarian incompatibilists believe that we do have free will and that causal determinism is false. Compatibilists claim that we choose and act freely when we are not constrained, coerced, or compelled. Free will can come in degrees, depending on the extent to which we control the mental states that issue in our actions. Because causal determinism does not entail constraint, coercion, or compulsion, free will is compatible with causal determinism.

Philosopher Robert Kane insists that the AP condition is too thin a basis on which to rest the case for libertarianism. Kane says that, in addition to the forward-looking AP condition, a backward-looking condition of ultimate responsibility (UR) is necessary for libertarian free will. UR consists in "the power of agents to be the ultimate creators (or originators) and sustainers of their own ends and purposes" (1996, 4). Kane emphasizes that this condition "puts the emphasis for being up to us not in the power to do otherwise, but on the *source* or *explanation* of the action that is actually performed: that source must be in us" (ibid., 34). We must be the ultimate, buck-stopping originators of our actions. But we cannot be the originators of our actions if the mental states issuing in them are causally determined by antecedent events. I take Greene and Cohen to be referring to a version of the UR condition when mentioning "people's common sense libertarian conception of free will." On their view, the threat to libertarian free will is not from natural laws and events in the past and the idea that they rule out alternative possibilities. Rather, the threat is from neuronal processes in the brain and the idea that they, not our mental states, are the ultimate and only effective source of our choices and actions. Neuroscience suggests that the UR condition cannot be met. Insofar as neuroscience implies that brain processes do all the work in the causal pathway leading to action, we cannot be ultimately responsible for our choices and actions because we are neither the source nor the authors of them.

Kane is an event-causal libertarian. He holds that the decisions and actions of human agents are physically caused. Free will requires only that these events are caused in an undetermined way. If decisions and actions are caused but not determined by antecedent conditions, then this may be enough for us to be the authors of at least some of our actions. Agent-causal libertarians claim that agents can initiate causal processes without any antecedent causes. Some events are caused not by other events but solely by agents (Clarke 2003). According to compatibilist versions of free will, at least some mental states and events can be within our conscious control and causally efficacious in action even if they are causally determined. The question is whether the idea that something is caused in a deterministic way implies that it has no causal influence of its own.

For a causal explanation of a voluntary action, we need to account for all the steps in the causal sequence resulting in that action. At the mental level, this would include desires to act, beliefs about the circumstances surrounding the action, the intention or plan to act, and the execution of that intention in the choice or decision to act. At the neuronal level, this would include all the cortical and subcortical regions that mediate thought and behavior. What occurs at the mental level depends on what occurs at the neuronal level. Although some philosophers identify intentions with decisions, I distinguish them as separate components of the mental process leading to action. An intention is a plan to do something (Bratman 1986). A decision or choice is the execution of that intention in action. One can change one's mind, alter one's plan, and execute a different plan in an action different from what one initially intended. The pathway from desire to action involves an extended process involving both unconscious brain events and conscious mental events. But the cognitive neuroscientists and psychologists I have cited claim that brain events are doing all the causal work. In that case, our conscious decisions and actions are not really up to us and have no impact on internal or external events.

Defusing the Threat

Libet's experiments to measure intention focus on a narrow time frame: the proximal urge or intention to act now and the wrist- or finger-flexing that immediately follows it. As philosopher Alfred Mele points out, Libet confuses proximal urges or desires to act with proximal intentions to act: "Failing to distinguish intending from wanting can lead to serious errors" (2006, 31). There could be an unconscious desire to flex, which could be followed by a conscious intention to flex. This would imply that the mental events of forming and executing the intention to flex causally influence the act of flexing. Or as a distal intention, a person could plan to perform a particular action not now but at a later time (Mele 2008, 2009, 2010). Even if the "act-now" event were an unconscious brain event, it would not rule out long-range planning leading up to the action as at least partly a conscious process. Also, Libet noted from his experiment that, although the intention to flex was unconscious, his subjects could "veto" this intention, suggesting that a conscious intention and decision not to flex would result in their not flexing (2004, 137-49). This seems to open a window of opportunity for free will. Still, Libet's notion of a veto only suggests that we can consciously refrain from performing some actions that would have issued from unconscious urges or intentions. It does not satisfactorily explain how or why one would translate a different conscious intention into a different action. Even if one accepts the notion of a conscious veto, it offers only an incomplete account of the will.

Mele takes issue with a different aspect of Libet's idea of a veto, asking how an agent simultaneously can be settled on A-ing at t and settled on not A-ing at t (2008, 115). This may not be a problem for Libet if we distinguish between forming intentions and making decisions as separate mental acts. For example, I may form an intention to take a certain route to the airport. Just before turning onto that route, I notice that the traffic is heavy and quickly form a different intention to take a different route. I can form but veto one intention and form and decide to act on a different intention, in which case I was not settled on the first. What *is* a problem for Libet is that this process does not only occur at the unconscious level. The fact that taking a different route is motivated by my conscious awareness of the traffic and by a more general conscious distal intention to go to the airport suggests that an important part of the process occurs within my conscious control. When I start to drive, my intention to go to the airport as quickly as possible is a conscious distal intention that influences the proximal intention about the best route to take now. One cannot draw general conclusions about willing and acting from Libet's experiments because wrist- and finger-flexing are not representative of most of the actions we perform in our lives. Many of these actions involve at least some conscious deliberation and formation and execution of conscious intentions, a process that extends over time.

The claims by Greene and Cohen (2004) and Farah (2005) that mechanistic processes in the brain determine behavior seem to imply that they completely explain my behavior. But consider the following example. Suppose that I have distinct desires to begin an essay and exercise at the same time. Each of these desires corresponds to a proximal urge in my brain. Whether I form and execute an intention to do one thing rather than the other cannot be explained satisfactorily in terms of unconscious neural urges. Each of these competing desires is influenced by distinct long-range plans of mine to be healthy and more productive in my scholarship. My decision to write or exercise at a particular time depends on how I respond to the reasons for performing these actions. My response to these reasons will be influenced by my conscious response to factors external to the brain, such as the weather, the volume of noise in my home, and the deadline for submitting the essay. These reasons involve more than proximal urges in my brain. They also involve conscious beliefs whose content reflects features of the external environment. As part of this environment, the reasons for performing either action reflect the fact that I live in a culture that values health and scholarship. Appeal to the brain alone cannot explain why I perform one action rather than the other.

Unconscious mechanical processes in the brain are part of the pathway leading to my decision and action. But one must not mistakenly infer from the fact that a decision has an unconscious cause that the decision itself is unconscious. Unconscious mental states may initiate an action. Yet this does not imply that conscious mental states play no causal role when an agent forms and executes a proximal intention in that action. An unconscious urge to act may itself be influenced by a conscious distal intention involving long-range planning. The brain is not doing all the causal work in the process leading up to and resulting in action but causally *under*determines it. At least some mental states are doing some of the causal work. In this and the preceding example, the fact that events in the external environment influence my plan of action shows that more than just the brain is involved in what I choose and do. Like the brain, though, the environment influences but does not determine what I do. Given the same environmental conditions, I may choose to perform a different action.

Daniel Wegner offers the most extreme version of the view that conscious intentions play no causal role in our action. He claims that "conscious will is an illusion ... in the sense that the experience of consciously willing an action is not a direct indication that the conscious thought has caused the action" (2002, 2). Our behavior is the result of a deterministic process that can be completely explained in physical terms. The intentions and other mental states we associate with conscious will are epiphenomenal. Wegner admits that we do have conscious intentions. If they are causally inert, then why would he claim that we have them? His reply is that conscious intentions give us a sense of responsibility for some of the things we do, albeit in a magical or supernatural sense: "Seeing one's own causal influence as supernatural is part of being human" (2008, 228). Free will is part of what Wegner calls a "magical self." In using this term, he appears to associate the self and free will with substance dualism and the idea of an immaterial mind or soul causally independent of physical events in the brain. Biologist Anthony Cashmore is more explicit in saying that "if we no longer entertain the luxury of a belief in the 'magic of the soul', then there is little else to offer in support of the concept of free will" (2010, 4499). Yet if conscious will is not real but magical, then we cannot attribute the property of agency to ourselves. Wegner posits a mysterious concept of agency based on an implausibly strong assumption about the extent of unconscious processes in the production of action. Responding to Wegner's position, Mele notes that "if one sets the bar for free will (that is, for the power or ability to act freely) ridiculously high, the thesis that people sometimes act freely should strike one as ridiculous" (2008, 124). Mele adds that "if the bar for the existence or efficacy of 'conscious will' is set so high that we have to be supernatural beings for conscious will to exist or be efficacious in us, then, of course, conscious will should be lumped together with ghosts, fairies, and the like" (ibid.).

Most cognitive psychologists and neuroscientists give more weight to libertarianism than it has in philosophical debates on free will. They also ignore the fact that there are different (agent-causal and event-causal) versions of libertarianism. More importantly, a significant number erroneously assume that free will presupposes substance dualism and the idea that mental states can operate independently of physical states and events in the brain. Libertarians are a minority among philosophers writing about free will. A very small number of these are substance dualists. The majority of philosophers working on free will are compatibilists. For most compatibilists, causal determinism just means that our mental states and actions are the products of antecedent physical events, such that, if it were not for the latter, the former would not occur. Mental states are necessarily generated and sustained by brain states. But this does not mean that the choices and actions that issue from mental states are coerced or compelled. This is consistent with what David Hume calls "liberty of spontaneity," which involves freedom from force or constraint. Hume argues that, since the existence of causal laws governing our actions does not undermine this type of liberty, there is no conflict between causal determinism and moral responsibility (1978, 407). Locke holds a similar view and presents the example of a man who finds himself in a room that he cannot leave because the door is locked. Since this fact does not affect his choice to remain in the room at that moment, he chooses freely even though he could not have done otherwise (1975, ch. XXI). This is a negative-default conception of free will. Many compatibilists offer a positive conception as well.

Philosopher Harry Frankfurt has developed one of the most influential positive-compatibilist accounts of free will. He defines persons as individuals with the capacity to form first-order desires to perform certain actions. They also have the capacity to form second-order desires to have certain first-order desires (1988, ch. 2). The will is the effective first-order desire that moves or would move a person all the way to action. One wills and acts feely when one's effective first-order desires align with one's second-order desires, and one identifies with both. There is a mesh between valuational and motivational mental states. Identification follows from a process of critical self-reflection after which the relevant desires become part of the set of a person's motivational states. The agent forms an unopposed second-order desire to make a particular first-order desire his will. In addition, the agent judges that no further consultation with even higher-order desires would result in a reversal of that decision. This process of reflective self-control is what enables one to make the mental springs of action one's own. It is a process with a phenomenological aspect because it involves the experience of control. Conscious reflection on the springs of our actions is what makes them self-generated and is essential for us to be autonomous agents. Still, the challenge to free will from cognitive neuroscience is not that brain processes interfere with identification or that they coerce or compel us to act. Rather, the challenge from Wegner and others is that brain processes alone account for all the events in the pathway leading to action. If so, then these processes render mental states epiphenomenal.

Our first-order desires may very well be causally determined in the sense that they are necessarily generated and sustained by events in the brain. But this does not put all these and other motivational states beyond our conscious control. Nor does it render all of them causally inert. Our capacity to make these desires conform to second-order desires, to identify with them, and to translate them into actions may provide us with enough conscious control of our motivational states to be the authors of them and to make them play a causal role in our actions. There is both brain–mind and mind–brain causal interaction. The underlying brain circuits are reentrant loops in which information is constantly recycled. The causal trajectories are best described as neither top-down nor bottom-up but circular (Spence 2009, 154). Cognitive behavioral therapy is just one example of how some mental states can be causally efficacious in altering brain states and influencing actions that issue from them. Reframing our beliefs about the world can have modulating effects on cortical and limbic regions of the brain. These effects occur because of the intentionality of beliefs, a property that neurons lack.

If the lower- and higher-level capacities in Frankfurt's model are intentional and part of circular causal trajectories, then these capacities may be sufficient for us to be ultimate, buck-stopping originators of some of our actions. They may also be sufficient for some of our conscious mental states to be causally efficacious in producing these actions. In these respects, Frankfurt's version of compatibilism can satisfy a condition analogous to UR. We do not need to endorse a libertarian rejection of causal determinism to satisfy it. If neuroscience threatens only libertarianism and not also compatibilism, then the threat to free will might not be so great after all.

Unlike libertarian incompatibilists such as Kane, for Frankfurt and other compatibilists what matters in having or lacking free will is not so much whether external *sources* influence the mental states issuing in our action – indeed, they do. What matters more is whether we have the internal *resources* to identify with our desires, beliefs, and intentions and execute them in actions. Just because these resources have physical causes does not mean that we cannot consciously identify with or act on them. Some would claim that social factors beyond our control have such a strong influence on our thought and behavior, that what we think and do is not up to us. These external sources play such a significant role in the causal history of our choices and actions that they preclude free and responsible agency (Strawson 1994, Pereboom 2001). This may be a legitimate challenge to free will and responsibility for a compatibilist. Some may question whether the process of identification can minimize the force of these external factors on one's motivational states. They may question whether one can integrate these factors into the autonomous springs of one's actions or whether they are alien to these springs and, thus, not one's own. Yet this is not part of the challenge to free will from neuroscience, which is not concerned with social factors but only events in the brain.

In Libet's model, unconscious brain events associated with the urges or intentions to act occur at discrete, measurable times. But it is difficult to see how a mechanistic model of the brain-behavior relation based on readiness potentials can account for the extended temporal process involved in deliberation and decision making leading to action. There is a similar weakness in Frankfurt's account, which fails to acknowledge that the process of identification extends into the past. Philosopher Michael Bratman defends a historical theory of practical reasoning and intention. An agent may reason and act in a nondeliberative and nonreflective way at a certain time. Yet there is often a rational link to prior deliberation: "it seems quite plausible to suppose that the relevant process is the *extended deliberation* that begins at t0 [some time in the past] and continues through to t1 [the present time of action]" (1986, 80). Further, "assessments of the rationality of agents are sensitive to how in fact the agent comes to have the intentions he has, not to how he might have come to have them" (Bratman 1986, 82). Bratman's historical theory of intentions supports the idea of distal intentions and their possible influence on the proximal intentions that directly issue in action.

It is debatable whether the influence of external sources on our motivational states threatens compatibilism. More importantly, if an intention is part of a deliberative process that extends into the past, then this casts doubt on Libet's claim that forming an intention occurs at a particular time or within a very narrow temporal interval. It also calls into question the claim that events and processes in the brain occurring at specific times determine the formation of an intention and its execution in action. By focusing on the current time-slice relation of a brain event to a mental event such as forming an intention, many neuroscientists ignore the critical role of the history behind this mental event.

In a study published three years ago, neuroscientist John-Dylan Haynes and colleagues used fMRI to monitor patterns of activity in the prefrontal cortex as subjects concentrated on choosing between two future actions (Haynes et al. 2007, Haynes 2010). The researchers reported that the cortical activity patterns corresponded to the subjects' different plans. This study seemed to show that the process of deliberating and decision making could be measured by brain imaging. It seemed to display brain activity corresponding not only to proximal intentions but distal intentions as well. While this study was an improvement over Libet's experiment, it had limitations of its own. The duration of the patterns of brain activity was relatively short. They did not correspond to plans that extended over many hours, days, or months. So, one can question whether the imaging could accurately measure distal intentions and their influence on proximal intentions. Moreover, the correspondence between the cortical activity and the plans did not rule out the possibility that conscious mental states influenced the plans and the execution of one plan rather than the other in action. Even if imaging could display the neural mechanisms underlying the choice between two future actions in the experiment, it could not explain why a subject entertains different plans of action in actual life. Nor could it explain why a subject forms and executes one plan rather than another. A satisfactory answer to these questions requires consideration of factors in addition to the brain.

There are seven main problems with the argument from illusion. This is by no means an exhaustive list. But these problems are enough to expose flaws in the argument.

First, claims about neuroscientific determinism or mechanism presumably are based on empirical evidence. Most of this evidence is in the form of neuroimaging. Functional brain-imaging experiments conducted by cognitive neuroscientists and psychologists show correlations between brain activity and behavior. Correlation is not causation. Yet the claim that every decision is a mechanical process completely determined by prior mechanical processes in the brain is a causal claim. Some correlations may be strong enough to suggest causation, especially if one can eliminate other factors in explaining the relation between anatomical and functional brain features and behavior. If a person loses control of impulses, a brain scan shows a tumor in the person's prefrontal cortex, and he or she regains impulse control with the removal of the tumor, then this would indicate a causal connection between the brain abnormality and the behavior. But this is an example of brain dysfunction. It does not support the claim that imaging establishes a causal connection between normal brain function and a particular action or pattern of behavior. Correlations between normal brain activity and behavior are not strong enough to support the claim that brain processes causally determine behavior. In the absence of a causal connection, the claim that brain processes determine behavior is an assumption lacking the necessary empirical evidence. Correlations between brain processes and behavior may leave room for some of our mental states to play some causal role in our actions.

Second, claims about a causal connection between brain events and voluntary actions are usually based on images of localized brain activity. They tend to focus on executive functions in the prefrontal cortex, the premotor cortex, and the motor cortex. Yet the neural activity that underlies decisions and actions is distributed throughout the brain (Glannon 2005, 2006). The anterior cingulate cortex also plays a critical role in behavior control by mediating cognitive and affective processing and the capacity to monitor and select plans of action. In subcortical regions, the basal ganglia and cerebellum not only enable voluntary movement but also influence such cognitive functions as planning, working memory, and attention. Psychiatrist Sean Spence explains that the neural circuits mediating action involve mainly basal ganglia-thalamic-cortical loops. These run between the cerebral cortex, basal ganglia, and specific thalamic nuclei, and then project back to the cortex (2009, 154). Functional brain scans may show activation in these regions when a person performs cognitive tasks in the scanner. But they cannot show how these regions project to and from each other or how these projections enable the coordinated brain functions that are necessary to plan and execute intentions in actions.

Third, many experimental settings using functional brain imaging and similar techniques involve artificial scenarios that cannot replicate real-world situations in which people choose and act. The techniques cannot diagnose *post hoc* what one was thinking when one performed a particular action and thus cannot explain why one performed that action. With the exception of some motor functions, imaging cannot predict how one would act in a given situation. When one gets into the driver's seat of a car or mounts a bicycle, the actions that follow are to some extent predictable. But their predictability and the fact that they are performed unconsciously do not mean that there is nothing voluntary about them and that they are beyond our conscious control. This further calls into question claims about determinism and mechanism based on neuroimaging. There was nothing artificial about Libet's experiments. Still, finger- and wrist-flexing are not the sorts of actions that make us candidates for attributions of praise, blame, and responsibility.

Fourth, the argument from illusion involves an invalid inference about causation. The fact that a mental state or event has a physical cause in the brain does not imply that it is not among the causes of an action. Just because an action is preceded by unconscious brain events does not mean that no conscious mental states and events have a causal role in the pathway leading to that action. As Mele points out, "[N]ot only is there no rule against causes themselves having causes, it is also the *norm* for causes to have causes (How many causal processes start with uncaused causes?)" (2009, 72). Libet, Haggard, Roediger et al., and Wegner all make this faulty inference. It is symptomatic of the view held by many biologists and psychologists that free will presupposes substance dualism and the idea that the soul or mind can function independently of physical states and events in the brain. Very few philosophers writing on free will hold this view. Greene and Cohen associate compatibilism with a materialist account of the mind: "However, in our estimation, even people who do or would readily endorse a thoroughly material account of human action and its causes have dualist, libertarian intuitions" (2004, 1779). Compatibilists would strongly disagree with this claim, and their writings would back them up.

Fifth, the idea that conscious mental states and events play no causal role in action and are epiphenomenal offers an impoverished account of human agency. It implies that we never do anything on the basis of our desires, beliefs, emotions, intentions, and decisions. All our behavior is the product of unconscious mechanical processes. It seems to explain away practical and moral reasoning and decision making. Indeed, if we define *persons* as essentially agents who act on the basis of conscious mental states, then on this account persons do not exist.

In addition to conscious desires and beliefs, interests are an important component of human agency in the way they shape the distal and proximal intentions that lead to our actions. Neither neurons nor unconscious urges have interests. Only persons do.

Sixth, the idea from Libet and other neuroscientists that we can explain how brain events cause mental events in a current time-slice ignores the history of our intentions and choices. Proximal intentions may be influenced by distal intentions. These, in turn, may be shaped by the cultivation of values and dispositions over a period of time. Because values, dispositions, and some intentions extend into the past, the neuroscientific time-slice view leaves out an important historical component of planning and acting.

Seventh, if an explanation of our behavior just consists of neurons up and down, then the motivation for the judgment that we should reject retributive punishment is unclear. This appears to be pulling a normative rabbit out of an empirical hat. There is a need to explain how to derive a normative "ought" from an empirical "is" (Greene 2003). Empirical facts about the brain may explain why we have certain intuitions about cases of moral conflict. These may involve intuitive responses to questions such as whether we can harm some people in order to save others. But the judgment that a person is responsible for his or her actions involves more than intuitions generated by neuronal processes. It requires justification based on reasons reflecting principles and rules of behavior constructed by human agents in a social setting. While information about the brain can inform moral judgments, the social construction of these principles and rules forms the basis of these judgments.

A Broad Conception of Free Will

Every human agent enlists unconscious and conscious mental states when he or she interacts with the environment. These are not discrete, isolated events occurring at specific times in the brain or mind. They are part of a broader process of agency that extends over time and involves the brain, body, and external world. Against Libet's view, neurosurgeon and philosopher Grant Gillett asserts that "a decision is … not a circumscribed event in neuro-time that could be thought of as an output, and an intention is not a causal event preceding that output, but both are much more holistically interwoven with the lived and experienced fabric of one's life" (2009, 333). Further, "the dynamic structure of normal human action makes such a posit look mistaken, an artificial construct bolstered not only by an experimental situation in which the actions are of a staccato and discrete kind" (2008, 115). Decisions, intentions, and actions are more than just a function of events in the brain. The interaction of the organism, or subject, with the environment influences the activity of billions of neurons and can change the morphology and function of the brain. Since the subject's actions influence brain function, this discredits the idea that particular brain states can predict particular choices and actions. Organism-environment interaction undermines neurobiological determinism, which assumes that there is only one causal direction in explaining action – from the brain to action. It ignores the fact that there is a second causal direction at work – from the environment to the brain. The causal process issuing in action is not linear but circular. It goes from brain to mind to world and then back again.

Some who endorse a mechanistic view of personhood employ a divide-and-conquer strategy to defend ontological reductionism and epiphenomenalism about the brain-mind relation. In a position similar to that of Wegner and Cashmore, Farah and theologian Nancey Murphy state that "brain processes ... are not mere correlates but are the physical bases of [the] central aspects of our personhood. If these aspects of the person are all features of the machine, why have a ghost at all?" (2009, 1168). The suggestion is that we are either machines identical to our brains or ghosts identical to mental properties that are independent of the brain. We can explain away the ghost by accepting the presumed fact that we are just machines. But from the fact that the mental aspects of personhood have physical bases in the brain, it does not follow that mental properties are nothing more than physical properties. We are neither machines nor ghosts defined essentially in terms of either physical or psychological properties. This is a mistaken picture because we are essentially constituted by both the brain and the mind. Brain and mind are interacting components of a person. They mutually influence each other in a nested series of feed-forward and feedback loops enabling human agency. Neither the brain nor the mind can account for agency on its own.

As noted, in his earlier work replicating results from Libet's experiments, Haggard makes a faulty inference about brain processes alone causing action. In a recent article, Haggard notes that networks in the presupplementary motor cortex, anterior prefrontal cortex, and the parietal cortex underlie voluntary action and responsibility. Yet Haggard suggests that mental states may causally influence the brain in saying that "responsibility might depend on the reason that triggered a neural process culminating in action, and on whether a final check should have stopped the action" (2008, 944). Reasons can be either external or internal to human agents (Williams 1981; Scanlon 1998). An external reason is associated with rules or norms recognizable by any rational person as a member of a social or cultural group. External reasons ground contractualist moral theories, where agents interacting in a social context agree on rules and principles to guide behavior. These reasons obtain independently of particular agents and provide objective grounds for the permissibility or impermissibility of any given action. An internal reason consists of a combined desire and belief of a particular agent. Internal and external practical and moral reasons motivate persons to perform some actions rather than others. Haggard appears to be using "reasons" in both senses. One can plausibly assume that internal reasons are emergent mental states that are dependent on but not reducible to neural processes. Insofar as these reasons can function as a "check" on our action, they can influence processes at the neural level. If so, then we have at least some control of our behavior because of processes operating at the mental level.

Haggard notes that our ability to respond to external reasons for or against actions can influence processes at the neural level:

> Interestingly, both decisions [to act or not to act] have a strong normative element; although a person's brain decides what they carry out, culture and education teach people what are acceptable reasons for action, what are not, and when a final predictive check should recommend withholding action. Culture and education therefore represent powerful learning signals for the brain's cognitive-motor circuits. ... Although neuroscientific detection of the brain circuits that generate actions and conscious awareness can contribute to an evidence-based theory of responsibility, it is unclear whether they can capture all the nuances of social and legal concepts of responsibility. (2008, 944)

Given the role that Haggard attributes to external reasons and associated normative practices in actions, it appears that neuroscience cannot capture these nuances.

There are three points that are worth making in the light of Haggard's claims. First, they suggest that the social environment can influence the brain and the way it mediates the mental states associated with voluntary action. Second, they suggest that mental states associated with internal reasons and one's response to external reasons can influence events in the brain. Third, the upshot of the first two points is that neural networks cannot satisfactorily explain human behavior. The brain alone does not decide what we do. Spence says that "ventral and medial brain systems seem to function 'as if' biology 'recognizes' valence, value, moral checks and balances. It doesn't necessarily 'do the right thing', but it does seem to 'represent' what is right and what is wrong. It is the agent who 'chooses' what 'to do' next" (2009, 306). This is because there is an essential subjective element in human agency that cannot be explained in terms of brain function. A description of cognitive-motor circuits cannot capture the first-person experience of deliberating and choosing what to do. Spence continues,

> we might conclude that no account of human action (and therefore human moral responsibility) is ever complete in the absence of a subjective report, a "view from within," provided by the agent ... So, when we wish to apportion responsibility, we are not merely identifying an organism ... we are saying something important about "its" underlying volitional processes: the symmetry pertaining between desires and deeds, intentions and actions. (ibid., 236)

A satisfactory explanation of behavior must include internal and external reasons, which reflect the subjectivity of the agent and the social and cultural environment in which the agent lives and acts.

These points indicate that free will and moral responsibility are not just empirically grounded metaphysical notions involving considerations of causation, possibility, and necessity. They are also normative notions reflecting the fact that we are social beings with expectations about what we can and should do. Some philosophers argue that free will should be construed even more broadly to include a political dimension. Jason Brennan and David Schmidtz argue thus:

> Freedom of the will is not an on/off switch, something you either have or not. Instead, real-world freedom of the will is an ongoing achievement. It is achieved in degrees, and not everyone achieves it to the same degree. Moreover, our wills can be freer in some circumstances than in others. Because our culture and system of government affect people's inclinations and ability to make up their own minds, the most interesting views of the free will problem today are personal, social, and political, not metaphysical. (2010, 208)

The most defensible model of voluntary action is one that includes complementary empirical and normative dimensions reflecting causal interaction between the brain and the mind of a human subject acting in the world. It is worth noting that, in contrast to Wegner, Haggard does not attribute anything magical to the normative dimension of human behavior. This dimension is a real function of our activity as social beings. This makes it difficult to understand how we could retain the normative concept of responsibility without the idea that willing and acting are at least partly within our conscious control. Otherwise, it would be magical.

Conclusion

Nothing about the normal structure and function of the brain or how it generates and sustains the mind implies that we are mistaken in believing that we have the capacity to form intentions and execute them in choices and actions. Neuroscience does not show that our conscious mental states have no causal role in our behavior. Nor does it imply that an action is compelled, coerced, or constrained if it is causally determined by brain events. Insofar as the relevant mental capacities ground our normative practices and institutions, and neuroscience does not show that we lack these capacities, neuroscience does not threaten these practices and institutions. It is possible that future advances in neuroscience will call into question our conviction that we have free will and can be responsible for our behavior. If they do, then it will still be unclear how empirical findings about the brain-mind relation will influence our normative judgments about moral and legal responsibility. This will require debate about the meaning of information about the brain, which will not be limited to neuroscientists but will include philosophers, social scientists, and, indeed, society as a whole.

Future discoveries in neuroscience may show that all our choices and actions are the result of mechanistic processes in the brain. This would challenge the assumption that we have conscious control over what we choose and do. It may turn out that free will is an illusion after all. Insofar as free will is one of the properties that define us as humans, this may lead us to redefine the sorts of beings we are. As matters now stand, however, neuroscience does not provide sufficient reasons for us to relinquish our commitment to free will. The conviction that we have the power consciously to control our choices and actions may seem precarious in a transhuman world in which human-machine interfaces and psychotropic drugs alter our mental states. But the reasons for retaining this conviction should make us question the idea that we will inevitably adopt a transhuman conception of ourselves.

References

Bratman, Michael 1986. *Intention, Plans, and Practical Reason.* Cambridge, MA: Harvard University Press.

Brennan, Jason, and David Schmidtz. 2010. *A Brief History of Liberty.* Malden, MA: Wiley-Blackwell.

Cashmore, Anthony. 2010. The Lucretian swerve: The biological basis of human behavior and the criminal justice system. *Proceedings of the National Academy of Sciences* 107: 4499-4504.

Clarke, Randolph. 2003. *Libertarian Accounts of Free Will.* New York: Oxford University Press.

Farah, Martha 2005. Neuroethics: the practical and the philosophical. *Trends in Cognitive Sciences* 9: 34-40.

Farah, Martha, and Nancey Murphy. 2009. Neuroscience and the soul. *Science* 323: 1168.

Frankfurt, Harry. 1988. *The Importance of What We Care About.* New York: Cambridge University Press.

Gillett, Grant. 2008. *Subjectivity and Being Somebody: Human Identity and Neuroethics.* Exeter, UK: Imprint Academic.

–. 2009. Intention, autonomy, and brain events. *Bioethics* 23: 330-39.

Glannon, Walter. 2005. Neurobiology, neuroimaging, and free will. *Midwest Studies in Philosophy* 29: 68-82.

–. 2006. *Bioethics and the Brain.* New York: Oxford University Press.

Greene, Joshua. 2003. From neural "is" to moral "ought": What are the moral implications of neuroscientific moral psychology? *Nature Reviews Neuroscience* 4: 847-50.

Greene, Joshua, and Jonathan Cohen. 2004. For the law, neuroscience changes nothing and everything. *Philosophical Transactions of the Royal Society of London* 359: 1775-85.

Haggard, Patrick. 2005. Conscious intention and motor cognition. *Trends in Cognitive Sciences* 9: 290-95.
–. 2008. Human volition: Towards a neuroscience of will. *Nature Reviews Neuroscience* 9: 934-46.
Haynes, John-Dylan. 2010. Beyond Libet: Long-term prediction of free choices from neuroimaging signals." In Sinnott-Armstrong and Nadel, eds., ch. 8.
Haynes, John-Dylan, et al. 2007. Reading hidden intentions in the human brain. *Current Biology* 17: 323-28.
Hume, David. 1978. *A Treatise of Human Nature*. Edited by P. H. Nidditch. Oxford: Clarendon Press.
Kane, Robert. 1996. *The Significance of Free Will*. New York: Oxford University Press.
Libet, Benjamin. 1985. Unconscious cerebral initiative and the role of conscious will in voluntary action. *Behavioral and Brain Sciences* 8: 529-66.
–. 2001. Consciousness, free action, and the brain. *Journal of Consciousness Studies* 8: 59-65.
–. 2004. *Mind Time: The Temporal Factor in Consciousness*. Cambridge, MA: Harvard University Press.
–. 2010. Do we have free will?" In Sinnott-Armstrong and Nadel, eds., ch. 1.
Locke, John. 1975. *An Essay Concerning Human Understanding*, P. H. Nidditch, ed. Oxford: Clarendon Press.
Mele, Alfred. 2006. *Free Will and Luck*. New York: Oxford University Press.
–. 2008. Recent work on free will and science. *American Philosophical Quarterly* 45: 107-30.
–. 2009. *Effective Intentions: The Power of Conscious Will*. New York: Oxford University Press.
–. 2010. Libet on free will, readiness potentials, decisions, and awareness. In Sinnott-Armstrong and Nadel, eds., ch. 3.
Pereboom, Derk. 2001. *Living without Free Will*. New York: Cambridge University Press.
Roediger, Henry, et al. 2008. Free will and the control of action. In *Are We Free? Psychology and Free Will*, edited by J. Baer, J. Kaufman, and R. Baumeister, 205-25. Oxford: Oxford University Press.
Scanlon, Thomas. 1998. *What We Owe to Each Other*. Cambridge, MA: Harvard University Press.
Sinnott-Armstrong, Walter, and Lynne Nadel, eds. *Conscious Will and Responsibility: A Tribute to Benjamin Libet*. New York: Oxford University Press,
Spence, Sean. 2009. *The Actor's Brain: Exploring the Cognitive Neuroscience of Free Will*. Oxford: Oxford University Press.

Strawson, Galen. 1994. The impossibility of moral responsibility. *Philosophical Studies* 75: 5-24.

Wegner, Daniel. 2002. *The Illusion of Conscious Will*. Cambridge, MA: MIT Press.

–. 2008. Self is magic. In *Are We Free? Psychology and Free Will*, edited by J. Baer, J. Kaufman, and R. Baumeister, 226-47. Oxford: Oxford University Press.

Williams, Bernard. 1981. Internal and external reasons. In Williams, *Moral Luck*, 101-13. Cambridge: Cambridge University Press.

Part IV:
Transhumanism as a Futuristic Vision

The (Un)Likelihood of a High-Tech Path to Immortality

Barry G. Ritchie

Immortality as the Ultimate Goal of Technology in Transhumanism

The array of technological human enhancements and therapies tagged for inclusion under the umbrella term *transhumanism* has proven contentiously flexible. Some argue that commonplace enhancements like contact lenses, knee replacements, and heart pacemakers fit into the "low end" of the spectrum of bodily additions or alterations qualifying an individual for inclusion in the new species of transhumans (Hames 2007, 162; Grundmann 2007, 85). Others counter that these same technologies merely represent medical progress and caution that claiming these advances fall within the definition of *transhumanism* amounts to a bait-and-switch strategy to legitimize the more fantastic and controversial ideas about the future of human enhancement (Hefner 2009; Nordmann 2007).

Regardless of the disagreements about what represents the "low end" of the technological territory for transhumanism, the upper limit of that realm is usually accepted as self-evident: immortality. Since that particular word is eschewed sometimes due to perceived religious overtones or fears that word choice may sound too audacious, some prefer terms like *indefinite lifespan, infinite lifespan, endless living*, and so forth. Nonetheless, what is meant is the removal of death as the (currently) certain outcome of human life, with the proviso that the particular life being extended indefinitely includes, at a minimum, an intact mind and personhood exhibiting the continuity of past experience we associate with being alive and conscious.

Much of the media attention devoted to transhumanism on television and in the popular science and technology press revolves around this particular hope for the unlimited technological extension of human lifespan. This goal is so audacious as to be inconceivable to some people, and a common response from them is that no one could seriously entertain such an idea. On the contrary, many transhumanists believe this specific goal is not only most certainly attainable but also inevitable. As examples of the latter view, a volume published by the Immortality Institute (2004) provides eighteen enthusiastic contributions espousing the tools, ethics, and prospects for limitless human existence. Aubrey de Grey argues in that volume that, rather than being a far distant technological goal, "it is probable that most of the first generation of 150-year-olds … – a group who are almost certainly already alive and may well be middle-aged – will not die unless at their own hand" (2004, 30-31); elsewhere, he further elaborates on this conclusion about the likelihood of "ending aging" and what he sees as the techniques necessary for doing so (de Grey and Rae 2007). James Hughes opines that "the many lines of converging sciences and technologies and the rapidly escalating pace of medical knowledge suggest that indefinite life extension will be possible in this century" (2004, 29).

For one of the better-known transhumanists, immortality may not only be close at hand but also may not even be the final goal: futurist Ray Kurzweil has seized upon the possibility of resurrecting the dead, presumably, one would suppose, as a prelude to being introduced to the new world of technological immortality:

> Using technology, [Ray Kurzweil] plans to bring his dead father back to life. … In a soft voice, he explains how the resurrection will work. "We can find some of his DNA around his grave site – that's a lot of information right there," he says.
>
> > "The [artificial intelligence] will send down some nanobots and get some bone or teeth and extract some DNA and put it all together. Then they'll get some information from my brain and anyone else who still remembers him."
>
> When I ask how exactly they'll extract the knowledge from his brain, Kurzweil bristles, as if the answer should be obvious: "Just send nanobots into my brain and reconstruct my recollections and memories." The machines will capture everything: the piggyback ride to a grocery store, the bedtime reading of *Tom Swift*, the moment he and his father rejoiced when the letter of acceptance from MIT arrived. (Kushner 2009)

This chapter briefly assesses the likelihood of attaining the goal of "indefinite human lifespan" (*immortality*, in other words) through advances based on extrapolations of several technological approaches commonly mentioned today. At the risk of giving the surprise away early, my primary argument is that the various approaches aimed at enabling infinite life spans are unlikely to be successful, a conclusion that becomes most evident when the brain is the focus for those approaches. Regardless of whether that goal is possible, the ethical and theological considerations for the pursuit, impact, and availability of indefinite-life-extension technologies are important and have been discussed elsewhere (Fukuyama 2002; Hefner 2003, 2009; Immortality Institute 2004, ch. 2; Kass et al. 2003; Overall 2009; Waters 2006). However, the focus in this chapter is solely on several scientific and technological issues related to the likelihood such a goal can be achieved by "immortalizing" the brain.[1]

---

1 My sincere appreciation for helpful and clarifying discussions and comments on this chapter is extended to Arizona State University (ASU) colleagues Jeff Drucker and Stuart Lindsay and to my colleagues in the seminar on transhumanism at ASU, particularly Brian Gratton, Michael Mobley, Kenneth L. Mossman, Norbert Samuelson, and Hava Tirsoh-Samuelson. This paper represents an expanded version of an invited presentation delivered at the 2009 Metanexus annual conference held in Tempe, Arizona, July 2009.

Common Age-Related "Failure Modes"

To assess the likelihood of a high-tech path to immortality, it is instructive to begin by noting the starting point for such a program: the lifespan of the "unenhanced" human. The process of natural selection, working over billions of years, has yielded each of us a body with robust mechanisms for cellular and systemic homeostasis and self-repair such that this body usually will survive in relatively good health through the years leading up to sexual maturity, when reproduction presents the first opportunity to bequeath our species' genetic heritage to the next generation. Since human offspring are born relatively fragile and defenseless for a decade or so, there is also likely an evolutionary advantage to having bodies that also remain healthy for a few decades or so after the onset of our reproductive years (Carey 2003).

Beyond that point, however, evolution becomes indifferent to the reliability of those bodies once our genetic legacy has been passed to our progeny. With that legacy transferred, the host of environmental challenges that have assailed the smooth functioning of the biochemical "wheels within wheels" throughout our lives begin to overwhelm the mechanisms for homeostasis and self-repair, mechanisms that themselves have begun to lose efficiency and accuracy. As a result, over time, our cells, our organs, and then our bodies succumb to those challenges and fail through one or more "failure modes." As Carnes and Olshansky have noted, "While bodies are not designed to fail, neither are they designed for extended operation" (2007, 374).

When those bodies break down such that death occurs, one or more failure modes – diseases and maladies – are said to be the cause of death. The likelihood that a person will die *primarily* of a particular cause – recognizing that more than one ailment may be present at death – varies in a relatively smooth way with age, as shown in Figure 1. With the exception of accidental death and liver disease, the variations seen for death rates in that figure show remarkably similar trends: for most causes of death, the death rate for a particular cause approximately doubles about every eight to ten years, a trend usually attributed to the actuary Benjamin Gompertz, whose studies in the early nineteenth century showed this doubling phenomena (Olshansky and Carnes 2001, 88-90). Curiously, some of the causes in Figure 1, such as influenza and septicemia, are microbial in origin, yet nonetheless follow the same doubling trend of eight to ten years. Correlation does not equal causation, but the similarity of the increase in the death rates with age for these microbial ailments to those from other sources that are likely degenerative (see below) suggests evidence for a linkage to a degenerating immune system.

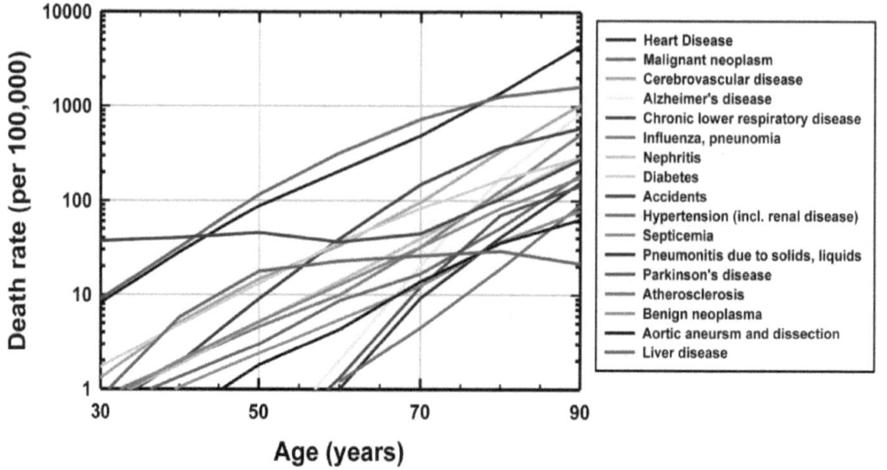

Figure 1: Death rates per 100,000 people for ages from 30 to 90. Only the data for the leading causes of death for U.S. citizens from 70- to 90-years-old are illustrated. *Source*: Data from National Vital Statistics Center 2006.

With the longer lifespans today brought about by the medical advances of the twentieth century (which, as noted above, some may already consider "enhancement"), another trend for another set of causes arises after around age seventy. That set of causes – including Alzheimer's disease and Parkinson's disease – becomes more significant in later life and exhibits a trend where the death rate nearly doubles in about five years, resulting in a much steeper trend in Figure 1 than for most of the causes shown there. If medical progress extends lifespan such that living to one hundred would be common, this steeper trend could bring that set of diseases close to the top of the causes of death for the longest-living people.

Though the exact pathways are not known, a rough consensus exists on the list of factors that arise as a person ages that are likely to lead to most of the conditions listed in Figure 1. Such a consensus would include, for example, accumulated genetic damage, damage wrought by reactive oxygen species, deleterious alterations in long-lived proteins, disruption and failure of genetic- and protein-repair processes, diminished immune system function, and untoward changes in epigenetic expression (cf. Hayflick 2004, 573; Holliday 2004, 568-69). Since these conditions arise in every person's cells over time, a "solution" to the "problem" of aging that immediately comes to mind would entail "simply" reversing all these. (The scare quotes in the previous sentence highlight the words that immediately provoke many specialists working in the field of biogerontology.) Though his list of factors is somewhat different, reversing these ubiquitous aging factors is, to a great extent, the strategy to "end aging" proposed by de Grey and his colleagues (de Grey 2003; de Grey and Rae 2007). Such a strategy presumes – to be most charitable – significant extrapolations of current genetic engineering and molecular biological techniques, if not wholly new approaches. Thus, the de Grey proposal has been met with both broad skepticism[2] and harsh criticism (Warner et al. 2005; Hayflick, Olshansky, and Perls 2005). (The discussion below of applications of gene therapy to a small subset of this list of factors may help explain part of that skepticism.)

Several further observations and comments related to this figure are pertinent to our assessment of the likelihood of extending the human lifespan indefinitely. First, though the graph shows the death rates for these failure modes as a function of age, the previous precaution not to link correlation to causation needs to be kept in mind, and simple interpretations need to be examined critically. Age alone does not specifically cause disease, as might seem the case in Figure 1; rather, the accumulation over time of the slings and arrows of environmental stresses, replication errors, and so on, serves to pile up problems in our cells, ultimately leading to woe. An additional wrinkle is that some of these failure modes are correlated with others, so selecting one as the primary cause of death can obscure the underlying important roles played in some cases by others.

A second observation with respect to Figure 1 comes from noting that we already live in a remarkable era of relatively long lifespans compared to other times in human history, a result of the tremendous gains earned from the medical victories over most causes of infant mortality during the last century, as well as other advances in medicine and public health. Pushing that lifespan higher still will be increasingly difficult. As the figure illustrates, if the leading cause of death at a given age could be magically eliminated, another cause of death then becomes just as prevalent within a year or so later. Thus, completely eliminating one or two causes will not extend human lifespan appreciably. For example, eliminating Alzheimer's disease as a cause of death would extend the average human lifespan in the U.S. only by about 19 *days* – days, not years (Hayflick 2004, 574). Elimination of both heart disease and cancer would push the U.S. life expectancy at birth out only to about eighty-five years (Carnes and Olshansky

2 Warner et al. contest the need to even debate the merits of de Grey's work: "It is, however, our opinion that pretending that such a collection of ill-founded speculations is a useful topic for debate, let alone a serious guide to research planning, does more harm than good both for science and for society." After then comparing de Grey's strategy to creationism, those same authors go on to say, "Treating arguments and proposals that are not backed up by scientific evidence *as though they were scientific ideas* carries the risk of making them impressive to laypersons, whose main way of distinguishing among hypotheses is to take note of those that are promoted in public media or presented to them by advocates whose style they like" [emphasis added] (2005, 1008).

2007, 368). To push life expectancy at birth from eighty-five years to, say, one hundred would require the near-eradication of every cause shown in Figure 1 (Olshansky, Carnes, and Désesquelles 2001, 1491).

Additionally, it is not unreasonable to suppose that there exists yet another set of presently unknown potential causes of death that could become prominent once a significant number of individuals live to ages beyond ninety or higher. These speculative unknown causes, currently masked by the other illnesses listed in Figure 1, conceivably could follow the death rate doubling time for Alzheimer's and Parkinson's diseases or could have an even shorter doubling time. Finally, since nature is not stagnant, the evolution and spread of new infectious lethal diseases might present formidable challenges that are absent today (as was the case with HIV, for example), particularly when those new challenges are coupled with the widespread and interconnected transportations systems woven throughout all parts of the world.

All these observations related to Figure 1 suggest tremendous (and conceivably insurmountable) barriers to any scheme at extending human life span indefinitely, with the possibility that other new barriers also may arise of which we are currently unaware. As will be noted below, this does not mean at all that there is no reason to pursue research that might eliminate or ameliorate any of the specific disorders and diseases tabulated in Figure 1. Rather, sober reflection on that list of ailments should give one considerable pause at the suggestion that they could *all* be eliminated someday, unless one is committed to such faith in progress that one subscribes to what I will call here "The Fundamental Principle of Futurism": at some time in the future, we will be so clever that we will be able to do *anything*.

For the sake of considering further the technological arguments for achieving immortality, we will set these reservations aside and look somewhat more closely at a set of possible strategies that might restrain or get around these failure modes.

"The Three R's": Several Technological Paths to Indefinite Lifespan

For some of the failure modes seen in Figure 1, the simplest technological quest for unlimited lifespan could be based on three "R's": *Replace, Repair, and Rejuvenate*. With the replacement strategy, if an organ wears out, then, like an old car, one can squeeze out a few more miles by swapping out an old part for a new one. Artificial tissues are already in use, and simple swap-outs of joints are common. There are certainly clear paths (or at least some generally accepted directions) forward in addressing some of the leading failure modes shown in Figure 1 via replacement strategies. The technologies associated with artificial hearts may over the next few decades reach the stage where the leading role of heart disease in limiting lifespan might be addressed. Stem cells may someday be harnessed to grow pieces of malfunctioning organs, and, in time, whole organs may be generated as replacements; perhaps this will be the path to eliminate heart and cardiovascular diseases as causes of death, for instance.

Yet, a key set of attributes in our definition of immortality – an intact conscious mind and personhood – rule out replacement as an option for achieving indefinite life spans, because the organ that undergirds those attributes cannot be swapped out for a new model. With fifty billion or so specialized cells, the adult human brain holds perhaps one hundred trillion synaptic interconnections.[3] The constantly changing pattern of those linkages defines for each human being that person's identity, a tapestry whose weaving reflects that person's distinctive history. To be worthwhile, then, one essential, nonnegotiable demand on any scheme for unlimited lifespan is that the brain must stay in good health so that personhood remains intact. Even if every other organ was swapped out to sustain a body indefinitely, immortality would be pointless if the purpose of that patchwork body was to sustain a hopelessly ravaged, minimally functional mind. The brain must be the ultimate strategic target for an immortality approach via repair and rejuvenation.[4]

Many changes take place as the brain ages, including the loss of neurons and reductions in neuron size, which reflect underlying molecular, metabolic, and genetic changes within those cells (Esin 2007). Some of the cells of the nervous system are among the largest cells in the human body, and all have prodigious energy requirements owing in great part to the need to maintain electric potentials along the axons; any changes that affect energy flow into the nervous system directly impact its function. All these changes affect the optimal functioning of neurons individually, as well as complexes of neurons as systems.

---

3 Estimates of the total number of neurons and synapses in the brain vary widely based on a number of factors, including which structures and parts of the brain should be counted toward the total. Estimates for the number of neurons present in the brain also explicitly ignore the similarly huge numbers of neurons in other parts of the body. For a popular level overview of the brain and brain research, see, for example, Rose 2005.

4 The topic under scrutiny here is personal immortality, not merely the simulation of some subset of aspects from a person's consciousness and experience. In some contexts, such as the scenario described in the first quote above from Kurzweil (Kushner 2009), the emphasis may subtly shift to *simulating* a particular individual, rather than actually giving that person an indefinite lifespan. If the goal is shifted to simulating only some aspects of an individual's consciousness and experience, then the intent is quite different from what is intended by the discussion here.

Using the Third "R" to Immortalize the Mind: Repairing Genetic Damage in the Brain

To stay within the limits imposed on this contribution, the focus here will look only at the genetic damage that mounts up in the brain with advancing years, ignoring other types of brain deterioration and all age-related damage to other organ systems that represent failure modes in Figure 1. By age seventy, most brain cells exhibit some of the hundreds of different genetic flaws impacting communication between neurons and the flexibility of the brain to learn and remember. This extensive damage has been convincingly sketched by a remarkable analysis of postmortem samples of brain tissues taken from the frontal cortex area for thirty individuals of ages from 26 to 106 (Lu et al. 2004). The study examined gene expression profiles in the tissue samples to determine the extent to which of more than eleven thousand different genes assayed in the tissues exhibited marked changes. That report found about 4 percent of those factors (over four hundred genes) showed significant (defined as 150 percent or more) increases or decreases in activity for those specific genes. A list of those genes exhibiting significant changes yields a steady drumbeat of bad news. Genes that affect, for example, memory, brain plasticity, and synaptic function had significantly decreased expression with age. Struggling to cope with these changes, genes responsible for repair, immune response, and stress coping showed significant increases. Further analyses in the same study of the promoters for thirty different genes important for brain function showed that all thirty indicated significant DNA damage by age seventy; the authors summed up the situation: "Thus, DNA damage is pervasive in the aging human cortex" (Lu et al. 2004, 885). With such widespread genetic damage, it is daunting to realize that much work has to be done to repair *even one* of the hundreds of types of defects. Myriads of microscopic repair agents would be needed to carry out a brain-wide restoration program via gene therapy, with each of those agents working with perfection, yet not triggering the body's immune system or causing other damage.

Despite their prominence in science-fiction movies and some transhumanist literature, those repair agents are unlikely to be nanoscale, rigid robotic machines with tiny cogs, wheels, and gears for manipulating molecules – the so-called nanobots, inspired by Eric Drexler (1986) and mentioned by Kurzweil in the quote above. Fundamental physical considerations strongly suggest rigid machines formed from assemblies of a few thousand atoms functioning collectively as molecular repair agents in cellular environments are unlikely. This is, in part, because the world within the cell is a vastly different environment from what our experience with mechanical devices in the macroscopic realm might lead us to believe. The warm, viscous interiors of cells are filled with a menagerie of frenetically jostling, sticky molecules, which make those interiors miserable places for tiny mechanical repair devices if they ever could be assembled. The atoms that make up the nanobots themselves would be in constant motion at the atomic level, and, depending on which atoms were used to make them, parts of them would be sticking fleetingly (or, worse, permanently) to passing molecules or molecular structures in the cell; they would not be the absolutely rigid, self-contained assemblies we associate with tools on a garage workbench. Thus, the concept of building little rigid machines moving within cell nuclei to fix genes runs counter to our expectations for the atomic realm. As Richard Jones (2008) has suggested, "It would be like making a clock and its gears out of rubber, then watching it tumble around in a clothes dryer and wondering why it doesn't keep time."

Independent of the complexity of the *mechanical* design of a nanobot is the issue of the complexity of its *operational* design:

> To function, a Drexlerian nanobot would have to store high-level instructional software on-board in large quantity. ... [T]he nanobot would also have to distinguish among many possible conditions, materials, and configurations, and then act instantly and appropriately in every case. It would have to sense distances to sub-angstrom accuracy and act in shavings of a picosecond. Given the absurdly tight dimensional constraints, there would literally be no room for error. (Atkinson 2005, 255)

The operational design for the nanobot, thus, must include the error-and-ambiguity-free specification and development of instructions for dealing with thousands of different scenarios the agent is likely to encounter within a cell or cell nucleus (assuming that it gets there to work at all) and the means to execute those instructions absolutely perfectly; if this seems overly demanding, recall, for instance, that there are over twenty thousand different genes in human DNA, and part of the mission of such an agent conceivably might be to find and fix one or more specific genes within the nucleus of a cell. Those time- and situation-dependent operational instructions must be (1) implemented mechanically somehow within the structure of the nanobot, or (2) some portion of the nanobot must be a tiny computer within the nanobot capable of processing information for those instructions (also stored within the nanobot), or (3) some portion of the nanobot must be allocated to a device that can receive instructions fed to it from outside somehow (presumably, in a way that does not interfere with the operations of the other thousands of nanobots in other cells) and use those instructions to operate the nanobot. The nanobot also would also need some means of navigation and directed propulsion.

All this complexity bumps up against the hard limits of how many atoms can be put into structures. Physically, if the nanobot was a precisely engineered spherical-diamond artifice 10 nanometers in diameter – which is roughly the size of each opening in the pores of the membrane that surrounds the cell nucleus

(Alberts et al. 2002, 670-71) – then all this mechanical and operation complexity would have to be accomplished in a device containing only about one hundred thousand carbon atoms. If each tiny individual subcomponent within a nanobot needed around one hundred atoms for its construction, then only around a thousand parts would be available for all the monstrous mechanical and operational complexity required to deal with the thousands of possible different events the device would encounter. Avoiding the use of the pores in the nuclear membrane so that larger nanobots could be used would require adding instructions and materials for drilling an entrance hole in the wall of the nucleus, as well as patching the hole up after transit.

This latter scenario would be feasible if one grants the First Principle of Futurism, but a near-term application – say, the next forty years – is not credible; there is no serious and clear way forward toward making such machines. A committee commissioned by the National Academy of Sciences to review the state of nanotechnology noted that the feasibility of molecular-manipulating technologies is difficult to assess "because of the lack of experimental demonstrations of many of the key underlying concepts. … Thus, this work is currently outside the mainstream of both conventional science (designed to seek new knowledge) and conventional engineering (usually concerned with the design of things that can be built more or less immediately)" (Williams et al. 2006, 107).

But dispensing with the pictures of rigid microscopic pliers and tin snips, nature has already solved the problem of working in such a messy environment. The cells of our bodies are filled with biomolecular repair agents that find and fix damage, though those natural agents become damaged and less efficient with age. In a form of molecular jujitsu, rather than work against the vibrational and sticky character of the cellular environment, these biomolecular agents instead have evolved to take advantage of (and depend on) those features of atomic and molecular physics in the cellular environment that make things so dauntingly difficult for nanobots. Thus, to fix the age-damaged DNA in our neurons, a plan using specialized biomolecular machines would probably be the likeliest path toward immortality.

A repair and rejuvenation plan for damaged genes in brain tissue based on biomolecular repair agents would then proceed predictably. Pick a particular type of genetic damage to be repaired from the hundreds of types present in the aging brain. Construct a specific biomolecular repair agent that can respond to that particular type of genetic damage by repairing or replacing the damaged stretch of genetic material. Embed that repair agent in an appropriate nanoscale transportation device – say, encapsulated in a nanoparticle. Transport the encapsulated repair agent across the blood/brain barrier[5] to a target cell within a reasonable amount of time, without having the repair agent altered or degraded during transit in the bloodstream[6] and without triggering a damaging response in or from the tissues. Finally, have the agent find and mend the damage within the target neuronal cell with absolute perfection, so as not to induce other problems by a botched repair. Repeat as necessary.

In this sketch of the genetic-repair strategy, the multiple concurrent hurdles of specificity, mobility, efficiency, efficacy, and reliability are apparent and profound at every step. For example, isolating and identifying a strategy for addressing a particular genetically based brain malady already is difficult since some important neurological disorders involve more than one gene. For each step in this simple sketch, the difficulties compound each other. For a given genetic intervention for a particular gene-based disorder in the brain, options that overcome one or even several barriers might be found. But there is no *a priori* reason, other than faith in the Fundamental Principle of Futurism, to assume that the *combined* requirements for specificity, mobility, efficiency, efficacy, and reliability would leave any options available for *every* single item in the currently known inventory of hundreds of types of genetic damage present in brain tissue (and ignoring, of course, any types yet to be discovered).

These formidable hurdles for any gene-therapy approach to repairing genetic damage in the human brain – the only age-related factor considered here for repair and rejuvenation, as we have been ignoring all the other factors noted above – are manifest in the understandably slim existing track record for human gene therapies for any disorder, despite great promise and herculean efforts. To date, gene-therapy research involving human subjects has resulted in only a small number of heroic trials at repairing a small number of genetic disorders, none related to the brain (Barlow-Stewart 2010). No therapeutic approach based on gene therapy has been approved anywhere in the world for treatment of age-related genetic neurological damage. For that matter, the brain aside, only China (Wilson 2005) and the Philippines (Pharma Projects 2009) have approved gene therapies for anything (in those cases, only for types of cancer). Realistically, then, achieving the level of repair needed for just the age-related genetic damage in our brains seems very remote within the next few decades, if ever.

5 The blood/brain barrier provides a major hurdle for any gene-therapeutic approach targeting the brain. See, for example, Saunders et al. 2008. The barrier blocks direct passage of all but the tiniest molecules; most compounds delivered across the blood/brain barrier rely on cooperative intracellular transport within the cells that make up the barrier.

6 Strands of DNA or RNA that might be carried by the repair agent to replace damaged stretches of genetic material will degrade rapidly in blood or simply clump up, so an encapsulating strategy is usually necessary. See, for example, Sanders et al. 2008.

A Fourth "R": Refrigeration – Cryonic Preservation of the Brain

An unwavering faith in technology, as represented in the Fundamental Principle of Futurism, can always translate the words "very remote, if ever" into "someday." If one is convinced that a usable 3-R's technology for repairing genetic brain damage will most certainly exist someday decades or more hence, a fourth "R" might be added to provide a form of "medical time travel" (a phrase used in Wowk 2004) to the future where that technology might exist: *Refrigerate*. In this approach, the plan is to vitrify (being extremely careful to avoid the damage that is attendant with freezing tissue) and store the brain at cryogenic temperatures today, awaiting the tomorrow when hypothetical new technologies for repair and rejuvenation of genetic brain damage would be available and reliable. At that point, one would resurrect the person by reanimating his or her brain (and perhaps vitrified body, too).

Developments in cryobiology have led to the ability to store human embryos and tissues for long periods of time without apparent harm to their functionality upon thawing. The extrapolation of this process to whole human beings is called *cryonics*, a field with a modern history of about a half century (Parry 2004). In cryonic preservation, first discussed extensively by Ettinger in the 1960s (Ettinger 1965), the body is partially dehydrated (to lessen the formation of damaging ice crystals) through the use of chemical solutions infused through the circulatory system. Special emphasis in the perfusion process is paid to the brain, the assumption being that the primary (or only) location of the individual's personhood lies in the brain. (For this reason, in some cases, only the head is preserved.) The body is then rapidly cooled to liquid nitrogen temperatures (-196° C) such that, rather than freezing, the tissues enter a glass-like state through vitrification.

Many obstacles are encountered that make this fourth "R" approach uncertain (Parry 2004, 406-8). These include problems in getting sufficiently high concentrations of the cryoprotectant into the organs to prevent ice formation, getting those same highly toxic chemicals out of the tissues upon thawing, and resolving the problems inherent in uniformly and quickly cooling and thawing large volumes of nonuniform tissue density without ice formation. The most severe problems are associated with fracturing due to thermal stresses. While small tissue slices and embryos have a relatively small surface-to-volume ratio, larger organs have comparatively far less surface area through which heat can be transferred or removed. Vitrification of a large organ like the brain inevitably generates thousands of internal cracks and fissures within the organ due to thermal stresses, despite whatever care one takes in cooling and thawing the tissue. In the brain, each of those cracks severs large numbers of synaptic interconnections. At the cellular level, the cracks are chasms exposing large numbers of broken synaptic connections. Perhaps a nanoscale technology will appear in the distant future that could generate a host of tiny repair agents (the First Principle of Futurism at work, again in the form of nanobots) to work their way along the faces of the myriad frozen canyons scattered throughout the damaged tissues of the vitrified brain, reconnecting the broken and damaged neural links by grappling a specific neural connection on one side of the chasm here and mating that synaptic connection to its counterpart on the other cliff there. As noted above for molecular-manipulation techniques, no such technology is even remotely possible today. Even if the technology was available, however, the broken connections between the neurons all look essentially the same even at the molecular level; there likely is precious little (if anything) in the synaptic linkages themselves analogous to the color-coded wiring inside electronic devices that helps sort out how connections are to be made. With no master map of the unique "wiring" of a person's brain, reweaving the brain's torn tapestry would demand an immense amount of guesswork and an irreducible, inevitable, and sizeable amount of error, resulting in an unavoidable scrambling of the original pathways for impulses to travel between cells. The personhood represented by that tapestry would be either seriously altered or substantially lost forever.

In a frank display of *caveat emptor*, one cryonic preservation firm candidly states on its Web site, "Cryonics cannot be reversed by any simple means" and "There is still no definitive proof that cryonics can preserve long-term memory or personal identity" (ALCOR Life Extension Foundation 2010). While this candor is refreshing, these stark warnings nonetheless still seem generous. More accurate would be saying that *no means at all*, simple or otherwise, are currently known for how this process applied to a human brain can be successfully reversed and that *no proof of any kind* exists that human-brain storage at cryogenic temperatures preserves any memories or identity at all. Schermer, while misunderstanding the cryonics process as simply freezing rather than vitrification, nonetheless commented accurately in *Scientific American* that cryonics "promises everything, delivers nothing (but hope) and is based almost entirely on faith in the future" (Schermer 2001, 29).

A Fifth "R": Replication – Uploading the Brain

The four R's considered thus far have shown little promise in gaining much ground toward the distant goal of immortality. Yet the four R's discussed up to now may have been handicapped by the blinkered vision that those strategies had to repair or rejuvenate the original brain material. Since those organic brains appear to be destined for eventual decay, perhaps a fifth "R" could open up another technological path to immortality: *Replication*. In this strategy, the trick would be to reproduce the entire "information-bearing pattern" of synaptic connections in a particular brain within a huge programmable array of electronic logic gates. Supposedly, then, the consciousness and personhood represented by that information-bearing pattern will have been replicated in a new nonorganic (and more permanent) structure. The person thus replicated will be as immortal as the substrate within which the consciousness has been embedded. (More accurately, we should say that any consciousness that resides within the replication will be "immortal," while the original person, embodied in organic tissue, is destined for death through one or more of the failure modes noted above.)

In the replication approach, then, a person's consciousness is "uploaded" to a device much like we would upload data files from a thumbdrive to one (or more) computers. Rather than fluctuating electrical potentials along neurons, the consciousness embedded in a person's brain is converted into the shuffling of bits between electronic memory locations in a large computer or array of computers. (Of course, multiple copies of the uploaded immortal would be possible, in principle.)

For this uploading approach to work, consciousness must be nothing more than the combined, moment-by-moment working out of the interactions of impulses within the vast assembly of neurons in the brain, both with each other and with their environment. Is consciousness ultimately simply calculation? If the "obvious" answer to that question is "Yes," then one should be honest and admit that such a glib answer already assumes much. To get to that point, one must, for instance, forget (or forego) full consideration of a vast literature devoted to the longstanding debates about what precisely is meant by the words *person*, *mind*, and *consciousness*. Assuming that affirmative answer also sets aside the host of physiological and neurological contributions that the neural structures distributed throughout a person's body (see footnote 2) makes to their consciousness and sense of self. Finally, assuming this consciousness-computation equivalence to be true ignores all the ways a brain is different from a computer, or, for that matter, if Lucas's theorem is correct (Lucas 1961), how a brain *cannot* be like a computer.

In the case of the present discussion, however, let us assume the consciousness-computation-equivalence argument is correct. If that is the case, one approach to assessing the feasibility of uploading consciousness boils down to the question of how practical it will be accurately to replicate a brain within large electronic logic arrays and/or computers. Earlier, the number of synapses in the brain was estimated to be roughly one hundred trillion. Using that estimate, if each synapse and its associated complex and nonlinear signaling functions could be replicated with electronic logic circuits embodying as few as one hundred transistors, then a single computer chip with the equivalent of ten quadrillion transistors could be sufficient for the job. Such a chip would have about five million times more transistors than the current record of around two billion transistors per chip. If the number of transistors per chip doubles every two years (as suggested by, e.g., Kurzweil 2006, 66) according to Moore's Law (Moore 1965), then simple extrapolation predicts a single chip containing enough transistors to simulate the brain should be available by mid-century. At that point, the information-bearing pattern stored in a person's brain can be transferred into this enormous programmable array of electronic logic gates so as to replicate that person's consciousness, thereby creating the world's first immortal. (As noted above, the uploaded consciousness will become immortal in its new substrate, but the original person embedded in flesh and bone will die.)

Completely ignoring, in the interest of space limitations here, all the many software issues involved with what it means to upload memories of, say, a person's first kiss, more important is the observation that Moore's Law is at root an *economic* observation about market forces in the semiconductor industry; it is not derived from fundamental science. Indeed, what science *does* forecast is that Moore's Law is approaching the end of its applicability to silicon-based semiconductors; even Moore himself gives the trend no more than fifteen additional years (Gruener 2007). A few more doublings may occur over the next decade, but twenty or more doublings over the next four decades almost certainly will not happen, if for no other reason than a handful more doublings will take the length scales of elements of electronic logic gates close to the size of an individual atom or two, a hard limit on miniaturization using standard principles of chip design. Other materials may be developed for semiconductor devices, but various issues (including cost considerations) suggest those materials likely will not move things far toward the five-million-fold increase in component densities needed.

If quadrillion- or quintillion-transistor chips are not going to be available for the replication approach, a new computational paradigm might offer another implementation path. However, at present, few options seem credible. Quantum computing, sometimes mentioned in uploading discussions, may prove useful for a number of applications that require algebraic computations that are too costly by brute-force methods, such as quickly determining the multiplicative factors generating a given integer, a tool useful for cryptography (Childs and van Dam 2010; Stoneham 2009) or solving large systems of equations (Harrow, Hassidim, and Lloyd 2009). Quantum computers take advantage of the simultaneous coherence and interference between discrete quantum elements of a circuit, called *quantum bits* or *qubits*. In principle, the quantum elements themselves (e.g., electron spins) can be smaller than an atom, so this offers, at least in theory, the possibility of getting around the size limits noted above for semiconductor electronics.

While applicable as a novel approach to computations that classical computing approaches find intractable or impractical, the ability to scale up the particular computational processes associated with quantum computing to sizes appropriate for anything approaching even the computational power available in silicon for typical computational problems today is uncertain. In an experimental *tour de force*, the first programmable quantum computer was demonstrated in 2009 (Hanneke et al. 2009); but that device had *only two* qubits available for manipulation, a far cry from the perhaps millions that might be needed to achieve even the computing power for problems similar to those handled readily by the silicon-based computers of today. Further, quantum-computing approaches require special environmental considerations for implementation that would make them unattractive for replicating a brain should they ever prove practical; for example, quantum computers likely will always need cryogenic environments (Stoneham 2009).

As a final observation on the overall feasibility of uploading method of implementing the replication approach using any computing approach, consider that many of the speculative trend diagrams about chip density, speed, and so forth that are associated with those advocating the consciousness-calculation equivalence imply that computer chips *already* commonly exist that are more than capable of replicating the computing power of insect brains. From such a plot (e.g., Kurzweil 2006, 70), one would infer that we have exceeded the single-chip computing power equivalent to that present in the brain of a dragonfly, for example. If this hardware equivalence is really true, an obvious and worthwhile demonstration project for the consciousness-computation equivalence principle is apparent: upload a dragonfly's brain into a computer now – and I mean *today* – and convincingly replicate the consciousness (such as that might be) of the insect. While there is no burning need in the world for immortal dragonflies, the ethical and technical barriers presented by such an experiment are nowhere near as formidable as would be encountered in transferring human consciousness. Since the necessary computer hardware would appear to be available today, then, until the solutions to the problems of hardware interfacing and software design make practical and routine the successful uploading of a dragonfly brain (such that it convincingly demonstrates the transfer of that insect's consciousness to a computer), it is unreasonable for anyone to anticipate success with uploading the far more complex human brain. Until that "simple" demonstration, the replication approach is not a credible method of achieving personal immortality.

Conclusion

As the only species on our planet capable of deeply pondering questions about both life and death, each of us lives with the knowledge that we will suffer pain and eventually die. The desire to eliminate pain and the longing for immortality are universal and as old as our ability to ponder. As but one example, John of Patmos's vision from two millennia ago of the New Jerusalem foretold for its inhabitants that God "will wipe every tear from their eyes. Death will be no more; mourning and crying and pain will be no more, for the first things have passed away" (Rev. 21:4, New Revised Standard Version).

It is not surprising, then, that dreams of a technological new world encompass the elimination of pain and death, with those visions firmly and faithfully rooted in the First Principle of Futurism. However, having examined five different "R's" – replacement, repair, rejuvenation, refrigeration, and replication – some basic considerations in each case imply that every one of these fails as a credible technological path to indefinite human lifespan for the foreseeable future. I am personally unaware of any strategies for extending indefinitely human lifespan that are not variations on one or more (or hybrids of one or more) of the themes considered above. Thus, the likelihood of extending the duration of any individual's consciousness and personhood indefinitely via technology appears to be negligible.

The usual caveat for such a statement applies, of course: predictions with regard to progress in science and engineering are always fraught with the danger they may appear foolish when an unanticipated and revolutionary advance offers a new pathway to solving an old problem by exploiting a previously unknown physical phenomenon. A common rejoinder from those who believe in the Fundamental Principle of Futurism to the negative conclusion of the preceding paragraph is a repetition of famous instances where such confident pronouncements about the limits of progress have proved wrong. But less often repeated (and, thus, less well appreciated) are the cases where expansive predictions related to new technologies have never come to pass, such as predictions that radiation would prolong life, fast electric ocean liners would complete trans-Atlantic trips in two days, and that cities would be built under enormous domes – all predictions that were to have come to pass by now (Seidensticker 2006, 23-24). The permanent moon outposts, the lifelike and informative human-computer spoken conversations, and the use of suspended animation for humans undertaking long journeys that were envisioned in the motion picture *2001: A Space Odyssey* were not seen as impossible in 1968, as humanity was preparing to land on the moon for the first time, even though those first theater audiences were only looking a mere third-of-a-century into the future. Those visions of bases, conversations, and "travel conveniences" remain as futuristic and as unfulfilled today, nearly a decade *after* 2001.

So, from our vantage point at the end of the first decade of the twenty-first century, it seems reasonably safe to surmise from this quick review that technology seems very unlikely ever to make us immortal. This negative assessment for technological approaches to achieving indefinite human lifespan is completely consistent with a position statement signed by fifty-two researchers in human aging which, after considering many possible approaches to stemming the effects of aging, said, "The prospect of humans living forever is as unlikely today as it has ever been, and discussions of such an impossible scenario have no place in a scientific discourse" (Olshansky, Hayflick, and Carnes 2002, 293).

This emphatically is not to say that there will be little further progress in dealing with the many ailments listed in Figure 1; there is, on the contrary, considerable hope for ameliorating the effects of many of those "failure modes" and, in some cases, perhaps even eliminating them. For that matter, the reason the "5 R's" are discussed at all as possible paths toward immortality is in part that, in contrast to the far-off goal of indefinite life span, the practical extrapolations to important near-term successes are readily conceivable. Practical extrapolation of today's replacement approaches means the list of replacement parts will be expanded to more and more organs and body parts, perhaps even including some brain tissues, but total replacement for *all* brain tissue is not a credible prospect. Realistically, one can expect that repair and rejuvenation stratagems for various health conditions via gene therapies will become available, addressing some illnesses and conditions associated with abnormal gene function, but it is nearly certain that there will not be approaches that address most of the genetic damage accumulating in the aging brain. Cryopreservation techniques in use now for tissues and organs will continue to improve, but reanimation of cryopreserved brains (and, for that matter, whole bodies and heads) will remain outside mainstream medical discussions. Improvements in brain/computer interfacing may possibly lead beyond the therapies to address brain and nerve damage to encompass some level of cognitive enhancement, but the replication of individual personalities in computers likewise is unlikely ever to fall within discussions in mainstream science, engineering, and medicine.

Thus, while immortality is unlikely be achieved through technology, we can reasonably expect progress on many fronts in our battle with the ailments of aging. The declines and deficits to be faced with aging will be ameliorated or softened but not altogether eliminated. While those achievements fall far short of immortality, they are still eminently worthy and (more to the point here) plausible pursuits.

References

Alberts, Bruce, Alexander Johnson, Julian Lewis, Martin Raff, et al. 2002. *Molecular Biology of the Cell.* 4th ed. New York: Garland Science.

ALCOR Life Extension Foundation. 2010. Scientists' Cryonic FAQ: http://www.alcor.org/sciencefaq.htm, accessed July 17, 2011.

Atkinson, William Illsey. 2005. *Nanocosm: Nanotechnology and the Big Changes Coming from the Inconceivably Small.* New York: AMACOM.

Barlow-Stewart, Kristine. 2010. Gene therapy. *Australian Genetics Resource Book, Fact Sheet 27*: http://www.genetics.com.au/pdf/factsheets/fs27.pdf, accessed July 17, 2011.

Carey, James R. 2003. Life span: A conceptual overview. *Population and Development Review* 29, Supplement: Life Span: Evolutionary, Ecological, and Demographic Perspectives: 1-18.

Carnes, Bruce A., and S. Jay Olshansky. 2007. A realist view of aging, mortality, and future longevity. *Population and Development Review* 33: 367-81.

Childs, Andrew M., and Wim van Dam. 2010. Quantum algorithms for algebraic problems. *Reviews of Modern Physics* 82: 1-52.

De Grey, Aubrey. 2003. The foreseeability of real anti-aging medicine: Focusing the debate. *Experimental Gerontology* 38: 927-34.

–. 2004. The war on aging. In Immortality Institute, 29-45.

De Grey, Aubrey, and Michael Rae. 2007. *Ending Aging: The Rejuvenation Breakthroughs That Could Reverse Human Aging in Our Lifetime.* New York: St. Martin's Press.

Drexler, Eric. 1986. *Engines of Creation.* New York: Anchor Books.

Esin, M. M. 2007. Ageing and the brain. *Journal of Pathology* 211: 181-87.

Ettinger, R.C.W. 1965. *The Prospect of Immortality.* New York: Sedgwick and Johnson.

Fukuyama, Francis. 2002. *Our Posthuman Future: Consequences of the Biotechnology Revolution.* New York: Picador.

Gruener, Wolfgang. 2007. Gordon Moore says Moore's Law will hit "fundamental barrier" in 10 to 15 years. http://www.tgdaily.com/hardware-features/33924-gordon-moore-says-moores-law-will-hit-fundamental-barrier-in-10-to-15-years, accessed July 17, 2011.

Grundmann, Melanie. 2007. Transhuman arts. Aesthetics of the future? Parallels to 19th century dandyism. In *Tensions and Convergences: Technological and Aesthetic Transformations of Society*, edited by R. Heil, A. Kaminski, M. Stippak, et al., 83-92. Piscataway, NJ: Transaction Publishers.

Hames, Richard David. 2007. *The Five Literacies of Global Leadership: What Authentic Leaders Know and You Need to Find Out.* West Sussex, UK: John Wiley and Sons.

Hanneke, D., J. P. Home, J. D. Jost, J. M. Amini, et al. 2009. Realization of a programmable two-qubit quantum processor. *Nature Physics* 6: 13-16.

Harrow, Aram W., Avinatan Hassidim, and Seth Lloyd. 2009. Quantum algorithm for linear systems of equations. *Physical Review Letters* 103: 150502.

Hayflick, Leonard. 2004. "Anti-aging" is an oxymoron. *Journal of Gerontology: Biological Sciences* 59A: 573-78.

Hayflick, Leonard, S. Jay Olshansky, and Thomas T. Perls. 2005. Guest editors' response. *Journal of Gerontology: Biological Sciences* 60A: 140-41.

Hefner, Phillip. 2003. *Technology and Human Becoming.* Minneapolis: Fortress Press.

–. 2009. The animal that aspires to be an angel: The challenge of transhumanism. *Dialog* 48 (2): 158-67.

Holliday, Robin. 2004. The multiple and irreversible causes of aging. *Journal of Gerontology: Biological Sciences* 59A: 568-72.

Hughes, James. 2004. *Citizen Cyborg: Why Democratic Societies Must Respond to the Redesigned Human of the Future*. New York: Basic Books.

Immortality Institute. 2004. *The Scientific Conquest of Death: Essays on Infinite Lifespans*. Buenos Aires: LibrosEnRed.

Jones, Richard A. L. 2008. Rupturing the nanotech rapture. *IEEE Spectrum* 45: 64-67: http://spectrum.ieee.org/semiconductors/nanotechnology/rupturing-the-nanotech-rapture, accessed July 17, 2011.

Kass, Leon, Elizabeth H. Blackburn, Rebecca S. Dresser, Daniel W. Foster, et al. 2003. *Beyond Therapy: Biotechnology and the Pursuit of Happiness*. New York: Harper Perennial.

Kurzweil, Ray. 2006. *The Singularity Is Near: When Humans Transcend Biology.* New York: Penguin Books.

Kushner, David. 2009. When man and machine merge. *Rolling Stone*, February 19, 56-61: http://www.kurzweilai.net/when-man-and-machine-merge, accessed July 17, 2011.

Lu, Tao, Ying Pan, Shyan-Yuan Kao, Cheng Li, et al. 2004. Gene regulation and DNA damage in the ageing human brain. *Nature* 429: 883-91.

Lucas, John. 1961. Mind, Machines, and Gödel. *Philosophy* 36: 112-27.

Moore, Gordon E. 1965. Cramming more components onto integrated circuits. *Electronics* 38: 114-17.

National Vital Statistics Center. 2006. Deaths, percent of total deaths, and death rates for the 15 leading causes of death in 10-year age groups, by race and sex: United States, 1999-2006: http://www.cdc.gov/nchs/data/dvs/LCWK2_2006.pdf, accessed July 17, 2011.

Nordmann, Alfred. 2007. If and then: A critique of speculative nanoethics. *Nanoethics* 1: 31-46.

Olshansky, S. Jay, and Bruce A. Carnes. 2001. *The Quest for Immortality: Science at the Frontiers of Aging*. New York: W.W. Norton.

Olshansky, S. Jay, Bruce A. Carnes, and Aline Désesquelles. 2001. Prospects for human longevity. *Science* 291: 1491-92.
Olshansky, Jay, Leonard Hayflick, and Bruce A. Carnes. 2002. Position statement on aging. *Journal of Gerontology: Biological Sciences* 57A: B292-97.
Overall, Christine. 2009. Life enhancement technologies: The significance of social category membership. In *Human Enhancement*, edited by Julian Savulescu and Nick Bostrom, 327-40. New York: Oxford University Press.
Parry, Bronwyn. 2004. Technologies of immortality: The brain on ice. Studies in History and *Philosophy of Biological and Biomedical Sciences* 35: 391-413.
Pharma Projects. 2009. Therapy analysis – Gene therapy – Still the next best thing?: http://www.pharmaprojects.com/therapy_analysis/genether_current_0409.htm, accessed July 17, 2011.
Rose, Steven. 2005. *The Future of the Brain: The Promise and Perils of Tomorrow's Neuroscience*. New York: Oxford University Press.
Saunders, Norman R., C. Joakim Ek, M. D. Habgood, and K. M. Dziegielewska. 2008. Barriers in the brain: A renaissance? *Trends in Neuroscience* 31: 279-86.
Schermer, Michael. 2001. Nano nonsense and cryonics. *Scientific American* 285: 29.
Seidensticker, Bob. 2006. *Futurehype: The Myths of Technology Change*. San Francisco: Berrett-Koehler Publishers.
Stoneham, Marshall. 2009. Is a room temperature, solid-state quantum computer mere fantasy? *Physics* 2: 34-40.
Warner, Huber, Julie Anderson, Steven Austad, Ettore Bergamini, et al. 2005. Science fact and the SENS agenda. *EMBO Reports* 6: 1006-8
Waters, Brent. 2006. *From Human to Posthuman: Christian Theology and Technology in a Postmodern World*. Burlington, VT: Ashgate Publishing.
Williams, James C., Cherry A. Murray, A. Michael Andrews II, Mark J. Cardillo, et al. 2006. *A Matter of Size: Triennial Review of the National Nanotechnology Initiative*. Washington, DC: National Academies Press.
Wilson, James M. 2005. Gendicine: The first commercial gene therapy product. *Human Gene Therapy* 16: 1014.
Wowk, Brian. 2004. Medical time travel. In Immortality Institute, 135-49.

Converging Technologies, Transhumanism, and Future Society

Daniel Barben

In public as well as in academic debates, converging technologies and transhumanism are often assumed to be vanguards of transformative change in the near or more distant future. Yet whether indeed such change will take place and in what form and with what consequences is at times a matter of intense dispute. If one day it turns out that neither converging technologies nor transhumanism is all that powerful – e.g., because they have proven to be rather unspectacular technologies or, respectively, have remained a set of beliefs at the fringe of mainstream culture in the scientifically most advanced countries – it would still be worthwhile to ask why both of them were at the center of quite some attention early in the twenty-first century and why they have mostly failed, at least with regard to the most ambitious aspirations associated with them. Nowadays, however, it is an important task to try to identify the various challenges brought about by converging technologies and transhumanism and to confront them from a broad range of disciplinary and interdisciplinary perspectives. Even more, as we struggle to come to terms with the significance of converging technologies and transhumanism, a particular challenge lies in the ability to combine critical reflection on past and contemporary developments and critical anticipation of possible and plausible futures.

In this chapter, I will mobilize analytical tools from the social sciences and science-and-technology studies to approach some of the substantive challenges posed by converging technologies and transhumanism, which entails a critical look at the evidence put forth by proponents of both. First, I will empirically explore different notions of converging technologies in science-and-technology (S&T) policy, i.e., the domain where important funding decisions about the future course of research and development are made. Second, I will portray the significant interest in converging technologies by transhumanists. In these two sections, I will show that transhumanist ideas provide an important resource for articulating technoscientific and sociotechnical visions relating to converging technologies but that nontranshumanist ideas also can serve that purpose. Third, I will focus on factors that determine the prospects of converging technologies or transhumanism in society, arguing that we need to adopt comparative perspectives and take into consideration cross-national differences to appreciate how converging technologies and transhumanist visions are conceptualized and practically pursued. Finally, from a social-science perspective, I will critique the way in which transhumanists inadequately conceive of the relationship between human nature, technology, and society.

Since the relationship between converging technologies and transhumanism is not self-evident – and the future impact of each of them on society is uncertain – this chapter aims at elucidating some key issues pertaining to the ways in which interdependent technological and societal change is being shaped. My main argument is that, although the influence of transhumanism on the overall configuration of converging technologies is still very fragmented and even precarious, transhumanism is (at least potentially) a powerful attempt at changing some of the foundations of human self-understanding, especially in regard to the place of human in nature and history.

Visions of Converging Technologies in S&T Policy

Some of the main ideas that transhumanism has come to articulate as its epochal goals are indeed not new but were articulated in different ways at different times before. On the one hand, various mythological sources have envisaged transmutations of human beings and their capabilities, including hybridizations of human and other forms of life or fusions between humans and machines. On the other hand, in particular the development of the life sciences since the nineteenth century has provided various opportunities for imagining – or practically experimenting with – radically new designs of how human beings are created and outfitted.[1] While myths occasionally may present inspiring ideas to those eager to push the frontiers of S&T, such mythical aspirations are also likely to put off people who perceive them as sacrilege or otherwise ethically or culturally undesirable. In any event, the progress of S&T initially determines which modifications of human biology become research targets and are ultimately rendered feasible. As regards the pursuit of transhumanist visions, an emerging set of interrelated fields of S&T – often simply referred to as "converging technologies" – has been presented as particularly promising for finally realizing those visions. For this reason, in this section, I will outline some key elements of the

1 A prominent example in this respect has been the famous – and to many infamous – Ciba Foundation Symposium on "Man and His Future", organized in London 1962 (Wolstenholme 1963). At this symposium, representatives of the international science elite – such as Julian Huxley, Gregory Pincus, Albert Szent-Gyorgyi, Hermann J. Muller, Joshua Lederberg, and J.B.S. Haldane – came together to talk about some of the big challenges facing humanity and speculate how they might be overcome, which included the exploration of approaches to design new kinds of humans that are resistant to stress, able to operate with only little sleep, or physiologically particularly fitted for space travel.

discourse on converging technologies in S&T policy, paying attention to the different ways in which these technologies are envisioned (1) in the U.S. and (2) in Europe.

In the United States

The idea of converging technologies was first featured in the proceedings of a conference sponsored by the U.S. National Science Foundation (NSF) and the Department of Commerce (Roco and Bainbridge 2002c) and became the subject of a series of subsequent conferences organized by the masterminds of the National Nanotechnology Initiative (Roco and Montemagno 2004; Bainbridge and Roco 2006a, 2006b). Based on recent advances in S&T, the report on "Converging Technologies for Improving Human Performance" envisions them as a fundamental force bringing about interrelated and far-reaching change to individuals and societies at various levels. The terms *converging* or *convergent technologies* refer

> to the synergistic combination of four major "NBIC" (nano-bio-info-cogno) provinces of science and technology, each of which is currently progressing at a rapid rate: (a) nanoscience and nanotechnology; (b) biotechnology and biomedicine, including genetic engineering; (c) information technology, including advanced computing and communications; (d) cognitive science, including cognitive neuroscience. (Roco and Bainbridge 2002a, ix)

Mihail C. Roco and William Sims Bainbridge claim that the convergence is "based on *material unity at the nanoscale and on technology integration from that scale*" (ibid.). Quite astonishingly, they hope that the convergence of the sciences – sometimes also referred to as "unification" (Roco and Bainbridge 2002b, 1, 2) – will embody "a holistic view of technology based on transformative tools, the mathematics of complex systems, and unified cause-and-effect understanding of the physical world from the nanoscale to the planetary scale" (Roco and Bainbridge 2002a, x). They thus aim for a comprehensive deterministic project that will allow for transformative interventions into an assumed hierarchy of systems, in order to design and implement massive improvements of perceived deficiencies at all levels of human life. Referring to the "Renaissance artist-engineers" who were "masters of several fields simultaneously," they hope for the "convergence of the sciences" to "initiate a new renaissance" (Roco and Bainbridge 2002b, 13).

"Enhancing human performance" builds the core concern in their vision of converging technologies and these technologies' role in transforming society. Imperfections in the constitution, together with insufficiencies in the exploitation, of human capabilities are seen as root causes for a broad range of personal and social problems. Consequently, improving the makeup and usage of those capabilities is presented as an approach to problem solving. The goal of enhancing human performance concerns capabilities that either already exist or should be created technologically. The meaning of human capabilities is, thus, ambiguous because of an underlying shifting boundary in the understanding of which capabilities can be considered given and which cannot. This situation is one of the reasons that the term *enhancement* often seems so hard to grasp.

Roco and Bainbridge's description of what they deem problematic in humans starts out with a couple of simple observations, such as that the "level of human thought varies greatly in awareness, efficiency, creativity, and accuracy", that our "physical and sensory capabilities are limited and susceptible to rapid deterioration in accidents or disease and gradual degradation through aging," and that "we communicate poorly with each other, and groups fail to achieve their desired goals" (2002b, 4). Accordingly, they portray the tools rooted in the Nano-Bio-Info-Cogno fields of S&T as promises "to increase significantly our level of understanding, transform human sensory and physical capabilities, and improve interactions between mind and tool, individual and team" (ibid.). They thus regard converging technologies to be transformative powers that mesh biological, physical, psychological, and social elements. The workshop engaged with numerous examples of how applications of convergent technologies "could benefit humanity in a time frame of 10 to 20 years":

- Fast, broadband interfaces directly between the human brain and machines will transform work in factories, control automobiles, ensure military superiority, and enable new sports, art forms and modes of interaction between people.
- Comfortable, wearable sensors and computers will enhance every person's awareness of his or her health conditions, environment, chemical pollutants, potential hazards, and information of interest about local businesses, natural resources, and the like.
- Robots and software agents will be far more useful for human beings.
- Individuals and teams will be able to communicate and cooperate profitably across traditional barriers of culture, language, distance, and professional specialization.
- The human body will be more durable, healthier, more energetic, easier to repair, and more resistant to many kinds of stress, biological threats, and aging processes.
- A combination of technologies and treatments will compensate for many physical and mental disabilities and will eradicate altogether some handicaps that have plagued the lives of millions of people.
- National security will be greatly strengthened by lightweight, information-rich war fighting systems … and effective measures against biological, chemical, radiological, and nuclear attacks.

- Anywhere in the world, an individual will have instantaneous access to needed information … in a form tailored for most effective use by the particular individual.
- [T]he ability to control the genetics of humans, animals, and agricultural plants will greatly benefit human welfare; widespread consensus about ethical, legal, and moral issues will be built in the process.
- The vast promise of outer space will finally be realized by means of efficient launch vehicles, robotic construction of extraterrestrial bases, and profitable exploitation of the resources of the Moon, Mars, or near-Earth approaching asteroids.
- Agriculture and the food industry will greatly increase yields and reduce spoilage through networks of cheap, smart sensors that constantly monitor the condition and needs of plants, animals, and farm products.
- Formal education will be transformed by a unified but diverse curriculum based on a comprehensive, hierarchical intellectual paradigm for understanding the architecture of the physical world from the nanoscale through the cosmic scale (Roco and Bainbridge 2002b, 4-6).

Roco and Bainbridge claim that pursuing many of these paths simultaneously could lead to "a golden age" providing "world peace, universal prosperity, and evolution to a higher level of compassion and accomplishment" (2002b, 6). Searching for an appropriate metaphor to describe the new state of things, they liken humanity to "a single, distributed and interconnected 'brain' based in new core pathways of society" (ibid.). Oddly, in my view, this vision appears to forego notions of freedom and democracy, instead rather following notions of efficiency-oriented managerialism. Moreover, this metaphor and some of the above statements about the future significance of converging technologies in society even implicate connotations of technocratic totalitarianism. However, by using these quite strong words, I do not want to suggest that we have come across the hidden agenda of Roco and Bainbridge's NBIC project – and certainly even less so of NSF's or the U.S. government's. I would assume instead that the two visionaries' excitement about imagined S&T-based futures has gone overboard, leading them to neglect the social and political implications of their visions.

In a follow-up workshop and publication, the NBIC proponents introduce some new language in an attempt to respond to concerns about lacking ethical and social considerations in their vision of converging technologies, hereby trying to generate greater appeal for human enhancement, among other things. Key terms reflecting greater attention to these criticisms and demands to better embed converging technologies in society are "responsibility," "deliberate choices," and "democratization" (Roco and Montemagno 2004). But in light of Roco and Bainbridge's enthusiastic projection of the potentials resulting from the NBIC convergence, it is questionable whether they would indeed be willing to engage in a fundamental debate about the desirability of human enhancement.

In Europe

Mainly in response to the bold promotion of converging technologies in U.S. science policy, the European Commission's Directorate General Research in 2003 set up a High Level Expert Group on "Foresighting the New Technology Wave." The group was charged with exploring the opportunities and risks of converging technologies, as well as with developing a distinctly European approach toward this set of emerging S&T. The expert group's report presents a definition of converging technologies that is different from Roco and Bainbridge's: "Converging technologies are enabling technologies and knowledge systems that enable each other in the pursuit of a common goal" (European Commission 2004, 14). While enabling technologies are understood to "prepare the ground for a wide variety of technical solutions," converging technologies are said to point to "the convergence on a common goal by insights and techniques of basic S&T" (ibid., 19). After elaborating on how nanotechnology, biotechnology, and information technology enable other technologies both conceptually and instrumentally, the report expands the list of enabling technologies and knowledge systems by adding – besides cognitive science – "environmental science, systems theory, and social science, including philosophy, economics and the law" (ibid., 15). In what seems like an ironic comment on the American NBIC project, the report subverts that project's S&T-driven aspirations by complementing Nano-Bio-Info-Cogno with "Socio-Anthro-Philo-Geo-Eco-Urbo-Orbo-Macro-Micro" (ibid., title page). Unlike the NSF reports, the European report does not put forth a general idea of what the common goal of convergence might be – unless one identifies the overarching perspective of converging technologies that advance a European path toward the knowledge society as the common goal of S&T convergence. This interpretation is quite plausible, however, as the report establishes a new acronym, CTEKS, which stands for Converging Technologies for the European Knowledge Society.

The expert group argues that the opportunities and risks brought about by converging technologies require tackling their ambiguities in a systematic manner. The social sciences and humanities are hereby expected to take on the important role of providing orientation for better assessing and embedding emerging fields of S&T in society. The report lists four characteristics of converging technologies that contribute to their specific profile of opportunities and risks. These characteristic challenges are labeled as follows: "*embeddedness,*" which refers to the fact that unlike "distinct technical devices or products in the classical sense, converging technologies can be spatially distributed, pervasive and inconspicuous"; "*unlimited reach,*" pointing to the tendency of converging technologies "to expand the engineering paradigm into areas that were thought to be immune to engineering"; "*engineering the mind and the body,*" meaning that "fundamentally different approaches to converging technologies" are pursued by engineering the "hardware" as well as the "software" of mind and body; and "*specificity,*" indicating that converging technologies may help address and achieve "very specific tasks" (European Commission 2004, 20-21).

Against this background, the report explores scenarios for converging technologies as regards the future of Europe, economic and technological opportunities, various kinds of risks, and research and policy challenges. Furthermore, the expert group outlines strategic steps for generating and shaping converging technologies in accordance with European priorities. Thus, the supranational framework of governance in the European Union is supposed to spur converging technologies, as well as to make sure that their potentials are developed and applied responsibly.

A report on "Nanoscience and Nanotechnologies" by the British Royal Society defines convergence as "the multiple ways in which nanotechnologies will combine in the future with other developments in new technology (reflecting its genuinely interdisciplinary nature)," assuming that convergence "probably presents some of the biggest uncertainties, with respect to what is genuinely plausible and when new technologies might actually come into use" (Royal Society and Royal Academy of Engineering 2004, 54). The report does not share the unanimous enthusiasm found in the NSF reports on converging technologies. Rather, it states that the NSF volume presented above

> provides a very good example of the difficulty some commentators find in drawing an appropriate line between hope and hype. The authors contributing to this report are almost universally optimistic about the potential of convergence for the human condition, and provide very little critical discussion of potential drawbacks. The report also makes strong assumptions about the social acceptability of some of its implications. … The book also places some very concrete and beneficial developments that converging technologies will shortly bring (non-invasive diagnostics for example) alongside more fanciful visions of the future (for example, of human society as one single interconnected "brain"). Many of the papers also advocate a highly mechanistic view of people and society, where machines and biological systems are intersubstitutable, with very little consideration of some of the ethical challenges that the more radical enhancement proposals (such as the development of direct neural-to-computer interfaces) might encounter. (Ibid., 55)

In light of its critical assessment of both the scientific and societal significance of the prospects presented in the NSF report, the Royal Society report goes on to despise much of it as "science fiction": "One would be forgiven … for dismissing many of the papers as being less about sound science and technology than they are about science fiction (for example, the volume talks extensively about the "human cognome project" but contains little by way of mainstream neuroscience)" (ibid.). Overall, this report aspires to provide a balanced assessment of the opportunities and risks brought about by a set of emerging technologies, particularly nanotechnology. Unlike the initial NSF report, the Royal Society report pays considerable attention to the potential social and ethical implications of these technologies (for a similarly designed assessment, see the report on nanotechnology by the Office of Technology Assessment of the German Bundestag [Paschen et al. 2003]; and for a critical assessment report about human enhancement technologies commissioned by the European Parliament STOA [2009]).

Visions of Converging Technologies in Transhumanism

Having reviewed visions and notions of converging technologies in S&T policy discourses in the U.S. and in Europe, let me now examine how converging technologies are viewed from a transhumanist perspective and highlight some commonalities and differences among the S&T policy and transhumanist discourses on converging technologies.

As indicated above, aspirations to alter fundamentally the biological constitution of human beings were articulated long before the latest wave of emerging powerful technologies. In the past few decades, developments in informatics, robotics, biotechnology, and nanotechnology inspired far-reaching ambitions of overcoming what was presented as essential limitations of human beings. For example, Marvin Minsky has been a pioneer of supplementing human with artificial intelligence and of creating artificial neural networks and emotion machines (Minsky and Papert 1973; Minsky 2006). Hans Moravec (1988, 1999) has proclaimed that machines can become the embodiment of human cognition and consciousness and, even more, that machines can assume qualities of human beings. Eric Drexler, an early visionary of nanotechnology, has imagined this technology to provide powerful tools for "molecular manufacturing," which would enable the atom-by-atom assembly in many fields of application and offer great promises yet also be accompanied with considerable risk – e.g., if and when self-replicating nanobots get out of control (Drexler 1985).[2] Gregory Stock (1993) has speculated about the merger of telecommunications, trade, travel, and human beings into a plane-

2 "Coal and diamonds, sand and computer chips, cancer and healthy tissue: throughout history, variations in the arrangement of atoms have distinguished the cheap from the cherished, the diseased from the healthy. Arranged one way, atoms make up soil, air, and water; arranged another, they make up ripe strawberries. Arranged one way, they make up homes and fresh air; arranged another, they make up ash and smoke" (Drexler 1985, 3).

tary superorganism. He has also advocated radical interventions into human biology, including germline gene modifications and development of artificial chromosomes intentionally to design biological traits and performance (Stock 2002). Initially building on Minsky and Moravec, Ray Kurzweil has championed the idea that achieving immortality may be reached rather sooner than later (in about twenty years, that is), not only thanks to "uploading" our minds but also to "upgrading" our bodies through genetics, nanotechnology, and robotics (Kurzweil and Grossman 2009). He also predicted that humanity's future was characterized by a state of "singularity," i.e., exponentially accelerating innovation leading to a posthuman species and interrelated systems of surpassing performance and robustness as well as planetary reach (Kurzweil 2005).[3]

All authors just mentioned are either well-known scientists or claim scientific credibility even when speculating about the future and are linked to the transhumanist movement in one way or another, with Kurzweil probably being its most prominent representative. The notion of converging technologies was first elaborated in the context of the U.S. National Nanotechnology Initiative – and the projects and prospects of S&T convergence presented there have clearly communicated with transhumanist ideas (the fact that Bainbridge has been engaged as a member of the community of transhumanists can be seen as an indicator of close ties). While visions of NBIC-enabled human enhancement have resonated with transhumanist visions of artificial intelligence and artificial life, the official discourse on NBIC technologies has lent some legitimacy to transhumanist ideas, which are still at the fringe of society. The S&T policy discourse on converging technologies has also been helpful for transhumanists to package some of their key aspirations.

However, it is important to note that the S&T policy discourse on converging technologies employs a broader focus on their potential significance than the transhumanist discourse. While governmental S&T policy is interested in shaping and seizing new research and innovation opportunities across all potential sectors of the economy and of society, transhumanism is primarily interested in pursuing those opportunities potentially offered by S&T that help advance its particular goals. This is also true with regard to Roco and Bainbridge's NBIC agenda, which emphasizes human enhancement with a larger scope. "The Transhumanist FAQ," which was published by the World Transhumanist Association as a collective endeavor under the editorial leadership of Nick Bostrom, provides a useful overview of the overarching ambitions and various concerns characteristic for most if not all transhumanists. In the FAQ, *transhumanism* is defined as, first, the "intellectual and cultural movement that affirms the possibility and desira-

3 Kurzweil claims not only that both human life and the universe have a purpose but also that they share the same purpose: "The purpose of the universe reflects the same purpose as our lives: to move toward greater intelligence and knowledge. … [W]e will within this century be ready to infuse our solar system with our intelligence through self-replicating non-biological intelligence. It will then spread out to the rest of the universe" (Kurzweil 2005, 372).

bility of fundamentally improving the human condition through applied reason, especially by developing and making widely available technologies to eliminate aging and to greatly enhance human intellectual, physical, and psychological capacities" (Bostrom 2003, 4). According to the FAQ, the term *transhuman* "goes back to the futurist FM-2030 (also known as F. M. Estfandiary), who introduced it shorthand for 'transitional human'" (ibid., 7). Since transhumanists aim for "a whole new stage in the history of the human species," they suggest referring to those "possible future beings whose basic capacities so radically exceed those of present humans as to be no longer unambiguously human by our current standards" with the term *posthuman* (ibid., 4, 5):

> Many transhumanists wish to follow life paths which would, sooner or later, require growing into posthuman persons: they yearn to reach intellectual heights as far above any current human genius as humans are above other primates; to be resistant to disease and impervious to aging; to have unlimited youth and vigor; to exercise control over their own desires, moods, and mental states; to be able to avoid feeling tired, hateful, or irritated about petty things; to have an increased capacity for pleasure, love, artistic appreciation, and serenity; to experience novel states of consciousness that current human brains cannot access. It seems likely that the simple fact of living an indefinitely long, healthy, active life would take anyone to posthumanity if they went on accumulating memories, skills, and intelligence. (Ibid., 5)

However, it would be shortsighted for us to assume from a contemporary point of view that posthumans will still necessarily inhabit human bodies, but if so, these bodies would be fundamentally altered:

> Posthumans could be completely synthetic artificial intelligences, or they could be enhanced uploads … , or they could be the result of making many smaller but cumulatively profound augmentations to a biological human. The latter alternative would probably require either the redesign of the human organism using advanced nanotechnology or its radical enhancement using some combination of technologies such as genetic engineering, psychopharmacology, anti-aging therapies, neural interfaces, advanced information management tools, memory enhancing drugs, wearable computers, and cognitive techniques. (Ibid., 5-6)

As the goals of overcoming aging and even death, together with enhancing cognitive, physical, and emotional performance, are the top transhumanist priorities, these priorities shape the research and innovation agenda accordingly. In addition to genetics, pharmaceutics, robotics, informatics, cognitive science, and nanotechnology, cryonics plays a key role (see, for two seminal texts, Ettinger 1964, 1972). Cryonics predominantly serves as a rather primitive promise of eventual resurrection and thus immortality.[4] There are massive if not insurmountable obstacles

4 The Transhumanist FAQ portrays the reversal of death as saving live and the dead not as biologically but rather as only legally dead: "Cryonics is an experimental medical procedure that seeks to save lives by placing in low temperature storage persons who cannot be treated with current medical procedures and who have been declared legally dead, in the hope that technological progress will eventually make it possible to revive them" (Bostrom 2003, 15).

to realizing the dream of those who refuse to accept that all life on earth is of limited duration – i.e., to reverse freezing damage, to reverse the known or unknown original cause of exitus, and to reverse the state of an organism back to life.

Although the Transhumanist FAQ lists as the second distinctive feature of transhumanism the "study of the ramifications, promises, and potential dangers of technologies that will enable us to overcome fundamental human limitations, and the related study of the ethical matters involved in developing and using such technologies" (Bostrom 2003, 4), in transhumanist writings, one cannot find substantial engagement with probable or potential social and ethical implications and risks related to the future realization of transhumanist goals.[5] The likely reason for this gap is that transhumanists are positively convinced of the general desirability of their agenda. Thus, rather than articulating moral concerns, they tend to project an ethical superiority of and a "moral obligation" to transhumanist enhancements (Harris 2009).

Converging Technologies and Transhumanism in Future Society

In the previous two sections, I have elaborated on converging technologies and transhumanism as distinct yet interrelated sets of concepts. Since the future of both converging technologies and transhumanism will depend on much more than their success in the realm of ideas, I will now turn to the ways in which emerging technologies – together with nascent technocentric ideologies – become embedded in society.

I argue as follows: (1) the significance of converging technologies will be shaped by numerous factors concerning their generation, regulation, and enculturation, while (2) the impact of transhumanism will depend on its societal resonance and its ability to relate effectively to various institutional contexts relevant to the development of converging technologies.

Prospects of Converging Technologies

Emerging fields of S&T – or emerging processes among fields of S&T such as their convergence – are subject to manifold uncertainties. These uncertainties

5 Even at the very basic level of everyday life, an individual brought back to it after a long period of time, disconnected from the fabric of his or her previous life and unaware of the intricacies of societal change that has taken place since should feel fundamentally estranged and disoriented – a simple fact transhumanists do not even bother to contemplate as potentially problematic. Lepore (2010, 29) recounts the lead character's amazement in Woody Allen's 1973 movie *Sleeper*, when he awakens after a cryogenic sleep of 200 years to find that his friends are dead: "But they all ate organic rice!"

relate to different contexts of, as well as points in time in, the development of S&T. For example, in very early stages, the nature of the new and emerging potentials of S&T may be fundamentally unclear and thus be perceived in diverging ways even among experts; later on, the potentials of emerging and evolving S&T may be assessed very differently. Further, the potentials of S&T have to be realized, and it may be quite uncertain which approach to generating new knowledge, methods, processes, and products is the most promising – and ultimately successful. In addition to scientific and technological obstacles in the generation of S&T itself, new S&T is often also competing with already established procedures, which is particularly significant when it comes to large-scale industrial production in companies and commercialization on markets.

Moreover, emerging S&T may bring about regulatory uncertainties, such as those relating to health and environmental risks, domestic and international security, industrial or intellectual property, and significant ethical issues. The ways in which such uncertainties are perceived, as well as dealt with in different institutional contexts, determine whether and how new potentials, processes, and products are being pursued and finally realized.

Last but not least, uncertainties also relate to the enculturation of new S&T, for even the successful creation, production or provision, and commercialization do not guarantee that new applications of S&T are successfully implemented into society, i.e., welcomed and appropriated by users. Of course, there are different degrees of success – e.g., overall, sectoral, or fragmented. So, for a particular community (such as transhumanists) interested in using certain technologies, it may be sufficient if they simply become available. Once these technologies have been used and discussed more broadly, they may gain increasing appeal among other potential users – thus increasing the significance of markets and, eventually, contributing to social and cultural change. This kind of development is by no means unavoidable. It is also possible that new applications of S&T fail because they turn out not to deliver the benefits initially promised or they give way to uses hitherto not thought of.

Considering the divergent notions of converging technologies found in different national S&T policy contexts and considering the divergent political approaches toward converging technologies, it would be most appropriate to study the generation, regulation, and enculturation of converging technologies in a comparative fashion – i.e., from cross-national, cross-institutional, and cross-cultural perspectives. The history of those fields of S&T that are generally considered the main constituents of converging technologies – information technology, biotechnology, nanotechnology, and neurotechnology – provide ample examples that comparative studies are not only fruitful but necessary (Jasanoff 2005; Barben 2007). Otherwise, one may miss the specifics of both societal and technological developments.

It certainly depends on one's own perspective whether transhumanism is perceived as an oddity and as something to be contested or welcomed. Looking at contemporary mainstream culture, however, transhumanism without doubt is a fringe phenomenon, although some of its aspirations may enjoy a rather strong affinity with certain societal values, such as "competitiveness."

Similarly, neither transhumanism nor the transhumanist interpretation of converging technologies has been established among mainstream science or S&T policymaking. Rather, transhumanist ideas have been disputed by both academics and policymakers. To date, transhumanist ideas have failed to pass the test to conform to standards of sound science (see, for example, Barry Ritchie in this volume). This deficit should be a major obstacle for transhumanism to gain traction in the domains of science and policymaking. Furthermore, transhumanist visions of converging technologies have been fiercely criticized by some civil-society groups, such as the ETC group (ETC Group 2003).

It is important to note, however, that transhumanism seems to have gained some ground lately, appearing to be more influential and appealing than just a decade ago (Hayles 2008). Looking beyond the realm of mere ideas, we can observe some of the progress made by transhumanists. For example, a couple of the best-known transhumanists have served in prominent academic positions, even after becoming vocal proponents of transhumanism (e.g., Bostrom) or have won awards by well-regarded institutions (such as Kurzweil, winner of an Innovation Award by the *Economist* in 2009). In addition, transhumanists have managed to build key elements of an infrastructure needed to sustain their intellectual endeavors – in particular the World Transhumanist Association, which is now called Humanity+ or H+; a number of institutes and think tanks, such as the Institute for Ethics and Emerging Technologies (directed by Hughes), the Foresight Institute (founded by Drexler), the Singularity University (founded by Kurzweil), and the Future of Humanity Institute (directed by Bostrom); and the *Journal of Evolution and Technology*, among other publication forums.

A rich infrastructure to support the promotion and discussion of transhumanist ideas is a necessary – though not sufficient – prerequisite for any serious attempt to move these ideas gradually away from the fringes of culture toward the mainstream. However, in my view, it is a completely open question whether these ideas will ever gain the kind of appreciation the transhumanists are seeking. Even more, to become successful in everyday life, transhumanists need to be able to enter their visions into the complex fabric of societal institutions and practices. In the end, one might expect that transhumanists will be more successful in some countries, institutional contexts, and (sub-)cultures than in others –

and that some technological applications currently envisioned will turn out to work, while others will fail.

Outlook: A Social Science Critique of Transhumanism

In this chapter, I started out by outlining how the so-called converging technologies have been portrayed in U.S. and European S&T policy documents, as well as in transhumanist writings. I then turned to the ways in which both converging technologies and transhumanism are configured in society. To sum up, I have argued that, although the reports that originated in the domain of governmental S&T policy share a notion of converging technologies that refers to actual or expected processes of convergence among key areas of contemporary science-based technologies, each report articulates this common understanding in a rather different way. The NSF reports put together under the auspices of Roco and Bainbridge link the basic notion of converging technologies with a cosmology of hierarchical systems ranging from the nanoscale to the cosmic scale, which is envisioned to provide the basis for technological integration of interventions that will fundamentally enhance human performance at individual and societal levels. With this framework, transhumanist ideas of transforming the biological constitution of human beings encounter a rather sympathetic ground, largely unencumbered by ethical, legal, political, and social considerations.

In contrast to the reports published by the U.S. National Nanotechnology Initiative, the European report written up by the high-level expert group approaches converging technologies as a set of challenges that need to be met such that valuable opportunities are pursued – in particular, those that help advance both competitiveness and social and environmental justice – and precautionary measures are taken against certain detrimental risks. The report authorized by the Royal Society aims for a balanced assessment of the opportunities and risks engendered by converging technologies, hereby expressing criticism of the first NSF report on NBIC convergence about the lack of sound science and sensitivity toward the ethical and social implications of converging technologies. As the Royal Society report is certainly aware of the fact that emerging technologies need to meet acceptance to be implemented successfully in society, it aims at neutralizing those who attempt to obstruct – rather than shape – nanotechnology and other emerging technologies, while the NSF report is much more likely to instigate criticism by vocal civil-society groups such as the ETC.

While transhumanists acknowledge that their views are not yet shared by a majority of the population in various countries, they attempt to put forth persuasive arguments in support of ethical foundations of transhumanism. Hereby, they strive to cause a fundamental shift in how problems, or approaches to solve them, are commonly perceived and valued. For example, transhumanists like to claim that the fact of death that has characterized human life ever since it emerged is simply unacceptable. Thus, many of their aspirations, including their appreciation of converging technologies, aim at overcoming even limitations that evidently are an evolutionary given.

Adding to the arguments presented above concerning the factors that determine the prospects of transhumanism, which includes the transhumanist appropriation of converging technologies, I would now like to turn to the peculiar social theory transhumanism is proposing – as regards the relationship between human nature, technology, and society. It is a simple theory, one based on problematic – or, in my view, wrong – premises.

First and foremost, transhumanism focuses on human beings not as social beings but as biological organisms. Thus, its adherents portray the limitations of what they call the "human condition" as rooted in biology instead of society.

Transhumanists miss the basic fact that human life is primarily defined not by biological evolution but by historical development.[6] Human capacities are not limited as much by biological conditions as by societal conditions. Whether one is successful – however *success* is defined – depends on social conditions and equipment rather than biological conditions and equipment. Throughout human history, the vast majority of people have lived in ways far below what their biologically given potentials would allow them to achieve. The stage of historical development itself, plus various kinds of societal relations displaying power and exploitation, limits the opportunities for learning and thriving available to the broad mass of individuals and groups across the globe. Obviously, this does not preclude the possibility that exceptional individuals may achieve extraordinary things.

Of course, human potentialities are bound to biological capacities (e.g., those related to the human brain) because evolution has generated as an outcome human beings capable of a new kind of development – based on work, language, division of labor, technology, institutions, and culture.[7] But again, overcoming the limitations set by the conditions under which people live is essentially a problem of societal reform and not of human engineering. Even if human-enhancement technologies were to provide the performance-increasing effects advertised and

6 In the history of human thought, a wide variety of schools have shared this insight, ranging from early Enlightenment philosophy and idealistic or materialistic historicism to modern anthropology and (post-)structuralism (e.g., Foucault 1970; Godelier 1972; Hegel 1956; Marx 1998; Vico 1968).

7 Since concepts concerning the specific foundations of human societies can be articulated from divergent or even opposing (e.g., social vs. biological deterministic) perspectives, what is needed most are approaches that help overcome the nature/nurture dichotomy (Habermas 2003; Keller 2010).

even if these benefits were made available to a great number of people and not just a lucky few and the wealthy, the restrictions embodied in certain social conditions would most likely remain intact. Thus, improving the living conditions at a grand scale would still require pursuing the creation of appropriate societal institutions.

In consequence, the transhumanist emphasis on improving the human condition by enhancing physical, cognitive, or emotional performance isolates human beings from the particular societal conditions that, to a large extent, determine what being human means. Furthermore, the transhumanist focus contributes to neglecting the social quality of human beings in favor of their biological quality, thus essentially reducing them to their biological substrate.

In a similar vein, however, Roco and Bainbridge too approach issues of human performance such that they draw conclusions from biological capabilities to societal performance, i.e., by way of a shortcut. As a consequence, the specific characteristics of societal configurations, such as institutions, remain outside the focus. Thus, there is little analytical interest in the societal conditions and relations as they have an effect on how they impede, or further, the flourishing of human capacities.

References

Bainbridge, William Sims, and Mihail C. Roco, eds. 2006a. *Managing Nano-Bio-Info-Cogno Innovations: Converging Technologies in Society*. Dordrecht: Springer.

–. eds. 2006b. *Progress in Convergence: Technologies for Human Wellbeing*. Boston: Blackwell (on behalf of the New York Academy of Sciences).

Barben, Daniel. 2007. Changing regimes of science and politics: Comparative and transnational perspectives for a world in transition. *Science and Public Policy* 34 (1): 55-69.

Bostrom, Nick. 2003. *The Transhumanist FAQ: A General Introduction*. Version 2.1. Oxford: World Transhumanist Association.

Drexler, Eric. 1985. *Engines of Creation: The Coming Era of Nanotechnology*. London: Forth Estate.

ETC Group. 2003. *The Big Down: From Genomes to Atoms*. Winnipeg: The Action Group on Erosion, Technology and Concentration.

Ettinger, Robert C. W. 1964. *The Prospect of Immortality*. Garden City, NY: Doubleday.

–. 1972. *Man into Superman: The Startling Potential of Human Evolution – and How to Be Part of It*. New York: St. Martin's Press.

European Commission. 2004. Converging technologies – Shaping the future of European societies. Report of the High Level Expert Group "Foresighting the New Technology Wave" by Alfred Nordmann, Rapporteur. Brussels: European Commission, Directorate-General for Research.

Foucault, Michel. 1970. *The Order of Things: An Archaeology of the Human Sciences*. London: Tavistock.

Godelier, Maurice. 1972. *Rationality and Irrationality in Economics*. Translated by B. Pearce. London: NLB. Original edition, 1966.

Habermas, Jürgen. 2003. *The Future of Human Nature*. Cambridge: Polity.

Harris, John. 2009. Enhancements are a moral obligation. In *Human Enhancement*. Edited by J. Savulescu and N. Bostrom. Oxford and New York: Oxford University Press.

Hayles, N. Katherine. 2008. Wrestling with transhumanism. Paper read at Transhumanism and the Meanings of Progress, Arizona State University, April 24 and 25: http://www.metanexus.net/magazine/tabid/68/id/10543/Default.aspx, accessed July 17, 2011.

Hegel, G.W.F. 1956. *The Philosophy of History*. Translated by J. Sibree. New York: Dover Publications.

Jasanoff, Sheila. 2005. *Designs on Nature: Science and Democracy in Europe and the United States*. Princeton, NJ: Princeton University Press.

Keller, Evelyn Fox. 2010. *The Mirage of a Space between Nature and Nurture*. Durham, NC: Duke University Press.

Kurzweil, Ray. 2005. *The Singularity Is Near: When Humans Transcend Biology*. New York: Viking.

Kurzweil, Ray, and Terry Grossman. 2009. *Transcend: Nine Steps to Living Well Forever*. Emmaus, PA: Rodale.

Lepore, Jill. 2010. The iceman: What the leader of the cryonics movement is really preserving. *The New Yorker*, January 25, 24-30: http://www.newyorker.com/reporting/2010/01/25/100125fa_fact_lepore, accessed July 17, 2011.

Marx, Karl. 1998. *The German Ideology, including Theses on Feuerbach and Introduction to the Critique of Political Economy*. Amherst, NY: Prometheus Books.

Minsky, Marvin. 2006. *The Emotion Machine: Commonsense Thinking, Artificial Intelligence, and the Future of the Human Mind*. New York: Simon & Schuster.

Minsky, Marvin, and Seymour Papert. 1973. *Artificial Intelligence*. Eugene: University of Oregon Press.

Moravec, Hans. 1988. *Mind Children: The Future of Robot and Human Intelligence*. Cambridge, MA: Harvard University Press.

–. 1999. *Robot: Mere Machine to Transcendent Mind.* New York: Oxford University Press.

Paschen, Herbert, Christopher Coenen, Torsten Fleischer, Reinhard Grünwald, et al. 2003. *Nanotechnologie.* Berlin: Büro für Technikfolgen-Abschätzung beim Deutschen Bundestag.

Roco, Mihail C., and William Sims Bainbridge. 2002a. Executive summary. In Roco and Bainbridge, eds.

–. 2002b. Overview. Converging Technologies for Improving Human Performance: Nanotechnology, Biotechnology, Information Technology and Cognitive Science (Nbic). In Roco and Bainbridge, eds.

–. eds. 2002c. *Converging Technologies for Improving Human Performance: Nanotechnology, Biotechnology, Information Technology and Cognitive Science.* Dordrecht and Boston: Kluwer Academic Publishers.

Roco, Mihail C., and Carlo D. Montemagno, eds. 2004. *The Coevolution of Human Potential and Converging Technologies.* Annals of New York Academy of Sciences 1013. New York: New York Academy of Sciences.

Royal Society and Royal Academy of Engineering. 2004. *Nanoscience and Nanotechnologies: Opportunities and Uncertainties.* London: The Royal Society and Royal Academy of Engineering.

STOA. 2009. *Human Enhancement: Study.* Brussels: European Parliament, Directorate General for Internal Policies: Scientific Technology Options Assessment.

Stock, Gregory. 1993. *Metaman: The Merging of Humans and Machines into a Global Superorganism.* New York: Simon & Schuster.

–. 2002. *Redesigning Humans: Our Inevitable Genetic Future.* Boston: Houghton Mifflin Company.

Vico, Giambattista. 1968. *The New Science of Giambattista Vico.* Translated by M. H. Fisch and T. G. Bergin. Ithaca, NY: Cornell University Press. Original edition, 1774 (3d).

Wolstenholme, Gordon E. W., ed. 1963. *Man and His Future: A Ciba Foundation Volume.* Boston: Little, Brown.

Transhumanism and Obligations to Future Generations

Joan L. McGregor

I teach you the overman. Man is something that shall be overcome.
Friedrich Nietzsche, *Thus Spoke Zarathustra*

"Sustainability" has become a unifying discourse both nationally and internationally even though there is little consensus about the concept's exact meaning and implications. There is, however, some unanimity that sustainability obligates us to consider the effects of our actions, practices, and institutions on the future. Living sustainably commands that we preserve resources and/or the welfare of future generations of humans. The normative claim is that current generations owe future generations a world that is not fundamentally depleted of natural resources (or other necessary ingredients to satisfy their welfare interests), leaving a world where future people are capable of living satisfying *human* lives (Norton 2005).

Our technology, though it has led to marvelous transformations in our lives, freeing humans from many diseases and drudgery, has a darker side as well. Technology has also produced devastating global environmental damage that will continue into the future and threatens to change fundamentally and even destroy human life as we know it. Modern societies' effects on the globe pose significant challenges for the sustainability of the earth. Technologies' impact is also felt on humans. Emerging technologies, viz., nanotechnology, biotechnology, information technology, and cognitive science (NBIC), are creating the ability to enhance humans and possibly transform humans into entities that only bear a family resemblance to the current species. These technologies are predicted to extend human lives and make us healthy, smarter, more athletic, better looking, and happier. These changes in humans and to human nature raise questions about the effect of these changes on what we morally owe future generations. Presuming that current humans consent to the risks of the enhancements (and this, of course, is not so simple since many of the contemplated enhancements are ones to be done by parents to their children where the issue of consent is controversial) and that there are not moral objections based on unfairness due to competitive advantage or harm to currently existing others, then should not we ask how these enhancements will affect future generations? Would our duties to the future militate against or possibly for human enhancements? What does sustainability as a normative prescription require us to do now in terms of human enhancements, given that our current actions will affect the lives of future people? In fact, since our current actions will determine who will exist in the future and in what state, how does that affect our duties to the future (Parfit 1984)? Do future generations, for example, have a right to genetic/biological heritage? In other words, do we owe them the human genome in roughly the same condition in which we inherited it? If there is a human nature, will attempts to change it violate the right of future generations to have that human nature? Just as there are arguments that we should preserve some natural resources for future generations, are we required to preserve some human ones as well? Though there have been volumes of literature addressing the moral permissibility of human enhancements, there has been little attention to whether human enhancements violate our duties to the future.[1] The focus of this paper will be a preliminary exploration of whether the transhumanism project or human enhancements violates our duties to future generations. Does our duty to live sustainably prevent us from pursuing some human enhancements on the grounds that those enhancements will (or might) have detrimental effects on future humans?

What Do We Owe the Future?

We are now well aware of the catastrophic effects of our consumptive lifestyle on the resources of the globe and the possible resulting effects the depletion of resources will have on the conditions of existence for future generations of humans and the planet itself. Sustainability requires that our scope of moral consideration – that is, what entities we need to take into account in our moral deliberations – include the effects of our actions and practices on future people. A more robust moral theory of sustainability would include the effects on animals and the Earth itself. Without doubt, we are morally obligated to avoid harm that might be caused by our actions, practices, and institutions on currently existing people, institutions, and nations (again, for many, on animals and the earth too). We are responsible for the harm that results to others from our actions and should avoid any actions that harm other people. But are we required to go beyond currently existing humans and take responsibility for our actions on future people as well, as dictated by the sustainability norm? Of course, it is already standard for individuals to concern themselves with the future for their children and grandchildren. But beyond concern for one's family, most individuals have not thought much about what or whether they owe the future their moral concern and respect. Institutionally, politically, and economically, we (the "we" I am thinking about is Western society) have been notoriously bad about reflecting on and accounting for the effects on future generations as part of our deliberations for policies. Current deliberation on climate-change legislation and the recalcitrance to it

1 A notable exception is Hans Jonas (1974, 1984, 1985) who has addressed the question of technology's effect on the future and the effect of genetic enhancement of humans on the future.

illustrate the distance we have to go to integrate widening the scope of our moral consideration to include future generations (Houghton 2004; Solomon 2003).

Our actions and practices can quite radically affect future individuals' lives and well-being as illustrated by the effects of, among other things, the desertification of lands, the eradication of species, the overfishing and collapse of fisheries, the destruction of forests, and global climate change that threatens to displace millions of people. But are those effects of our lifestyle on future generations really our problem? Should we concern ourselves with what happens to distant strangers whom we will never meet or hear from? Since we do not know who they are (will be), we do not know anything about their likes or dislikes, we do not know what they will want and need, why should we concern ourselves with them? How can we owe them anything when their identity is opaque to us?[2] Furthermore, since future people cannot reciprocate these obligations – we would have obligations to them, but they would not have any toward us – does that lack of reciprocity undermine the claim that we have duties to them? As has been quipped before: What has posterity ever done for me?

Thinking within the framework of the liberal tradition, Joel Feinberg has attempted to answer the question whether we have duties to future generations in his influential essay "The Rights of Animals and Unborn Generations" (1980). He framed the question in terms of whether future generations are the kinds of entities who could have rights that we could violate. His argument has two parts. First, he argues that "the sorts of beings who *can* have rights are precisely those who have (or can have) interests" (Feinberg 1980, 167). He then goes on to argue that

> Whoever these [future] human beings may turn out to be, and whatever they might reasonably be expected to be like, they will have interests that we can affect, for better or worse, right now. That much we can and do know about them. The identity of the owners of these interests is now necessarily obscure, but the fact of their interest-ownership is crystal clear, and that is all that is necessary to certify the coherence of present talk about their rights. (Ibid., 181)

It is coherent to ascribe interests to future generations and, hence, acknowledge that they have rights to which we have duties. Future generations are, consequently, the sorts of beings who can have claims against us, although they cannot make

2 Derek Parfit (1984) addresses the "non-identity problem" in his *Reasons and Persons*. The nonidentity problem illustrates a counterintuitive conclusion to our actions or policies that affect future generations. It shows that which particular future people will exist is dependent on what conditions pertain when those individuals are conceived. Different parents, different times, different policies and conditions lead to different people. Since individuals are better off being born, even if born into a world of depleted resources with disabilities, or enhancements, than not existing at all, no one who is born in the future is worse off by our actions or policies. If we adopted alternative actions or policies (did not conceive a child while sick with rubella or did not deplete the resources of the world), the individuals born as a result of those actions and policies would not have been born at all.

them on their own behalf – cannot exercise them on their own. That latter fact, that they cannot exercise them on their own behalf, is not necessarily problematic since there are other entities that we are familiar with, for example, infants and incompetent persons, who cannot make claims on their own behalf but are still rights' holders. Nor can those persons reciprocate; consequently, ability to reciprocate is not a necessary criterion for being a rights-holder either.

From establishing that future generations have rights, we get a basic conception of intergenerational justice. Showing that it is intelligible to ascribe to future persons rights, however, does not tell us the substance and justification of those rights and what to do when there are conflicts of interests between the present generation and future generations. There are many questions about what their interests will be, what they will care about, what they will need, and what kind of circumstances they will live in. Even with the best scientific models, there are problems of ignorance and uncertainty. Some might be inclined to suggest that, given the ignorance about the identity and interests of future people and the uncertainty about the effects of current activity on them, we have no obligations to them since what they would be is just too remote and speculative to determine.

Even with uncertainty about future persons, we are quite certain that many of our actions will have deleterious effects on them, even if we do not know all the details with a high level of certainty and know what kinds of lives they will lead. We should, therefore, still acknowledge that we have responsibility to prevent some level of harm to others, even others who do not exist yet but will at some point. On the assumption that we do have moral obligations to the future, we still need to ask about the content and scope of those obligations.

Many of the recent accounts attempting to justify intergenerational justice claims have relied on liberal contractualist arguments, the most famous of which is John Rawls's 1971 version in *A Theory of Justice*. Rawls uses his model of hypothetical consent, the "original position", to derive the "just savings" account of intergenerational justice. Behind the veil of ignorance, all generations are represented, but the veil prevents the contractors from knowing what generation in history they are from; therefore, they are not able to give preference to their own generation (Rawls 1971, sections 24, 44; Rawls 2001, sections 49.2 and 3). The Kantian interpretation is that each person (or in this case, generation) would prefer that the previous one save resources for the next generation; then universalizing the rule would require that each generation save for the subsequent generations. Generations, then, ought to leave sufficient, just savings, for their descendents or the next generation. But Rawls notes that, on the Humean version of the theory, "Each generation will reason as follows: surely we wish that our predecessors had saved for us; but since we are all members of the same generation, making rules only for ourselves, we must simply take what they have done as a given; and however much or little they might have saved, we contemporaries will be better off now if we ourselves save nothing" (Goodin 1986, 171). Since the contractors do not know if the previous generations have saved for them and they are making rules only for themselves, they have no reason to agree to save for the future. Given these problems, it is not clear that intergenerational justice can easily be derived from the contractarian model, at least the Rawlsian one.

Even with these difficulties, there is no doubt we have duties of justice for future generations since their basic interests can be harmed by us and since they have a right not to have those basic interests harmed. Nevertheless, relying only on considerations of rights of future generations will not get us very far, not even getting some of the weaker claims of sustainability. At this point, the threshold of harm is fairly basic, and there is no requirement to ensure that future people enjoy even the same standard of living that we have or that they have the same resources and opportunities that we have. We do not, for example, harm our contemporaries by not ensuring them the same resources that we enjoy. Intergenerational justice duties establish a threshold of harm and the fact that future people are owed something from us. Since this threshold is not necessarily very high, consequently, if we believe that the future should have a better life than avoiding some basic threshold level of harm and that the norm of sustainability is for more than just avoiding that threshold, then the moral theory for intergenerational relationships will need to include more than justice considerations. Many of us believe that sustainability requires that the future generations should enjoy many of the things that we have enjoyed and have a life at least as good as we do. Under the "minimal sufficiency" threshold conception of harm, we would not violate the futures' rights if we did not leave them such a world (Meyers 2003).[3]

Moving beyond a basic threshold of harm, what exactly are we required to sustain for the future? In the sustainability literature, two notions of sustainability have been distinguished: so-called weak and strong sustainability (Norton 2005, 307ff). What these two notions represent are two ways of conceptualizing what we owe the future: (1) weak sustainability measures the welfare of the agents in the future, and (2) strong sustainability measures the "stuff" left in the world for the future (this includes pluralists who measure both welfare and stuff). On the welfare account of intergenerational obligations, weak sustainability (WS), we are required to maintain at least as much in terms of levels of individual welfare as we currently have (you could think of this as a Pareto requirement of not leaving

3 The threshold conception of harm avoids Parfit's nonidentity problem. The threshold notion is unaffected by the nonidentity problem, for here the finding of harm does not require that the person who is in the subthreshold state would be in a better state otherwise than would have obtained in the absence of the harming action.

anyone "worse off" than current agents are). However *welfare* is understood, namely, happiness or pleasure, preference satisfaction, or objective list of goods (knowledge, friendship, peace), we need to preserve for future generations at least the same level of welfare that we currently have. Weak sustainability puts no constraints on where the welfare comes from so that there can be trades between types of capital and other forms of wealth to achieve the welfare satisfaction. If certain natural resources are used up but the society has more economic resources that can compensate agents and "make up" any welfare decline, then that depletion of resources is justified. Whereas on the "stuff" account of sustainability, strong sustainability (SS) requires that we save stuff for future generations, for example, intact ecosystems, adequate supplies of natural resources, "natural capital." Strong sustainability puts limits on substituting natural assets with human-built ones. In other words, an increase or equivalence in welfare cannot be purchased with the destruction of other kinds of goods. Strong sustainability supposes that we cannot know for certain what future generations will want or need but that, whatever their interests, having certain natural resources will facilitate their ability to live fulfilling lives.

Weak and strong sustainability may lead to different conclusions about whether transhumanism violates duties to the future. Economists, who dominant much of the normative sustainability discussion, by and large accept weak sustainability since that conception fits in with the standard economic assessment that conceptualizes assets as fungible and the goal as maximizing welfare.

What Is Transhumanism?

The idea of transcending the human condition has a long history. Within the modern period, Friedrich Nietzsche's Zarathustra contends the following:

> I teach you the overman. Man is something that shall be overcome. What have you done to overcome him? … All beings so far have created something beyond themselves; and do you want to be the ebb of this great flood, and even go back to the beasts rather than overcome man? What is ape to man? A laughing stock or painful embarrassment. And man shall be that to overman: a laughingstock or painful embarrassment. You have made your way from worm to man, and much in you is still worm. Once you were apes, and even now, too, man is more ape than any ape. … The overman is the meaning of the earth. Let your will say: the overman *shall be* the meaning of the earth. … Man is a rope, tied between beast and overman – a rope over an abyss. … [W]hat is great in man is that he is a bridge and not an end. (Nietzsche 1961, Prologue §§3-4)

Always enigmatic, Nietzsche seems to be claiming that our current state – being human – is an embarrassment that we ought to strive to go beyond, that we ought to overcoming our present condition, to become "superman." Failure to do so is to exhibit weakness and a desire to escape life. In many ways, Nietzsche's words are the precursors of modern posthumanists who point us to a better future beyond our current human condition. For Nietzsche, however, overcoming the human is done through the will, his so-called will to power, which is the human fully creating himself and his values – a kind of self actualization, a mastery of the will. Unlike the current transhumanists whose methods of transformation (often they call it "evolution") are technological, Nietzsche relies on humans' internal power, their own will to transform themselves into something new. In Nietzsche, the goal achieved by overcoming the human is ridding society of the Christian values of good and evil that stifle our ability to create our own values (Solomon 2003; Young 2006). Modern transhumanists such as Max More and Nick Bostrom concur with Nietzsche's assessment of the condition of humanity; More (1994) says, "Our creativity struggles within the boundaries of human intelligence, imagination, and concentration." More also sees transhumanism as breaking from the oppression of religion:

> The concept of God has been oppressive: a being more powerful than we, but made in the image of our crude self-conceptions. Our own process of endless progression into higher forms should and will replace this religious idea. Humanity is a temporary stage along the evolutionary pathway. We are not the zenith of nature's development. It is time for us to consciously take charge of ourselves and to accelerate our transhuman progress. (1994)

The question of what is the end of enhancements for modern transhumanists is answered by Max More (1994):

> Why reach beyond ourselves and our humanity? Why seek to become posthuman? Why not accept our human limits and renounce transcendence? … The Enlightenment and the humanist perspective assure us that progress is possible, that life is a grand adventure, and that reason, science, and good will can free us from the confines of the past. … [W]e can attain higher peaks only applying our intelligence, determination, and optimism to break out of the human chrysalis. … Aging and death victimize all humans. … [T]o Extropians and other transhumanists, the technological conquest of aging and death stands out as the most urgent, vital, worthy quest of our time. Some fear that life will lose its meaningfulness without the traditional stages of life produced by aging the certainty of death. … Meaningfulness and value require the continual making and breaking of forms, a process of self-overcoming, not a stagnant state.

Transhumanists promote the view that human-enhancement technologies should be made widely available and that individuals should have broad discretion over which of these technologies to apply to themselves (morphological freedom) and that parents should normally get to decide which reproductive technologies to use when having children (reproductive freedom). "Ultimately, it is possible that such enhancements may make us, or our descendants, 'post human', beings who may have indefinite health-spans, much greater intellectual faculties than any current human being – and perhaps entirely new sensibilities or modalities – as well as the ability to control their own emotions" (Bostrom 2005, 203).

Whether transhumanism is consistent with our duties to future generations depends on a number of factors. To begin, is the current transhumanism project fundamentally different from other ways we have been changing ourselves for centuries? Vaccines and other medical developments are good examples of human advancements that have enhanced our lives. Where there is widespread access to them, vaccinations have extended the average life span of populations. Agricultural advancements that have lead to a steady supply of nutritious food have significantly increased many human characteristics such as the height of those populations. These are kinds of "enhancements" over our ancestors' living conditions. These enhancements, extending life spans and increasing height, have changed humans but arguably not so fundamentally as to make us not human, a different species from earlier versions. Many of the developments that led to these changes were designed as "therapeutic" correctives of diseases or disabilities in humans, as opposed to being intended as improvements of humans. Cures for diseases return individuals to the "species norm," some statistical average of conditions of health and capabilities (which itself moves over time). Prescription eyewear and Lasik, for example, are corrections that return the individual to the species norm of appropriately 20/20 vision. Some "enhancements" – increases in height and lifespan, for example – are unintended consequences of improvements from food availability and medical treatment. Extending life spans was a welcome but unintended consequence of a convergence of technological improvements. To a large extent, medical and other technological developments have not been conceptualized as improving human beings or changing human beings but as corrective and therapeutic of conditions that cause suffering to humans. Nevertheless, the line between therapy (correctives) and enhancement (improvement) is not a bright one, and some of these advancements that resulted in "better people" probably fall on the enhancement side of the fence.

Are the human enhancements that are being contemplated by the current proponents different from the enhancements of the past? According to Michael Bess, they are:

> Biotechnological modifications are likely to come in discrete, incremental packages, each offering a slight improvement in some aspect of our bodies or minds, along a steadily increasing gradient of potency and sophistication. ... [The] net result will be a social context in which the very meaning of the word "normal" is constantly shifting. ... The enhancements of the mid-twenty first century will be far more potent than anything witnessed thus far in human history. They will affect the qualities we deem most centrally and deeply human. Personality, emotions, cognitive ability, memory, perception, physical sensation, the boundaries between one person and another – all these will be subject to deliberate manipulation. It is hard to see how such an unrelenting succession of profound changes would not produce a disorientation – a continually destabilized identity – among the citizenry of the coming era. (2008, 123)

Some of the most ardent critics of transhumanism raise the following types of alarms about the prospects of human enhancements. For example, Francis Fukuyama (2002) claims that it is the "world's most dangerous idea," Bill McKibben (2002) contends that enhancement would undermine the necessary context for human experience and, hence, render human life meaningless, and Michael Sandel (2007) argues that proposed enhancements undermine the dignity of the human being. Those critiques characterize enhancements as so dangerous and encompassing that their use would most certainly impinge on our duties to the future.

Proponents of transhumanism, such as James Hughes, Nick Bostrom, and Max More (Savulescu and Bostrom 2009), agree that there is something different in what they are proposing from the earlier therapeutic improvements in human health. They argue, agreeing with Nietzsche's advocacy, that transhumanism should be embraced. Hughes says, "[T]echnologies that push the boundaries of humanness, can radically improve our quality of life, and ... we have a *fundamental right* to use them to control our minds and bodies" (2004, xii; italics added). Hughes is incredibly sanguine about the prospects of transhumanism, carving up the world into those advocating "liberal democracy, science, and modernity" (ibid., xiii) and the bio-Luddites whose misplaced fears put them on the wrong side of human progress guided by human reason. Included in their failings are the rejection of democracy and equality. That characterization of the critics of transhumanism is hyperbolic and unjustified, but the question remains whether the transhumanist project undermines our moral obligations to the future. Bostrom and other transhumanist defenders pay very little attention specifically to what the effects will be on future generations. Bostrom, for example, when defending transhumanism focuses on responding to the arguments that transhumanism will undermine our dignity (of current humans) and that it will have detrimental effects on the unimproved (2005, 204-12).

Does Transhumanism Undermine Our Duties to the Future?

What are the arguments against transhumanism from the perspective of our obligations to the future? If, at minimum, we are proscribed from harming the future, then we can inquire into whether transhumanism harms future generations? Under the model proposed by contemporary transhumanists, human enhancements are done by individual agents to themselves or their children. Their model is based on personal freedom or autonomy – individual agents deciding to utilize these technologies to advance their own good. This characterization distinguishes the current enhancement movement from earlier attempts such as the eugenics movement of the last century wherein it was the state imposing its coercive measures on often-unwilling individuals. Eugenicists' aim was for the state's benefit or the so-called public health for the society. The current enhancement agenda is raised under the banner of individual freedom and welfare, often with a distinctly libertarian favor. Transhumanists are framing access in terms of fundamental rights against government interference of one's reproductive and morphological freedom. Parents' reproductive choices, designing their offspring, are motivated to help, not harm, their offspring. A parent's motivation is his or her children's welfare so that they will lead healthy, more successful, and happier lives. It should be noted that there has been considerable debate in the literature about the moral appropriateness of genetic alterations of children for enhancement purposes due to the potential risks of those procedures to healthy children. Subjecting one's child to risks for therapeutic reasons is justifiable, all things considered, but not, so the argument is advanced, for enhancements reasons. Assessing the risk/benefit ratio when correcting a defect that can radically diminish the quality of a child's life prospects is different from assessing the risk/benefit ratio of an enhancement to make a child "better than normal." Let's assume for the sake of this argument that all those risks of enhancement to one's progeny will be reduced or eradicated as the technology advances thereby reducing the moral concerns to immediate offspring. Here we want to consider the negative effects on generations downstream where there may be harmful unintended consequences of particular enhancements or harmful unintended consequences of the cumulative effects of the enhancements. Currently, future generations' interests are not factored into the assessment of risks and benefit in the same way that one's own or one's children's interests are taken into account in the decision-making process for enhancements. That is understandable, but since these technologies can have profound effects on the future generations' interests, they should not be entirely discounted.

What are the arguments against human enhancements to current people on the basis of the interests of future people? Hans Jonas argues that human enhancements – designing future people – objectionably dictate the state of existence for future humans:

> Technological mastered nature now again includes man who (up to now) had, in technology, set himself against it as its master. … But whose power is this – and over whom or over what? Obviously the power of those living today over those coming after them, who will be the defenseless, other side of prior choices made by the planner of today. The other side of the power of today is the future bondage of the living to the dead. (Jonas, quoted in Habermas 2003, 47, 48)

Jonas argues for a "right to ignorance" as "condition for the possibility of authentic action." The "ethical command" Jonas claims is "to respect the right of each human life to find its own way and be a surprise to itself" (Jonas 1974, 163).

Current generations can dictate the lives of future people in a fashion that objectionably limits their power to make their authentic choices.

Bostrom responds to Jonas's objection that human enhancement, specifically genetic enhancement, would "constitute a kind of parental tyranny [previous generation's tyranny] that would undermine the child's [future generations'] dignity and capacity for autonomous choice" (Bostrom 2005, 211). Bostrom's argument is that our descendents will be much more technologically advanced than we and that, if they do not like our expansion of their capacities, they can reverse them: "If, for some inscrutable reason, they decide that they would prefer to be less intelligent, less healthy, and lead shorter lives, they would not lack the means to achieve these objectives and frustrate our designs" (ibid.).

Bostrom misses the point of Jonas's objection that the earlier generation will dictate what those future people are like. Joel Feinberg's raises a similar objection to certain interferences of parents on their children, what Feinberg calls the violation of the right to an "open future." An argument against various enhancements, including genetic modification of one's offspring is that individuals have a right to an "open future." The idea is that parents must not constrain children (and, by extension, future generations with human enhancements that can continue well into the future) too much and should provide children with opportunities so that, when they grow up, they will have choices about the kind of life they want to live. Others have suggested that the right to an open future requires children to acquire to the fullest extent possible the capacity to choose between "the widest possible variety of ways of life" (Arneson and Shapiro 1996, 388; Habermas 2003, 79). In other words, children have a right not to have all the details of their lives mapped out in advance as has been projected with "designer babies." Parents would violate this right if they dictated all the characteristics of their children, viz., height, weight, career path, athletic and intellectual abilities, traits and dispositions. Whether this right is violated with any given modification is open to dispute (Coady 2009, 170). For instance, genetic therapy to correct for genetic diseases such as cerebral palsy would not violate the right since the child's opportunities would be expanded rather than constrained with that therapeutic intervention. Genetically engineering offspring so they will be taller may not in the long run confer any advantage if the trait modification is widespread – everyone will be taller – so it does not detrimentally affect the prospects of the future (although it could affect resources use). Altering the human genome so as to eliminate certain feelings such as sadness might well preclude human emotions such as compassion or empathy that expand our understanding of ourselves and others and ultimately enrich our lives. That alteration does seem to violate the right to an open future since it limits the experiences of those people and constrains their lives on the basis of previous generations' views of what is good.

Our current decisions to eliminate traits that are determined to be inconvenient or bad or add ones that are thought to be good could violate the future generations' rights to an open future. Whether they do is a matter of the degree of the characteristics changed and on the basis of what characteristics are changed. Slight increases in life span do not radically constrain the opportunities of future generations (in fact, they increase them) or fundamentally change the nature of human life. But eradicating emotions that we might suppose are foundational to human existence or constitutive of the human experience as we have known it might well violate the right to an open future or as Jonas discussed dictate too much the kind of life we lead, forcing future people into bondage from the past. Which human enhancements violate the right to an open future is still a significant question that needs more nuanced and detailed analysis than can be tackled here. Because of the long-term downstream effects, germ-line genetic alternations (modification of germ cell or gametes) have come under much more criticism than somatic cell alterations (somatic cell modifications are to any cells other than the gametes and thereby is not passed on to progeny). If the alterations are of the genome or other permanent changes, then there is more reason to suppose that they will have long-term effects that might undermine our responsibility to the future.

It is facile to say that we should not even worry about fundamental changes to humans since the future generations can easily reverse the traits if they wanted to do so. Some changes are not easily reversible or not reversible at all or, since those "reconstructed" people might not experience the loss or disadvantage, they would not seek the change or reversal. For example, on our hypothesis that the elimination of the feeling of sadness might result in a loss of the emotions of empathy and compassion (since emotions require a belief and a feeling), those people without those emotions do not have a conception of what they are missing and, hence, would not seek to get back the feeling of sadness. A world without the emotions of compassion and empathy would be a more impoverished one and one that constrains the experiences of humans and thereby reduces the opportunities of future generations. Additionally, assuming that a world without those emotions, even though people with those emotions are sad, is a worse world than one with them, then it would be a bad to eradicate those emotions from the human experience.

Bostrom's response also presupposes that there will be no unintended consequences of these alterations, that is, they will all be "good" changes, making us smarter, better looking, and longer lived. That response begs the question about the predictability of the long-term effects of human enhancements. One significant concern to any emerging technology, including ones that we apply to ourselves, is that the technology, although designed to have beneficial consequences, may have unwanted and/or unanticipated bad consequences. A brief reflection on the history of technology bears out this concern, making it one that should not be summarily disregarded.

Depending on whether weak sustainability or strong sustainability is the correct account of what we owe the future (and exactly how those are fleshed out), there are different answers as to whether transhumanism violates our obligation to the future. Remember that weak sustainability commands us to ensure that future generation's welfare is at least as good as our own. On a happiness (hedonist account) account of welfare, transhumanism might fare pretty well in advancing human welfare. This is particularly true since, on the WS account, it does not matter what the source of the welfare improvement (or equilibrium) is. Neuroenhancers, for example, created by pharmacology, implants, or genetic manipulation, designed to enhance our mood and eradiate our negative emotions, should make people happier (on the hedonist conception of happiness). If what we are required to ensure is that future generations' subjective states are as good as or better than ours and new drugs or implants can eliminate depression and make people "happier," then we will have satisfied our obligation to them by creating a world with widespread access to neuroenhancers. This is true even if those future generations are denied many of the natural resources that we currently experience, viz., relatively clean air and abundance of water, wild lands, and biodiversity since the neuroenhancers might guarantee that the people still experienced pleasure. Some predictions of the posthuman world have humans merging with machines; consequently, these merged humans presumably would not experience any deprivation from the depletion of natural resources (including the human resources) since their "experiences" will be in the virtual world and not as we currently experience the world (Kurzweil 2005).

We have been assuming that enhancements can and will sustain the level of welfare (happiness) of future generations and, hence, since they will make future generations happier, smarter, and longer lived, that human enhancements will satisfy WS. Even though many natural assets, for instance, natural resources and human characteristics, are gone, we will have satisfied our duties to future generations if their welfare is maintained through whatever means possible. This assumes, however, that we can predict all (or most) of the consequences of enhancements. This assumption is particularly problematic as we move further downstream in time and our ability to predict consequences is more tenuous. Consider the case of the mice that were enhanced to make them "smarter," i.e., able to run mazes better, but researchers found they were more susceptible to pain (Lehrer 2009; Tang et al. 1999). Similar outcomes might occur with large-scale mood or cognitive enhancements and thereby would violate our duties under weak sustainability. The point is that, unless we can assume that we know with a high level of certainty what the long-term consequences will be of the humans enhancements we impose on the future, we could very well violate duties to future generations and that, if we have "traded off" natural resources for the enhanced traits, they would not have the other options that natural resources might have provided them for their welfare.

Suppose, on the other hand, relying on some version of SS that we have responsibilities to future generations to ensure some "natural resources" and other stuff (might include preservation of art, valuable institutions, and practices) as well as welfare. It is not only because we are ignorant of the future's interests that we are obligated to leave them natural resources that will ensure they can satisfy their interests, whatever they turn out to be, but because we believe that some things are valuable and we want to preserve those things for the future, for example, wilderness areas, national parks, biodiversity, treasures of art, democratic institutions, and so. Some of those natural resources that we are responsible to preserve would be human ones too, for example, human genetic heredity and human nature. Any and all changes cannot be stopped since there are changes to the human genome occurring "naturally." But genetic changes to the extent of "transforming humans" into another species might well violate our responsibility to future generations to genetic heredity under SS.

Fiction writers have dealt with versions of this issue, portraying various dystopias with genetic engineering of humans, most notably Aldous Huxley's *Brave New World.* Margaret Atwood's *Oryx and Crake* (2004) includes genetically engineered "humans" – the "Children of Crake" who are genetically engineered to be peaceful, polite, and happy and feel no jealousy. They have thick skin that is impervious to the damaging sunlight, and they are naturally insect-repellant vegans "perfectly suited" to their environment. There are probably good reasons for excluding each of these characteristics: skin that is not damaged by sunlight means that people would not have to worry about prolonged sun exposure and the fact that "Crakers" turn a certain color when they are fertile and ready to copulate eliminates all the problems of romance and interpersonal sexual relationships! Whether these fictional depictions of the future of genetic engineering are accurate and plausible scenarios is, of course, difficult to say. The Children of Crake were created by Crake to address the "problems" of humans, to make them better than current humans. The eugenics program at the beginning of the last century in its fullest articulation tried to do something similar. Current posthumanist theorists argue that there is a vast difference between the current conceptions relying on the reproductive choices of individual actors focused on the best interest of their children and the draconian forces of the state aiming toward some goal. The eugenics movement as instituted, at least in Germany, was imposed by the state for the good of the nation-state.

Transhumanists emphasize that their plan for human enhancements will result from individual actions aimed at improving the lives of oneself or one's offspring and not a totalitarian imposition from the state on the population at large. Disability theorists are not convinced by the supposed differences between historical eugenicists and modern transhumanists; they argue that even under "liberal eugenics," the message is clear that disabled lives are not worth living and "good parents" should make the "right decisions" for their children and ensure that they are not born in the "natural lottery." These theorists remind us of John Stuart Mill's argument about the oppressive force of the "tyranny of the majority" dictating views and actions based on the majority's moral beliefs. Disability theorists worry that what starts out as voluntary individual decisions can rapidly move to societal pressure to perform some enhancements, leading to government coercion that the enhancement be preformed (Asch 1995). Slippery-slope arguments need to be evaluated carefully, but this one may have credence given the competitive disadvantage of those who are not enhanced in a world of the enhanced (think of the disadvantages of the unenhanced in the movie *Gattaca*) and the possible costs to insurance companies and the government of those not enhanced (think of the arguments for preimplementation genetic diagnosis for disabilities currently in populations where those diseases are present).

The plausibility of picking traits that we believe are good and eradicating those that we think are bad, like the fictional characters in Atwood's book, is already occurring at some levels. Parents currently do make decisions about characteristics that they suppose will improve their children's lives. For instance, currently some children who are statistically short in stature, but not deficient in human growth hormone, are given artificial human growth hormones so they will grow taller. Short stature is one among many characteristics that parents can decide is detrimental for their children and alter through artificial means. Other characteristics considered detrimental and alterable include shyness, attention deficit disorder, and physical characteristics such as big noses and small breasts. It is plausible that the decision to alter a person's morphology and psychology will move from individual decisions to do what is in your child's best interests to societal pressure to do so to ultimately other sorts of coercive pressures from insurance companies or the government.

Even if the changes that individuals make are not found to have downstream detrimental effects, the cumulative effects of enhancements on future generations might well be detrimental and limiting to their opportunities to live flourishing human lives. We are familiar with the "logic of collective action" that illustrates how individuals acting in their own self-interest, when others do so as well, can result in disaster for the collective. Individual changes or effects in isolation are not harmful but collectively might have harmful effects. This is what happened with Atwood's Crakers. In that case, the individual characteristics sounded beneficial to Crake (the genetic engineer), yet the combination of them left these individuals in a state that they could not fully care for themselves and only vaguely resembled humans.

Can human enhancements change or destroy human nature and, consequently, violate a right to human nature? It certainly is plausible to suppose that future people have an interest in preserving human nature if what we mean by that is to preserve many of the characteristics and dispositions that "define" us as human. What makes great literature engaging to us, for instance, is the exploration of human emotions and paradigmatic themes, for example, unrequited love, which are part of the human experience that is based (loosely) on some conception of human nature. Human nature connects us with the past and the future since we assume that humans have and will react to many experiences in the same way that we currently do. What exactly do we mean by human nature? It has been thought of in a number of different ways; for example, there have been religious, psychological, "folk," and evolutionary biological understandings of the condition. The following were taken as claims of human nature: "all humans are sinful," "all humans are egoists," "all humans care for their young," and "all humans are sociable." If we think of human nature as traits or characteristics or dispositions that all humans share, then it may be difficult to define human nature unless one believes in a human essence. If, rather, we define human nature as a cluster of those characteristics and dispositions and we need to investigate which ones are parts of the cluster, supposing that all humans have most of them but that none is necessary for being human, then we have a plausible account of human nature. Given this understanding of human nature as a cluster of characteristics that are typically found in humans, could transhumanism destroy human nature, and would it violate our duty to future generations?

Allen Buchanan is his recent article entitled "Human Nature and Enhancement" takes on some of the arguments raised against changing human nature, arguing "that that there is nothing wrong, per se, with altering or destroying human nature, because, on a plausible understanding of what human nature is, it contains bad as well as good characteristics and there is no reason to believe that eliminating some of the bad would so imperil the good as to make the elimination of the bad impermissible" (2009, 141). Looking at our experience with so-called enlightened management of the natural environment where we thought we could remove the "bad" animals (predators) and leave only the "good" ones (animals that hunters wanted to hunt) and livestock, we should be less sanguine about our ability to make those judgments about what are the bad characteristics versus the good ones (Leopold 1949, 129-33). Over a hundred years later, we are still facing environmental destruction from our implementing policy that attempts get rid of the "bad" animals. If we suppose that some version of SS is true and that we ought to leave as a legacy human nature, then we should be cautious about deep tinkering that can destroy human nature for future generations. Since it is not clear that there is a human essence or necessary characteristics for being human, what we owe to the future as a legacy is difficult to define. But arguably there is a threshold of characteristics that if all of those were destroyed or radically altered, human nature would be destroyed.

Upshot: Does Transhumanism Violate Our Duties to Future Generations?

Many theorists have been concerned about modern technology's power to change the planet radically and even destroy humans. Jonas's *Imperative of Responsibility* focuses on the effects of modern technology. It argues that modern technology, unlike earlier eras' technology, is significantly more powerful and has the ability fundamentally to change our environment and the world that the future lives in: "Modern technology has introduced actions of such novel scale, objects, and consequences that the framework of former ethics can no longer contain them" (1984, 6). Jonas's insights are important because of the potential downstream, long-term destructive impacts of modern technology. Since these global effects are unprecedented, we need, according to Jonas, to have a new ethical framework to think about it – we need to acknowledge our responsibility for those far-reaching impacts. This power over future generations, of changing human nature and human genetics, even of becoming a different species in a short period of time, has never been seen in history. As Lawrence Troster has written, "For Jonas, the lengthened reach of our deeds moves the principle of responsibility into the center of our ethical stage. His theory of responsibility, which he saw as the correlate of power, must therefore be proportionate to the range of modern power" (2008, 387). Jonas thought we should be attempting to predict the possible outcomes of technology, but he was aware that we could not always predict those effects. As he succinctly put it, "[A]s long as the danger is unknown, we do not know what to preserve and why" (1984, 27). Jonas was advocating in the face of uncertainty, where the risks are high and far-researching, an ethic of caution and responsibility. This ethic of caution and responsibility for our actions is found in the current "Precautionary Principle" (PP), which states an ethical norm for the introduction of new technology: "Where an activity raises threats of harm to the environment or human health, precautionary measures should be taken even if some cause and effect relationships are not fully established scientifically. In this context the proponent of an activity, rather than the public, bears the burden of proof" (Wingspread Conference 1998). Theoretically, there are a number of interpretations of the Precautionary Principle. Kerry Whiteside writes, "PP is understood to imply a broad range of possible measures – measures calibrated to the degree of uncertainty and the seriousness of the consequences that are feared" (2006, 53). In many of the cases of technologies used in human enhancement, the risks are not even known; consequently, it would be reckless to proceed with the technology without further knowledge. PP requires anticipating risks and reducing the uncertainty of risks (Allhoff 2009). It also places the "burden of proof" on the advocates of the technology, as opposed to the critics. Jonas would have endorsed PP, namely, that we should not rush ahead with unknown risks of harm for the future but rather proceed with much more caution and awareness of our responsibility to the next generations. Applying PP to human enhancements and focusing on the risk to future generations would be fulfilling our responsibilities to the future. Fiction writers, such as Atwood, and conservationists, such as Aldo Leopold, remind us of the hubris of the past where we supposed we could predict all the implications of our actions and practices and understand all the various harm caused to unknown entities.

References

Allhoff, Fritz. 2009. Risk, precaution, and emerging technologies. *Studies in Ethics, Law, and Technology* 3 (2): 1-27.

Arneson, R. J., and I. Shapiro. 1996. Democratic autonomy and religious freedom: A critique of *Wisconsin v. Yoder*. In *Political Order*, *Nomos XXXVIII*, edited by I. Shapiro and R. Hardin, 1:365-411. New York: New York University Press.

Asch, Adrienne. 1995. Can aborting "imperfect" children be immoral? In *Ethical Issues in Modern Medicine*, edited by John Arras and Bonnie Steinbock, 317-21. 4th ed. Mountain View, CA: Mayfield Publishing Co.

Atwood, Margaret. 2004. *Oryx and Crake*. New York: Anchor Books.

Bess, Michael. 2008. *Icarus 2. 0:* A historian's perspective on human biological enhancement. *Technology and Culture* 49 (1): 114-26.

Bostrom, Nick. 2005. In defense of posthuman dignity. *Bioethics* 19 (3): 202-17.

Buchanan Allen. 2009. Human nature and enhancement. *Bioethics* 23 (3): 141-50.

Coady, C.A.J. 2009. Playing God. In Savulescu and Bostrom, eds., 155-80.

Feinberg, Joel. 1980. The rights of animals and unborn generations. In Feinberg, *Rights, Justice, and the Bounds of Liberty*, 159-84. Princeton, NJ: Princeton University Press.

Fukuyuma, Francis. 2002. *Our Posthuman Future: Consequences of the Biotechnology Revolution*. New York: Farrar Straus & Giroux.

Goodin, Robert. 1986. *Protecting the Vulnerable*. Chicago: University of Chicago Press.

Habermas, Jürgen. 2003. *The Future of Human Nature*. Maldon, MA: Polity.

Houghton, John. 2004. *Global Warming: The Complete Briefing*. 3d ed. Cambridge: Cambridge University Press.

Hughes, James. 2004. *Citizen Cyborg: Why Democratic Societies Must Respond to the Redesigned Human of the Future*. Boulder: Westview Press.

Jonas, Hans. 1974. Biological engineering – A preview. In Jonas, *Philosophical Essays: From Ancient Creed to Technological Man*, 141-67. Englewood Cliffs, NJ: Prentice-Hall.

–. 1984. *The Imperative of Responsibility: In Search of an Ethics for the Technological Age*. Chicago: University of Chicago Press.

–. 1985. *Technik, Medizin and Ethik: Zur Praxis des Prinzips Verantwortung*. Frankfurt am Main: Suhrkamp.

Kurzweil, Raymond. 2005. *The Singularity Is Near*. New York: Viking Singularity.

Lehrer, Jonah. 2009. Neuroscience: Small, furry ... and smart. *Nature* 461: 862-64.

Leopold, Aldo. 1949. *A Sand County Almanac*. London: Oxford University Press.

McKibben, Bill. 2002. *Enough: Staying Human in an Engineered Age*. New York: Times Books.

Meyers, Lukas. 2003. Past and future: The case for a threshold conception of harm. In *Rights, Culture and the Law: Themes from the Legal and Political Philosophy of Joseph Raz*, edited by L. Mayer, S. Paulson, and T. Pogge, 143-59. Oxford: Oxford University Press.

More, Max. 1994. On becoming posthuman: http://www.maxmore.com/becoming.htm, accessed July 17, 2011.

Nietzsche, Frederick. 1961. *Thus Spoke Zarathustra*. Translated by A. M. Ludovici. London: Penguin Classics.

Norton, Bryan. 2005. *Sustainability*. Chicago: University of Chicago Press.

Parfit, Derek. 1984. *Reasons and Persons*. Oxford: Clarendon Press.

Rawls, John. 1971. *A Theory of Justice*. Cambridge, MA: Harvard University Press.

–. 2001. *A Theory of Justice*. Cambridge, MA: Harvard University Press.

Sandel, Michael. 2007. *The Case against Perfection*. Cambridge, MA: Harvard University Press.

Savulescu, Julian, and Nick Bostrom, eds. 2009. *Human Enhancements*. Oxford: Oxford University Press.

Solomon, Susan, Dahe Qin, and Martin Manning. 2007. Technical Summary. In *Climate Change 2007: The Physical Science Basis. Contribution of Working Group I to the Fourth Assessment Report of the Intergovernmental Panel on*

Climate Change, edited by Susan Solomon et al. Cambridge: Cambridge University Press.

Solomon, Robert C. 2003. *Living With Nietzsche: What the Great "Immoralist" Has to Teach Us*. Oxford: Oxford University Press.

Tang, Ya-Ping, Eiji Shimizu, Gilles R. Dube, Claire Rampon, et al. 1999. Genetic enhancement of learning and memory in mice. *Nature* 401: 63-69.

Troster, Lawrence. 2008. Caretaker or citizen: Hans Jonas, Aldo Leopold, and the development of Jewish environmental ethics. In *The Legacy of Hans Jonas*, edited by Hava Tirosh-Samuelson and Christian Wiese, 373-96. Leiden: Brill.

Whiteside, Kerry. 2006. *Precautionary Politics. Principle and Practice in Confronting Environmental Risk*. Cambridge, MA: The MIT Press.

Wingspread Conference. 1998. Wingspread Statement on the Precautionary Principle: http://www.gdrc.org/u-gov/precaution-3.html, accessed July 17, 2001.

Young, Julian. 2006. *Nietzsche's Philosophy of Religion*. Cambridge: Cambridge University Press.

Against Species Extinction Transhumanism and Contemporary Technological Culture

Jerry Coursen

Dinosaurs are extinct. Their fate is not unusual. It is, in fact, the norm for the vast majority of all biological species that have existed on this planet. More than 99 percent of all biological species have vanished. Species extinction *is* the norm.

Species extinction occurs for a variety of reasons. Sometimes it is the result of a special-cause event, such as the massive meteor that is thought to have struck earth and ended the reign of the dinosaurs. More often, it is a series of incremental events that alter the environment in which a species exists. These alterations may render its environment unfit for continued habitation by that species. Ironically, often these environmental changes are the result of doomed species itself. There is also credence to the popular notion that similar species compete in a winner-take-all contest for a given environmental niche where the fittest survive. However, competition between similar species does not necessarily result in the immediate extinction of the less successful species. In some instances, similar species have coexisted for long periods of time before one species fades into oblivion. Such has been the case with species with human characteristics. The forerunners of humans have included temporally overlapping species such as *Australopithecus*, *Homo habilis*, and *Homo erectus*, all of which have passed into extinction. One of the questions raised by transhumanism is whether *Homo sapiens* now or soon will coexist with a similar species that will persist as *Homo sapiens* becomes extinct.

Based, then, on the history of biological species, the likely ultimate fate of the current human species is extinction. Species extinction, however, is not obligatory. Species of scorpions, for example, similar or identical to current species of scorpions are believed to have existed unchanged for hundreds of millions of years. In so doing, scorpions existed long before the emergence and long after the extinction of dinosaurs.

It is, thus, a statement of the obvious to say that, as a species, humans will either continue to exist or will become extinct. The transhumanist philosophy believes that there is a third alternative. Humans may find a way to engineer their own evolution and, in so doing, cause the emergence of a new species. Thus, there are two potential routes by which the human species could thwart or at least significantly delay its extinction. It could survive by using its unusual capacity for self-reflective thought, a capacity that seemingly separates it from other biological species and that arguably could be used for species preservation. It could also produce an ensuant species for which current humans are the antecedent. Humans could design and create a posthuman species.

So long as whatever will happen occurs before the human species becomes extinct, it may not matter whether humans learn how to survive where other species fail or transform its species into a posthuman species that will allow the continuation of human-like existence after the extinction of the *Homo sapiens*. Survival of the human is the ultimate issue. The solution to the impending extinction of the current human species postulated by transhumanism is thus important. Is it a viable alternative? If it is, then humans have but one option with which to stave off their species' extinction. If it is not, does the energy spent in the pursuit of the false hope raised by the transhumanist solution diminish the likelihood of *Homo sapiens* finding a self-reflective species solution to prolongation of itself?

From Homo sapiens to Homo technicus

In 1735 Carl Linnaeus published *Systema Naturae*, which formed the basis for biological taxonomy. The terms he used to describe the various taxa were based on what he thought were common sense descriptors. Humans were said to be *Homo sapiens*, a modification of the word *sapience*, which Linnaeus took to mean "wisdom." The classification of humans as such hearkens back to Aristotle's definition of humans as "rational animals" and the identification of human nature with the capacity to reason. Today, more than 250 years after Linnaeus, the concept of human nature and identification of humans as animals – or, more precisely, primates – continues to generate a healthy debate. Yet those who advocate transhumanism perpetuate the age-old notion of "man the animal."

The proponents of transhumanism base their vision on yet another contentious notion: the theory of evolution. Although evolution is a central theory in biology, the theory is historical and not predictive. In fact, recent advances in complexity science suggest that the principles of evolution (especially natural selection) are subordinate to more fundamental comple-system properties. Transhumanists hypothesize that the human species can and will intercede in its own evolution to such an extent that, over time, human beings will create a new hominoid species. The mechanism for this intercession is technological and is based on knowledge acquired through scientific exploration.

The transhumanist vision has generated a healthy debate (Grassie and Hansell 2011). Yet, it is important to note that the acceptance or rejection of this vision is an act of the individual and that the *decision* to accept or reject the vision is culturally influenced and varies by geographic location, as well as by social, religious, and ethnic factors. Arguments concerning the validity of the concept of transhumanism based on the foregoing are, thus, ones based on epistemological differences.

Evolution is not just a theory in biology; it has also been applied to the social sciences, giving rise to the concept of social evolution (Kidd 1898; Dawkins 1976) whose fundamental soundness is nearly without contention (Hallpike 1986; Breed and Page 1989; Pluciennik 2005). Given our historical awareness, we take for granted that human societies have changed over time and that, in the past, humans have lived differently than they live today, although variations depend on geographic location. For example, currently people living in the so-called first world enjoy a very different lifestyle from people who live in the third world or in geographically isolated and technologically underdeveloped areas.

The mechanism by which social evolution has occurred is also not contentious. Technology underlies the evolution of human cultures from primitive to current first-world twenty-first century societies (Morowitz 2002). Initial change in human cultural structure came with the technology that produced tools. Subsequently, technology produced artifacts for other purposes.

Transhumanism posits that technology will create objects that will provide the means for *Homo sapiens* to evolve into a new species. Proposed mechanisms that could provide a means for this evolution include separation of information from the corporeal body and technology that will produce cyborgs. Combine these with molecular and synthetic biology and "the human is giving way to a different construction called the posthuman" (Hayles 1999, 2). Envisioned are humanoid entities with enhanced thinking abilities, total-recall memory, bodies that are physically perfect, beautiful, possibly immortal, and more – all the consequence of scientific discovery (Garreau 2005, 8-9). Transhumanists envision the rise of a new posthuman species, which we may call the *Homo technicus*.

Garreau sums up the debate about this shift in three main scenarios: the "heaven scenario" considers this in utopian terms; the "hell scenario" regards it a dystopia; and in between, there is the more pragmatic "prevail scenario." But all three scenarios share one thing: they presuppose the validity of the notion of a posthuman future. It may, however, be that the most likely scenario does not involve species-generated evolution of itself and that the question of "heaven" or "hell" is moot. Humans may be faced with the same issue all biological species must face – extinction. Can we prevail if we are not able to engineer our species into a new one populated with posthumans?

It may be that the public debate about transhumanism is important in and of itself but that the belief in the reality of the emergence of an engineered species, of *Homo technicus*, is faulty. But how has that belief come about? Why have we become so convinced that transhumanism and posthumanism are imminent scenarios? Could it be that scientists and engineers have unwittingly marketed the concept to a public that wishes it so? Why are we so willing to believe that humanity is on the verge of a new phase in its evolutionary development? This chapter argues that the transhumanist vision is a cultural construct that reflects the assumptions of our current technological culture. Only if we understand the interplay between technology and culture can we realize that the transhumanist future is neither determined nor necessary.

What is really at stake in the emergence of the *Homo technicus*? If *Homo technicus* does not emerge to salvage humanity or to be the blame for the demise of the human species, can *Homo sapiens* still prevail? The belief in the eventual arrival of a new human species could be devastating to the ability of *Homo sapiens* to prevail in a future created by biotechnological innovation. A prevail scenario written with the belief that biotechnology will generate a new and better human would be quite different from one written with the awareness that biotechnology, like all technology, creates as well as solves problems. The latter prevail scenario would focus not on the emergence of *Homo technicus* but on the ongoing survival of *Homo sapiens*.

The debate about transhumanism focuses on the impending evolution of *Homo sapiens*. The transhumanist vision emerged as a result of the confluences of developments in science, engineering, technology, and medicine during the twentieth century, all of which are culturally bound. Thus, the transhumanist vision carries the imprimatur of the cultural practices that gave rise to it. Indeed, the transhumanist vision and the transhumanist movement focus the attention of a learned population on future issues which are arguably important to the human species. The following highlights the cultural embeddedness of the main strands of transhumanist thought.

Perpetual Youth and the Possibility of Immortality

Transhumanism is preoccupied with radical life extension (De Grey 2007) and claims that attainment of immortality is, in principle, technologically feasible. There is little novelty in the human desire to restore youthful vigor, enhance physiological performance, or attain immortality; these desires have been expressed in many cultures of the ancient worlds. For example, in the fifth century BCE, Herodotus (1998) reports of a fountain containing restorative natural water that was possessed by the Ethiopians and that "their constant use of the water" made them "long-lived." In the Middle Ages, alchemists sought to discover the recipe for creation of the philosopher's stone, an object that could transmogrify base metals into precious ones, rejuvenate the sick, and provide a means for achieving immortality. The publicly shared belief in the existence of these mechanisms was so strong that governments and other social organizations supported searches for their discovery. Numerous explorations were commissioned, financed, and carried out in their pursuit. For example, Ponce de Leon searched for the fountain of youth as a part of his exploration of the Americas, and Isaac Newton pursued the formula for the creation of the philosophers' stone while he was the Lucasian Professor of Mathematics at Cambridge (White 1997).

As cultural beliefs changed over time, so did the perception in the likelihood of discovering the fountain of youth or the philosophers' stone. The rise of modern scientific thought also transformed cultural attitudes toward magical thinking, although, during the early modern period, there was no clear-cut separation between the "scientific" and the "magical." Newton, the father of modern physics, was an avid practitioner of alchemy, which at the time was considered a "science" but later will be relegated and discarded as "magic" (Osler 2000; Henry 2002 [1997]). Eventually, with the rise of modern science, the quests for the fountain of youth or the philosophers' stone came to be dismissed as rationally untenable. In other words, beliefs that are taken to be valid in one period are dismissed as foolishness in subsequent periods. To wit, beliefs about the world are necessarily culturally bound, and this is true even about modern science.

The pursuit of immortal life, however, seems to be more resilient. In fact, the emergence of modern science in the second half of the seventeenth century led to greater optimism about the potential for physiological rejuvenation and hopes for immortality became even more widespread. A good case in point is Mary Shelly's *Frankenstein* (1831), which was read as fiction but the underlying thesis of which – that science would tease out the transformative immortality mechanism – entered the collective social consciousness as reality.

In the late twentieth century, scientific progress in genomics, stem-cell research, biomedical technology, pharmacology, computer technology, nanotechnology, and other advancements led to a revitalization of interest in mechanisms for restoration of youthful vigor, physiological enhancement, and immortality. The progress of modern science also added a new wrinkle. Charles Darwin's concept of species evolution gave rise to a new presumption that became comingled with the notions of perpetual youth and immortality. Ardent followers of Darwin in the 1920s and believers in the ideology of scientific progress gave rise to the belief that humanity is the first species endowed with the ability to evolve volitionally – in the Darwinian sense of *evolve* – into a new species. H. G. Wells' fantasy *The Time Machine* (1922) about the Morlocks and Eloi fused with new beliefs and technologies in the opening years of the twentieth century. Today, some people hypothesize that *Homo sapiens* will soon evolve into a superior, new species (Hughes 2004; Bostrom 2005). The imagined descendents of *Homo sapiens* have been dubbed *posthumans*, and the process that will bring about their presumed evolution constitutes *transhumanism*.

The very naming of this future state of affairs and the process by which transformative human evolution will presumably occur gave social credibility and academic stature to concepts that are still rather dubious. Whereas the fountain of youth and the philosophers' stone have become unacceptable to the scientific mind, the educated elite today discuss transhuman and posthuman futures as if they were already real. Unknowingly and unconsciously, twenty-first century cognoscenti have taken up discredited beliefs of previous generations, compelling us to believe in unproven fantasies.

Thomas Kuhn (1970) has shed light on the process by which beliefs that are accepted in one era are dismissed as untenable in a subsequent time. For example, the emergence of the scientific paradigm associated with quantum physics arose as a part of a search to elucidate small failures of explanation associated with the scientific paradigm related to Newtonian physics (Kuhn 1970, 98-110). Another of Kuhn's tenets notes that emergent paradigms do not invalidate older ones. Physicists living in the twenty-first century live with the reality that Newtonian and quantum physics coexist. Quantum physics does not undo the utility of the scientific paradigm associated with Newtonian physics. In other words, with new knowledge about the world, beliefs of previous eras are judged to be erroneous or foolish, but the reasonableness or epistemic validity of a given belief is always a product of judgments by future generations and is always culturally sound. There is no way to determine in advance which belief will be deemed reasonable by future generations and which belief will be invalidated.

In the last quarter of the twentieth century, a new scientific paradigm has been established, recognizing the phenomenon of emergent, self-sustaining, far-from-equilibrium, dynamical systems. Unlike the Newtonian/Cartesian paradigm, this scientific paradigm is nonlinear. While rhetoric associated with this dynamical, nonlinear paradigm has entered the twenty-first century cultural lexicon, a general understanding of its fundamental concepts has not. In fact, it has been argued that, at an intuitive level, artists and systems scientists understand this complex paradigm much better than do geneticists and engineers who are more committed to previous linear scientific paradigm. The changes from one scientific paradigm to another and the interplay between technology and culture are most evident in the field of medicine.

Medicine as a Social Practice

The quintessence of the amelioration of pathologies, enhancement of physical and mental capabilities, and immortality throughout history – and prehistory – has been associated with doctors and physicians (Nuland 1988). In premodern societies, the physician was entrusted with healing the sick, reassuring those who suffered loss, and, occasionally even resurrecting the dead. Potions, incantations, blood lettings, quicksilver cocktails, and surgery in nonsterile environments all have been acceptable medical practices. That such practices are no longer acceptable is due to the emergence of a new scientific paradigm that altered the understanding of disease etiology.

The scientific practice of medicine began in the late nineteenth and early twentieth centuries. A convergence of technological innovation with developing theories of basic medical science helped physicians know for the first time the cause of many diseases: micro-organisms. Vaccines and antibiotics, anesthesia and aseptic techniques, laboratory tests and radiology – the scientific physician practiced medicine in a Newtonian paradigm and was finally able to act with knowledge of cause-and-effect. The results seemed miraculous. Diseases of germ etiology (such as pneumonias, plague, cholera, and small pox) were no longer the causes of suffering and death that they had been. Scientific medicine had taken on pathological micro-organisms and won.

Scientific medicine transformed the delivery of healthcare and its practitioners (Starr 1983). The hospital, hitherto a dreaded place rightfully believed to be a foul location where the impoverished or those without family went to die, was reenvisioned as a place people went to be healed. Likewise, the perception of the abilities and competencies of physicians changed dramatically and positively. As the efficacy of their practices rose so did the social stature of physicians.

Stimulated at least in part by two world wars, substantial medical advances were made in diagnostic and therapeutic technologies, pharmacological agents, and biomedical devices. Thus, concomitant with the rise in the social status of physicians was the rise in the belief in the efficacy of artifacts associated with the profession. Societal beliefs changed with regard to the mechanisms responsible for the physicians' capabilities. Facilitated by science and technology, the perception of medicine transitioned from an art to a science. The cultural perceptions of the physician changed from an individual who could divine a cure from a combination of knowledge, intuition, and spiritual guidance to an individual who used tools provided by science and technology to uncover the cause of pathology and to effect a repair that would restore or improve the patient's physiology.

Not surprisingly, this mechanistic view of medicine matched the Cartesian machine model of the human that was applied as well to anatomical/physiological systems. Thus, the heart was thought of as a pump, the lungs as a bellows, and the brain as a computer. Since muscle and nervous tissues functioned through the use of electrical current, they became studied using the methods of electrical engineers. Resistors, capacitors, and batteries were used metaphorically to understand electrophysiology. This linear, mechanistic understanding of the human continues to dominate the transhumanist discourse.

Yet the body is *not* a machine. The electricity that flows in it is not movement of electrons that flows down a metal wire but the sequential movement of ions in and out of electrically gated protein channels. Biological electricity, unlike the electricity in machines, travels at different rates of speed dependent on the diameter of the biological wire-like thing down which it travels and the wire-like thing's insulation or lack thereof. Biological contacts are, for the most part, not transmitting nodes as would be found in a radio or a computer but diffuse, modulating connections. Moreover, the couplings in the biological system are dynamic. They change their properties continually and do so within fractions of a second. In a computer, once the connections are manufactured on a silicone chip, they are there essentially forever. The connections in the body do things with space and time that are impossible in manufactured devices.

Nevertheless, as Herodotus and Newton had done in prescientific cultures, learned people in the twentieth and twenty-first centuries envisioned the future of biomedical progress using scientific paradigms with which they were familiar. Possibly because of the unprecedented progress made by medicine in the previous century and because continued progress is inevitable, twenty-first-century people share once again the same dreams that people living in prescientific eras had: namely, the dream about the discovery of a mechanism that will restore youthful vigor, enhance physiological performance, and bestow immortality. Once again, these fantasies are presented as realizable dreams that lie just around the corner. In turn, these presumptions lead people today to postulate a human-facilitated, new, hominoid species about to evolve from *Homo sapiens*.

The systems dictum, "every system is perfectly designed to produce the results it gets," is attributed to W. E. Deming (Pauker, Zane, and Salem 2005). The reemergence of the belief in the imminence of perpetual youth and immortality and the newly created belief that the biomedical and technological industries underlie a current evolution of a posthuman species are the result of the interacting systems that make up our culture. These beliefs are, however, false. They are as false now as they were in the seventeenth century or in antiquity. The development of artificial intelligence, biomedical devices, genomics and proteomics, autopoetic sets, nanotechnologies, synthetic biology, and a gamut of other scientific and technological advances do not change biological reality. Indeed, when the notions of perpetual youth and immortality and species evolution have been put forward by the academic community, it has been from social, not biological, science and from technological and humanities disciplines.

Credence for these ideas also came by way of the medical-legal system. Twentieth-century medicine began for reasons appropriate to the social mores apropos to the early 1900s. Accordingly, the patient-physician relationship that developed was paternalistic. In this situation, the physician became the individual who was responsible not only for diagnosis and treatment but for making decisions on the patient's behalf. Technological and pharmaceutical advances were made as the century progressed. These gave physicians abilities undreamed of before. The physicians' having assumed the role of the decision maker on their patients' behalf with genuine medical prowess unheard of only years earlier made the physician a target for litigation. Errors, which earlier had been taken for granted because expectations of positive outcomes were low as was the social status of the physician, became intolerable. Suits were filed, malpractice insurance came into existence and a positive feedback loop was created. Medical litigation became a normal component of the healthcare industry.

An unexamined cultural perception, which accompanied this rise in the prevalence of malpractice, was that death could be defeated by physician competence. For purposes of malpractice litigation, death was often treated as an unacceptable outcome. Thus, not only has malpractice litigation altered for many in medical professions their perception of healthcare culture as a whole, but it has also distorted the concept of death in American culture. That death can be considered an unacceptable and potentially a nonnecessary outcome changes the culture psyche. It creates the shared belief on a subconscious cultural level that the science and technology associated with modern medicine have the ability to defeat death.

While the beliefs in a fountain of youth and immortality imparted by the philosophers' stone sought by alchemists are dismissed by modern cultures, those same concepts have reemerged as attainable goals of modern bioscience. Naysayers are dismissed for several reasons. They are sometimes seen as individuals mired in the past who are unaware of the recent advancements made in biomedical technology. The perceived unknowability associated with the future, particularly with the more distant future, is also invoked as a rebuttal to naysayers. It is against this latter argument that culturally induced, unexamined beliefs come into play. If death has been deemed an unacceptable outcome and something that reasonable people might view as potentially defeatable, it is then argued that immortality through science and technology is potentially attainable.

The Alcor Life Extention Foundation, founded in 1972, is a case in point. Situated on the southeast side of the Scottsdale Municipal Airport, not far from the runway, this company engages in cryonics: in other words, people whose hearts have ceased to function but who are not truly brain dead lead a vitrified existence. There, brains in heads with or without bodies wait for their resurrection by scientists from the future; the vitrified entities are unfazed by the passing of time and the probability that the scientists they await reside far, far into the future … if at all. Meanwhile, the Alcor Life Extension Foundation advertises job opportunities, issues memberships, and solicits donations.

In a study of the lifespan of organizations conducted by Royal Dutch Shell, its corporate planning director Arie De Geus concluded that even large, multinational businesses survive for a duration equal to only about half the expected lifetime of a twentieth-century human being (De Geus 1997). Pushing forty, by the metrics suggested by De Geus, Alcor is likely approaching the end of its life. This might worry its inhabitant patrons, were their not truly dead brains more active.

The future postulated by those engineering a brave new biological future for twenty-first-century humans is somewhat unwittingly marketed in the same manner Alcor markets cryonics. Without a financially blessed subpopulation with a shared belief in revival of the long frozen, Alcor could not have come into being and could not continue to exist. The illusion of a posthuman future plays no small part in the ongoing financing of biotechnology said to be facilitating transhumanation. However, unlike Alcor's subpopulation of like-minded, financially able benefactors and clients, the constituent base supporting the industry built to bring the posthuman into reality seemingly includes almost everybody in the modern world. Governments of most first- and second-world nations ascribe to the notion of creating better humans through biological engineering: pharmacology, genetics, and biotechnology. Computers and other information technology also play a role in transhumanism, although whether the role is a supporting or starring one is uncertain.

The undeniable support for the belief that sees humankind fated to a transhumanistic trip that leads to posthuman beings lies in large part with an interpretation of history that points to such an evolution, as well as from reassurances by scientists from nearly every quarter that the transition from human to cyborg is just a matter of time. In fact, the implication is that, with a substantial ramping up of financial resources, this destination is temporally very near. Politicians and populations are susceptible to such exhortations based on widely shared fantasies. For example, not long ago, nearly the whole of the free world felt compelled to act – consequences and costs be damned – because Saddam Hussein was only months if not just days away from developing weapons of mass destruction. Political ideologies were united and pocket books were emptied because of a shared vision of a fictional future.

Future Scenarios Are Fiction

Whether the scenarios being spun are visions from cutting-edge research scientists, think-tank social strategists, political futurists, or crackpot prophets, images of the future are imaginary. It cannot be otherwise. However, those with the ability to create novel technology actually have an advantage when it comes to predicting the future. Technology shapes the future in ways that are sometimes predictable, sometimes not, but that are almost always irreversible. Attributed to Abraham Lincoln, Peter F. Drucker, and Alan Kay, the statement "the best way to predict the future is to create it" is occasionally accomplished by the creators of novel technologies who have the wisdom to wonder if/how what they have engineered into existence will alter humankind's future. An audience that wants more and wants it sooner frequently seduces those involved in the creation of novel technology unwittingly into overstatement, especially in the pursuit of securing funding.

More often than not the creators of new technology are oblivious to the social impact of their creations. It is left to philosophers, politicians, and artists to predict altered trajectories of social evolution that will arise with technological novelty. Often these predictions show up in popular literature. In fact, the creators of fictional works that find wide audiences at times themselves create a future into which society seems to grow. For example, in the latter part of the nineteenth century, Jules Verne anticipated submarines and space travel, with the result that his writings influenced their eventual manifestations. In 1984, William Gibson's science fiction in *Neuromancer* (1984) anticipated the evolution of the Internet and introduced us (some would say that he led us) to "cyberspace." In 1962, Hanna-Barbera introduced the 2062 technological society of the Jetsons. In many ways, the future predicted by *The Jetsons* popularized the notion that technology would be a boon to humanity, a goal to which humankind strove.

The Jetsons played to an American belief prevalent in the 1950s and 1960s: technology would enhance the quality of life. In the animated ABC television series, George Jetson worked a three-hour day, three days a week. His total job duties were the pushing of a single button connected to technology with artificial intelligence. In fact, the machine whose button he pushed was so advanced that it was a part of a technological network that had preservation of the human species as its primary goal. George Jetson's community, thanks to technology of the twenty-first century, was virtually utopian.

American society embraced a Jetsonian vision of a much more desirable future state made possible by technological society and pushed forward with a shared belief that things would improve incrementally with each technological advance. Toward that end, the public embraced the emergence of a new discipline, biomedical engineering that was tasked with retrofitting defective humans with mechanical devices that would compensate for a slew of pathological problems. By 1964, the National Institutes of Health had initiated the Artificial Heart Program with the expectation that, within ten years, artificial hearts could be used as replacements for defective human hearts. Biotechnological advancement had become an important component of humanity's technological future.

The future anticipated by *The Jetsons* in 1962 has already been incompletely realized a half century later. There are, however, deviations such that the technological utopia it predicted for 2062 seems much less likely now than it did when the show first aired. Ubiquitous computing and artificial intelligence exist. Robotics has greatly reduced much of the physical burden the manufacturing industries used to place on their employees. But the work week has not dropped to three days/three hours per day nor has there been an equal distribution of benefits parceled out to the public.

Biotechnology has created diagnostic and therapeutic tools that were not dreamed of when *The Jetsons* began its run, but overall access to healthcare has decreased and costs associated with healthcare have skyrocketed, while the overall quality of medical care has gone down relative to that provided in many other first-world countries. Rather than to a utopia, technology seems to be taking America toward a fate where huge socioeconomic differences will exist throughout its population. Or worse, the pursuit of technological advancement may ultimately be responsible for pushing the nation into bankruptcy.

There are, in the trajectory of time, bifurcation points. Complexity science sometimes calls these "frozen accidents" (Gell-Mann 1994). One such bifurcation point has apparently occurred that leads the trajectory of the future away from the future of George Jetson. The three-day work week, once a culturally agreed-upon component of the American dream, seems unlikely, despite the development of technology that would permit it. Instead, those with above-average income are likely to be working much more than forty hours a week. Things are actually worse than this appears at first blush, for technology has enabled many in the workforce to live considerable distances from their place of employment. The automobile has facilitated urban sprawl and with it increased the time spent on the commute to and from work.

The choice to move to an expanded rather than a shorter work week was facilitated by technology. Technology would have also facilitated the opposite choice. At the fork in the road to the future, societal mores, not technology, made the choice. Why, did we chose to work more hours? There was no vote or discussion about these monumental social changes.

Robotics, computerization, and artificial intelligence allowed the offloading of the existing specialized human workforce because robots with artificial intelligence and computerized programming could do the work of the specialized human workforce. This meant that the remaining human workforce could work less (that is, they could work fewer hours per week) or that fewer employees working a standard work week would be needed. Western industrialized societies chose the latter but without any substantive discussion. Aided by technology, fewer employees working the same hours as many workers without technology caused the costs related to human labor to fall. All other things being equal, this meant that profit margins rose. This financial windfall was then divided and distributed to the remaining workforce. Those in charge were thus rewarded for making the decision to reduce the workforce.

With regard to altering the demographics of the workforce, intelligent, labor-saving technology had a second effect. It could be used to reduce the average wage paid line employees by lessening the demand for specialized human skills. Thus, what could not be done by robots, computers, artificial intelligence, and other technological artifices could be done by a human workforce with fewer skills. Again, a bifurcation point: the need for a less specialized workforce opened up the possibility of outsourcing work to lower-cost providers. Technology assumed more and more of the functions previously done by human employees, and the domestic workforce was again significantly reduced in number. Again, technology was used to facilitate unemployment and a redistribution of wealth rather than to generate additional leisure time for the previously existing work-force in the form of a shorter work week.

Meanwhile, technological advancements associated with medicine initially postulated to improve the overall health of the nation grew rapidly, while the overall health of the U.S. population – relative to that of peer countries – declined. Abetted by hundreds or thousands of medical technological advances, healthcare costs soared. The mission of biomedical research and development became not to improve the overall health of the nation but to defeat death. So successful has the biomedical technology industry become that there are those who believe immortality is achievable within their lifetime (Kurzweil 2005). Humans are said to have become – or, at least, are becoming – cyberbeings. An imminent transhuman future is discussed by otherwise clear-headed people. The Jetsonian belief that technology will facilitate utopia has been revived.

Examined in the context of current events, the progress of the United States from 1962 to the present does not support the hypothesis that technology will relentlessly improve our lot. Widespread job loss and high levels of unemployment have become an accepted component of U.S. society. Lower-paying jobs (termed "Mac-jobs") are on the rise while the middle class shrinks. Healthcare expenditures have moved from 4.4 percent of the gross national product (GNP) in 1950 to 6.1 percent in 1965 to 10.6 percent in 1984 (Dougherty 1988) to 16.2 percent in 2008 just prior to the collapse of Wall Street (NHE Fact Sheet 2010). It will soon hit 20 percent of the GNP, and with the baby-boomer population poised to begin collecting Medicare benefits, before long, it could reach 25-30 percent. Nowhere else is such a large percentage of GNP spent on healthcare. Perhaps if U.S. citizens were enjoying health status that was the envy of the rest of the world, this excessively high rate of spending on healthcare might arguably be justified. However, by essentially all healthcare-outcome measures, health is worse for residents of the U.S. than it is for those of most other first-world countries (CIA World Factbook 2010).

Because of America's preoccupation with its perception of the benefits of technology, a shift in cultural values occurred. This shift has been supported by the marketplace in that a large percentage of the emerging non-Mac-job market is technology-related. The focus of many first-rate academic institutions has deliberately shifted from one celebrating a liberal-arts education to one that focuses on science and engineering. Engineering has become the new liberal arts (Epstein 2006; Roberson 2010). At many American colleges and universities, faculty not involved in mathematics, science, and engineering are asking whether their disciplines are relevant in today's world.

Consciously or unconsciously, our society has decided to pursue a technological future. This decision was made, at least in part, on the basis of the widespread shared belief that such a future would make our lot better. The creation of a technologic future became a national priority, and resources and social esteem were allocated in an effort to achieve it. Science and engineering were the beneficiaries. For example, whereas the physician of the 1950s enjoyed only mediocre social and financial status, specialty physicians today are among the most respected and highly compensated individuals in the country. While not treading such lofty heights as specialty physicians, the engineering faculty at many American universities are compensated at a substantially higher rate than many of their peers in other disciplines.

However, while technological enterprise has produced many results that outshine illusions created by *The Jetsons*, the present is rife with problems that had seemingly been solved when *The Jetsons* first aired. On a per capita basis in constant dollars adjusted for inflation, healthcare is about five times as expensive in 2009 as compared with 1962 and nearly eight times more than it was in 1950. Instead of creating a healthcare utopia, technology has created healthcare that is becoming more difficult to afford. This stands in contrast to many other technologies. For example, the first readily available color television cost about $1,300 in 1954 (equivalent to more than $10,000 in 2009.) By 1964, the price had dropped to $400 (about $2,700 in 2009 dollars) to $250 in 1972 (about $1,250 today), and is available for about $200 now (Powelson 2003). For that technology, there was an approximately fifty-fold decrease in cost.

Because the ultimate goal of biomedical technology is a shared conceptualization, it is able to demand resources in a manner different from the demands of other technologies. The emergence of the Internet, for example, was an unforeseen consequence of the development of the personal computer. The development of the mainframe and then the personal computer was not driven by a culturally shared vision of creating an Internet. By contrast, the impetus behind the development of biomedical technology is a culturally shared vision.

Technology and the Trajectory of Social Evolution

Fire, the wheel, pottery, metallurgy, glass (Macfarlane and Martin 2002), the printing press, the steam engine, the telegraph, and the personal computer – to mention a few – have been socially transforming entities. Not only has technology facilitated shifts from one cultural state to another, but technology has ensured that this movement has been in a one-way direction. Some people may long for a previous cultural state, may want a return to the "good-old-days," but technology's tangibility makes such a return impossible. Technology provides a one-way route out of Plato's cave.

Now enters biotechnology, which implies that it carries with it the possibility of engineering the posthuman and of immortality. Without a doubt, over time, biomedical science demonstrated its ability to understand and cure numerous pathologies and diseases and will continue to do so. In the 170 years since Matthias Schleiden and Theodor Schwann introduced cell theory (Turner 1890), numerous diseases have been eliminated or, at least, held at bay. Moreover, coupled with mechanical technologies, biomedical scientists have reengineered pathologically compromised individuals, giving them new joints, artificial kidneys, and heart valves. Bioscience developed the ability to photograph the inside of the intact body; more recently, dynamic, noninvasive bioimaging technologies have been able to observe the functioning of various physiological systems.

Until the emergence of biotechnology, technological novelty produced social transformations for the whole of the culture whether individuals in the culture had access to the technology or not (Arthur 2009). Biotechnology – especially biomedical technology – appears poised to prove the exception to that rule. While all the populous nations were affected by world-changing technologies, biotechnology by its very nature is personalized. Those with access to technologies of a biomedical nature benefit, while those out of its reach do not. This is made worse by the accelerating cost of biomedical technologies and, by extension, healthcare.

The ongoing creation of novel biomedical technologies may, however, not be the only reason healthcare costs are relentlessly increasing. It may be that this iteration of technological innovation plays a different game than do technologies that have come before. Earlier technologies often introduced surprising novelty into culture. The uses and consequences of these technologies often were not thought of before their introduction. As fire, the wheel, pottery, metallurgy, glass, the printing press, the steam engine, the telegraph, and the personal computer were developed, new and undreamed of uses for them were discovered. Biomedical technology fits a different paradigm. The uses for it are well understood at the outset. The purpose of this technology is to improve overall physical and mental health and to delay or prevent death. Biotechnology can also augment the normal functioning of our physical being and overcome limitations imposed by the human body created by nature.

The potential to enhance the human being through biotechnology has captured the attention and the imagination of many. Politicians and the military are keen to develop a population biotechnically enhanced for the national competitive edge such a population would provide. If it is possible to create biotechnically enhanced individuals who could self-sustain over time, these superhuman or posthuman individuals would be economically and politically important. Their scientifically enhanced abilities would set them apart from the human beings created by nature alone. Posthumans/superhumans would give competitive advantage to the nations they called home.

This postulated biotechnological creation of posthumans is the process of transhumanism. There appear to be several technologies "cranking up to modify human nature" (Garreau 2005, 4), including genetic, robotic, information and nano processes. There are drugs and chemical therapies that can alter immune-system functioning, mimic or neutralize neural and endocrine-system effects, and selectively poison human pathogens or malfunctioning cells. There are implantable biotechnologies that exist across a variety of scales. These can replace a defective joint, provide sound to the hearing impaired, improve vision, hold open arteries, and repair congenital malformations or lesions created by trauma. On the horizon are technologies that substitute cameras for eyes and robotic arms for flesh-and-blood limbs. Neural control of external mechanical devices is potentially possible by deciphering brain waves through the use of computer algorithms or through the use of microelectrodes permanently located in the brain.

The notion of genetic manipulation is another broad biotechnological area. If defective genes can be replaced in the genome of the affected, then diseases can be cured. Genetic manipulation targets the developing embryo. Through the use of stem cells, the possibility of providing cures for adult-onset disease is envisioned. Epigenetics (which looks at changes in inherited traits through mechanisms other than DNA sequence) and proteomics (proteins are produced by the information contained in genetic DNA and put that information into action; however, the translation of genetic information into proteins is affected by factors other than the genome) offer similar promise. And not only information management but the computer itself is seen by some as having the potential to house the information now housed in the DNA and the central nervous system of individual humans. As computer memory and processing speed continue to grow, some believe that there will come a time when the comuter will outstrip the memory and processing currently limiting human consciousness to the confines of the human brain. At that point, immortality seems possible.

Given this multipronged approach to technological enhancement of the human, transhumanists see posthumans as imminent. To many, the stage seems set for a momentous leap for humankind, and there are people all over the world who seek to facilitate this leap. Indeed, many nations, in the hope of substantially improving their fiscal futures, have made funding their nation's biotechnology development a priority. In many quarters, there is a globally shared belief in the impending ability of humans to transform natural humans into improved, engineered entities. This shared belief gives rise to a cultural intuition, which senses the eminence of posthumans. The likelihood of *Homo sapiens* using science and technology to evolve into *Homo technicus* differs with the methodology facilitating the evolution.

The promise that biotechnology will create enhanced humans in the near future enables the promoters of transhumanism to raise funds with which to proceed. In this regard, a positive feedback loop has been created. It is an amplifying feedback; it requires an increasing percentage of the gross national product of countries that consciously or unconsciously subscribe to a belief in process of transhumanism.

Whether a new species evolves or not, twenty-first-century technology will alter human culture, whether or not it alters individuals. Change at the individual level will also occur, however, because culture modifies individuals. While implantable medical devices, pharmaceuticals, and designer genetic manipulation may or may not produce *Homo technicus*, significant cultural transformation accomplished through the use of computer and communication technologies seems likely with or without conscious social facilitation. It is not unlikely that the individuals who comprise the whole of the human species will remain one kind of biological organism, *Homo sapiens*, but ongoing technological evolution makes us many kinds of psychological beings. Shared emergent psychological beliefs beget new culture. It could be that technology will provide the means for the emergence of *Homo sapiens* as a self-reflective species.

Medicine and the Promise of Biotechnology

Arguably, the oldest of the human professions is that of the physician. Characteristics attributed to the physician have included the ability to cure illness and overcome death, place and remove curses, and function as a conduit to immortality. Although at times some of the practices of the pre-twentieth-century physicians caused more harm than they did good, belief in the benefits associated with physicians persisted. The return of the population's faith in the promise of the physician took a long time to achieve. It was at least tens of thousands of years before aseptic technique, anesthesia, and antibiotics allowed physicians to deliver on even the most fundamental of their promises.

In the 1950s, the United States – flush with post-World-War-II earnings and impressed by the successes made by the scientific practice of medicine during the past half century – made a leap of faith. If the success trajectory for modern medicine continued, the U.S. had more than enough money to make everyone well. Medicine, funded solely by a fee-for-service compensation system, promised big. The medical-legal system interpreted the role of the medical system to be one that could defeat death. Medicine turned to applied science for the tools.

Even with the undeniable changes in efficacy made by medicine at this transition point, there were those who called for caution. In 1909, one of these critics was George Bernard Shaw (Shaw 2006, 1):

> That any sane nation, having observed that you could provide for the supply of bread by giving bakers a pecuniary interest in baking for you, should go on to give a surgeon a pecuniary interest in cutting off your leg, is enough to make one despair of political humanity. But that is precisely what we have done. And the more appalling the mutilation, the more the mutilator is paid.

As American medicine proceeded through the twentieth century, in many respects, Shaw was prophetic. Given the rewards provided the medical industry through the financing of healthcare based on fee-for-service compensation, there was virtually no downside for overpromising or for fantasizing. For example, a telethon begun in 1966 suggested that a cure for an incapacitating neuromuscular disease was right around the corner. More than forty years later, although millions of dollars have been raised and spent on research dedicated to finding the cure, it remains at least one more corner away.

The unflagging optimism of people hoping for medical help has been combined with the utopian vision of the future created by Walt Disney and Hanna-Barbera Productions, and the baton has been passed to biotechnology. Biotechnology has the potential to increase the species' life expectancy, enhance the functionality of the species, augment the beauty of individuals, and improve the prognosis of the pathologically impaired. Transhumanistic and medical objectives have become blurred.

Biotechnology and the healthcare industry are utterly intertwined and have been since the emergence of the era of modern scientific medicine. It began to seem that, in using science and technology, the human being could do what had hitherto seemed the ultimate but impossible goal. Through appropriate application of scientific knowledge, scientists could create technology that could be used to make human beings immortal. In the middle of the twentieth century, the economy of the United States was robust, and the decision to invest in the overall health of Americans was made. Medicare and Medicaid were two of the evidences of this decision.

In 1950 in the United States, per capita spending on healthcare amounted to about 4.5 percent of the gross national product (about $125 per person in 1950 dollars.) In 2009, U.S. per capita spending was 18 percent of the GDP (about $8,200 per person in 2009 dollars). Projections for healthcare spending put it at between 25 and 33 percent of the GDP within the next decade. The current rate of spending is approximately double that of peer Western-world countries and up to ten times more on a per capita basis when compared with other countries with which the U.S. trades. Healthcare outcomes for the U.S., however, are said to be thirty-seventh best when compared with healthcare outcomes of other countries.

Is Transhumanism the New Jetsons?

Technological progress creates sustainable, irreversible transformations in human culture. Iterations of technological novelty have allowed for the emergence of a number of cultural phenotypes. Historically, these emergences have not been continually sustainable but have been discontinuous. The discontinuity has been caused at least in part by competing emergent technologies. The spear, the bow-and-arrow, the wheel, domesticated livestock, folk-lore transmission of agricultural practices, the evolution of various forms of mathematics, monetary economies, metallurgy, gun powder, glass, the printing press, electricity, telegraph, steam and gasoline engines, telephone, airplane, computers, cell phones, and the Internet have underlain cultural emergences and social evolution.

There is an obvious disconnect between the future made possible by current technology, the future envisioned in the 1950s by a substantial part of the American public that would arise from technological advances made in the next half century, and that future as it actually exists as the present. The three-day work week and the expansion of the middle class and the benefits provided to it by the twenty-first-century technology envisioned by the Jetsons – a present state that could have been realized – does not exist. Instead, the percentage of the population in the middle class has fallen because jobs have become scarcer. Those who do have middle-class status and jobs are likely to be working more rather than fewer hours as compared with their Jetson-watching counterparts of fifty years ago.

The concept of transhumanism or posthumanism may have emerged as an alternative vision of a technologically created future. It may have emerged to answer the unasked question, "If not the future suggested by the Jetsons, then what?" If so, then it may be that one vision made up of attainable and of fanciful elements has been replaced by another vision of the same composition. Probable and improbable elements are intertwined in both visions. The Jetson's future included a substantially altered workforce made possible by robotics, as well as floating cities and flying cars. Transhumanism offers biotechnical solutions to a number of current pathological conditions as well as *Six Million Dollar Man*-like physical enhancements and immortality. These visions offer both realistic hopes to concerns of mature humans as well as pandering to the childlike fantasies of others. By not understanding the qualitative differences in the promises being made, society squanders financial resources and time.

Becoming Posthuman or Maturing As Humans?

For the human species, the issue is not immortality of individuals but continuation of the species. Science and technology are potentially components of a unique mechanism that might allow *Homo sapiens* to self-sustain itself past its otherwise looming species-extinction date. The critical issue is not the evolution of posthuman individuals but using the unique intellectual and communication abilities possessed by the human species to become – if not an immortal species – a maximally surviving species.

Physical and biological sciences have and can continue to provide a philosophical framework that will allow humans to mature as a species. Its work now is to become – as a species – self-reflective. In so doing, it will come to realize that, although species, like individual organisms, have a finite life span, the human species with its ability to think not only as individuals but as a collective has the potential to delay its extinction.

It must not be content with species homeostasis but make the decision to become cognitively allostatic. (The term *allostasis* is a physiological term that was introduced by Bruce McEwen to describe the ability of zoological organisms with hormonal and autonomic nervous systems to respond in such a way as to survive stressful changes [McEwen and Lasley 2002]. It differs from homeostatic mechanisms, which are feedback systems that preserve the internal status quo. Allostasis is accomplished through evolved complex physiological systems that alter homeostatic parameters in preparation for response to a perceived future threat.) It could be that *Homo sapiens* has evolved complex social systems (the ability to formulate theory, the intellectual tools with which cognitively to alter its evolutionary trajectory, the communication skills that result in synergistic accomplishment) that will allow it to prepare for ongoing and future threats to its existence.

New, novel technology transforms society. However, in this transformation, the human species has been – to date – essentially a passive participant. The transformations occur over time and new forms of culture ultimately come into existence. The process, though, is discontinuous. Historical political and philosophical structures and explanations intermingle with emergent social transformation. Allostatic thought intermingles with homeostatic thought.

While the current debate over concern for the direction that a potential posthuman future may take might be a debate over a purely fictional outcome, it is, nevertheless, a self-reflective internal monologue conducted by the human species. The conversation about transhumanism has stirred the imaginations of many and has attracted an interdisciplinary conversation. Academic disciplines not directly affiliated with applied science-and-technology creation are involved. It could be that the conversation surrounding the notion of transhumanism will serve as the strange attractor for a new – an emergent – form of collective human consciousness.

The public debate about transhumanism is about our technoculture, but this debate must also include the humanities and the arts, disciplines that have intellectually and historically engaged in this sort of conversation. Scientists and engineers must also play an active role in this discussion where they must help define the possible and eschew the fanciful. They cannot as individuals pander to the fanciful whims of an as-of-yet still-immature species. Rather science and engineering must join with the humanities, arts, and other traditionally self-reflective disciplines for the sake of the future of the human species.

References

Arthur, W. Brian. 2009. *The Nature of Technology: What It Is and How It Evolves*. New York: Free Press.

Bostrom, Nick. 2005. A history of transhumanist thought. *Journal of Evolution and Technology* 14 (1): 1-25.

Breed, Michael D., and Robert E. Page. 1989. *The Genetics of Social Evolution.* Boulder, CO: Westview Press.

Central Intelligence Agency. 2010. *The World Factbook*: https://www.cia.gov/library/publications/the-world-factbook/rankorder/2102rank.html, accessed July 18, 2011.

Dawkins, Richard. 1976. *The Selfish Gene*. Oxford: Oxford University Press.

De Grey, Aubrey. 2007. *Ending Aging: The Rejuvenation Breakthroughs That Could Reverse Human Aging in Our Lifetime*. New York: St. Martin's Press.

De Gues, Arie. 1997. *The Living Company: Habits for Survival in a Turbulent Business Environment*. New York: Basic Books.

Dougherty, Charles J. 1988. *American Health Care: Realities, Rights, and Reforms*. Oxford: Oxford University Press.

Epstein, David. 2006. The technology mosaic. *Inside Higher Ed*: http://www.insidehighered.com/news/2006/05/25/engineering, accessed July 18, 2011.

Garreau, Joel. 2005. *Radical Evolution: The Promise and Peril of Enhancing Our Minds, Our Bodies – and What It Means to Be Human*. New York: Broadway Books.

Gell-Mann, Murray. 1994. *The Quark and the Jaguar: Adventures in the Simple and the Complex*. New York: W.H. Freeman & Company.

Gibson, William. 1984. *Neuromancer*. New York: Ace Books.

Grassie, William. J., and Gregory Hansell, eds. 2011. *H+ Transhumanism and Its Critics*. Philadelphia: Metanexus Institute.

Hallpike, Christopher Robert. 1986. *The Principles of Social Evolution*. Oxford: Clarendon Press; New York: Oxford University Press.

Hayles, N. Katherine. 1999. *How We Became Posthuman: Virtual Bodies in Cybernetics, Literature, and Informatics*. Chicago: The University of Chicago Press.

Henry, John. 2002 [1997]. *The Scientific Revolution and the Origins of Modern Science*. 2d ed. New York: Palgrave.

Herodotus. 1998. *The Histories / Herodotus*. Translated by Robein. New York: Oxford University Press.

Hughes, James. 2004. *Citizen Cyborg: Why Democratic Societies Must Respond to the Redesigned Human of the Future*. New York: Basic Books.

Kidd, Benjamin. 1898. *Social Evolution*. New York: G. Putnam's Sons.

Kurzweil, Ray. 2005. *The Singularity Is Near: When Humans Transcend Biology*. New York: Viking Adult.

Kuhn, Thomas. 1970. *The Structure of Scientific Revolutions*. 2d ed. Chicago: University of Chicago Press.

Macfarlane, Alan, and Gerry Martin. 2002. *Glass: A World History*. Chicago: University of Chicago Press.

McEwen, Bruce, and Elizabeth Norton Lasley. 2002. *The End of Stress As We Know It*. Washington, DC: Joseph Henry Press.

Morowitz, Harold J. 2002. *The Emergence of Everything: How the World Became More Complex*. New York: Oxford University Press.

NHE Fact Sheet. 2010: https://www.cms.gov/NationalHealthExpendData/25_NHE_Fact_Sheet.asp, accessed July 18, 2011.

Nuland, Sherwin B. 1988. *Doctors: The Biography of Medicine*. New York: Alfred A. Knopf, Inc.

Osler, Margaret J. 2000. *Rethinking the Scientific Revolution*. Cambridge: Cambridge University Press.

Pauker, Stephen G., Ellen M. Zane, and Deeb N. Salem. 2005. Creating a safer health care system. *Journal of the American Medical Association* 294: 2906-8.

Pluciennik, Mark. 2005. *Social Evolution*. London: Duckworth.

Powelson, Richard. 2003. First color television sets were sold 50 years ago. *Pittsburgh Post-Gazette*, December 31: http://www.post-gazette.com/tv/20031231colortv1231p3.asp, accessed July 18, 2011.

Roberson, Mary-Russell. 2010. What's the big idea? Engineering – the new liberal arts? *Duke Engineering News*: http://prattpress.pratt.duke.edu/duke_summit_big_idea, accessed July 18, 2011.

Shaw, George Bernard. 2006. *The Doctor's Dilemma: Preface on Doctors*. Lenox, MA: Hard Press Editions.

Shelley, Mary Wollstonecraft. 1831. *Frankenstein, or, the Modern Prometheus*. London: H. Colburn and R. Bentley.

Starr, Paul. 1983. *The Social Transformation of American Medicine*. New York: Basic Books.

Turner, William. 1890. The cell theory, past and present. *Journal of Anatomy and Physiology* 24 (Pt 2): 253-87.

Wells, H. G. 1922. *The Time Machine: An Invention*. New York: H. Holt.

White, Michael. 1997. *Isaac Newton: The Last Sorcerer*. New York: Basic Books.

Technology and Transhumanism: Unpredictability, Radical Contingency, and Accelerating Change

Braden Allenby

Introduction

As with many arguable cultural constructs, transhumanism is highly contested ground.[1] Much of this dialogue, however, is replete with category confusion, and virtually all of it is based on a somewhat weak understanding of the power and unpredictability of technology and technological systems. Moreover, the complexity introduced by the accelerating conversion of *the human* – however one chooses to define it – into a system subject to intentional human design (a "design space") is profound and suggests a fundamental inadequacy in the way transhumanism debates are framed. Perhaps the most important source of confusion occurs, in fact, when one fails to understand *transhuman* as a cultural project carrying significant normative implications, as opposed to already advanced science-and-technology activity affecting human design through, for example, pharmaceutical manipulation of cognitive functions such as concentration and memory. Because "transhuman" is a normative concept, it encourages the sort of culture wars that are discussed in many places throughout this volume; the ongoing redesign of humans has, in fact, been going on for some time and is a quite different phenomenon (e.g., elements of medicine).

Accordingly, this chapter will try to do several things. I will begin with a discussion of the anthropogenic Earth, the context within which transhumanism as a cultural construct has arisen. Second, I will briefly touch on technological change, using both past examples and noting the truly transformative wave that towers above us, ready to crash down, with technology understood as a cultural, even an existential, force, not just things. Third, I will suggest the need to reconstruct our world. In this, I am not just suggesting that we are moving to a level of complexity and integration of human, natural, and engineered systems that we at present can at best barely glimpse through the fog of our outdated preconceptions and ideologies. That, I take to be a given. Rather, I am suggesting that, without a new and difficult ascension to a rationality suitable for a world in which "all that is solid melts into air" (in Karl Marx's words), we forfeit our

1 Much of this chapter is drawn from Allenby and Sarewitz (2011) and Allenby (2007a).

already tenuous hold on responsibility and on ethics. In this light, the current state of the discussion surrounding transhumanism is not encouraging.

The Anthropogenic Earth

We live in a world that is fundamentally different from anything that we have known in the past. In one sense, we have simply begun to perceive that which thousands of years of human history have created, although the Industrial Revolution undeniably accelerated the process (Thomas 1956; Turner et al. 1990). It is a world increasingly defined by the activities and products characteristic of one species, from automobiles to cities to the creation of vast new cyberspaces. It is a world where the critical dynamics of major Earth systems, be they atmospheric, oceanic, or biological, or for that matter cultural, economic, or technological, increasingly bear the imprint of the human (Allenby 2005). As the journal *Nature* put it in an editorial in 2003, "Welcome to the Anthropocene," roughly translated, the Age of the Human.

A few examples provide a glimpse of what we have already wrought. Perhaps most fundamentally, every planetary body has a characteristic radiation-emissions spectrum, which usually depends on the body's temperature. The Earth's spectrum, however, is not just a matter of reflections from clouds, emitted infrared radiation, and the like. Rather, it includes television and radio broadcasts and leakage from all sorts of technologies. Recall that picture of the Earth from space at night and the electric lights spread over North America, Europe, and Asia. In the Anthropocene, one of the most fundamental physical aspect of our planet, its radiation spectrum, carries our signature on it.

Another familiar example is the issue of global climate change, which vies with terrorism for existential catastrophe billing. Stand away from the Kyoto Protocol and the surrounding hysterics pro and con, however, and take a longer perspective. What that process represents, fitful and ad hoc as it is, is the dawning of a realization that, regardless of what the international environmental community accomplishes with the climate-change negotiating process, the human species will be engaged in a dialogue with climate, atmospheric chemistry and physics, and the carbon cycle so long as it exists at anywhere near current population numbers on the planet. Even if humans reduce – more likely, redistribute – some of the anthropogenic impacts on these complicated and interrelated systems, it is impossible to eliminate the growing human influence because these particular perturbations, and others as well, are all part of interconnected global systems and because a population of some seven billion humans, each seeking a better life, ensures that the overall human role in global systems will increase, absent some sort of population crash (Smil 1997). Indeed, although the tendency is to think of climate change as a problem to be solved, it is in fact a chronic condition of the anthropogenic Earth: it can be managed to some degree, but it cannot be solved (Allenby and Sarewitz 2011).

Yet another example comes from conservation biology. Among the currently most accepted "truths" is the idea that we are experiencing a "crisis in biodiversity" as human activity causes extinction levels to skyrocket. But some note that, even if the decrease in evolved biodiversity is as steep as alleged – something that the underlying data are surprisingly sketchy on, because we really do not even have a good idea of how many species there actually are – this may not be true given the rise of what scientists call "synthetic biology." Over the past decades, scientists and engineers have begun the project of understanding and designing new forms of life. These efforts, from genetics to agricultural science, have coalesced into a new field called "synthetic biology." Synthetic biology merges engineering with biology by, among other things, creating standard biological components that can be mixed and matched in organisms to provide desired functions. This allows researchers to treat biological pathways as if they were components or circuits and to create biological structures, including viruses, from scratch – not to mention extending beyond existing biological systems by, for example, creating life based on different genetic codes than those found in the wild (Ferber 2004; Check 2005). MIT, for example, has established a Registry of Standard Biological Parts ("BioBricks") that can be ordered and plugged into cells, just like electronic components, and holds an Intercollegiate Genetically Engineered Machine (iGEM) competition every year, where devices such as bacterial etch-a-sketches, photosensitive t-shirts, and bacterial photography systems, thermometers, and sensors are displayed. Somewhat controversially, a number of viruses have been assembled from scratch, including the viruses for polio and the 1918 flu epidemic. Other researchers have engineered the genes of *Escherichia coli* to incorporate a twenty-first amino acid, opening up an option space for design of biological organisms that has been unavailable to evolved biological systems for billions of years. Commercialization of these biotechnologies continues to accelerate, led by the introduction in agriculture of genetically modified organism (GMO) technology, which continues to accelerate in terms of acreage planted and new genetically engineered cultivars, despite strong European and environmentalist opposition. Reflecting the ongoing commoditization of life, figures for biotechnology patent filings in OECD countries continue to rise sharply.

At larger scale, the degree to which humans have over time created anthropogenic landscapes is somewhat disguised by people's strong cultural and psychological tendency to interpret landscapes with which they are unfamiliar, and which do not display the technological artifacts they are used to, as "pristine" and "natural," despite the fact that virtually all landscapes at this particular point in the evolution of our species are products of human intentionality. For example, even though arriving Europeans perceived the Amazon as "wild" and unaffected by the endogenous tribal cultures, research increasingly demonstrates that, in fact, large areas had been transformed through the construction of raised fields, large settlement mounds, earthen causeways, fish weirs, and large-scale soil enhancement for agricultural purposes; large human settlements existed in the Amazon well before Europeans arrived (Erickson 2000; Mann 2008). In the case of Hawaii, as with many previously inhabited landscapes "discovered" by Europeans, the human restructuring of Hawaiian ecosystems began well before Europeans reached the islands; it was the Europeans' Enlightenment romanticism that perceived that island, long modified by human action, as "natural" (Redman 1999). In fact, Europeans often labored under

> a widespread and important misconception [that] a natural landscape, untouched by human hands, exists; and that societies before European contact lived in a utopian paradise guided by an unselfish conservationist ethic. This European premise that an Eden-like nature existed was based largely on the belief that native peoples, particularly in the Americas, did not share in the biblical fall from grace. (Ibid., 12-13)

For example, Redman cites research that "suggests that the North American landscape at the time of Columbian contact was almost everywhere a humanized landscape and that the view of it as pristine was to a large extent an invention of nineteenth century romantic writers" (ibid., 196). In short, "wilderness" is not a characteristic of "natural" environments but a projection of a mental model arising from the Enlightenment romantic tradition (Abrams 1971), informed in particular by the emotionalism of the Rosseauean "noble savage."

In fact, at virtually all scales, few biological communities can be found that do not reflect human predation, management, or consumption. As Gallagher and Carpenter remarked in introducing a special issue of *Science* on human-dominated ecosystems, the concept of a pristine ecosystem, untouched by human activity, "is collapsing in the wake of scientists' realization that there are *no places left on Earth that don't fall under humanity's shadow*" (1997, 485; emphasis added). Initially trade and then transportation systems of various kinds have distributed invasive species around the world; as Kaiser notes, "The world's ecosystems will never revert to the pristine state they enjoyed before humans began to routinely crisscross the globe" (1999, 1836). Even those considered "natural" almost inevitably contain invasive species, frequently in dominant roles. Modern technological systems continue to increase the scale of these impacts: writing in *Science*, Palumbi notes that "[h]uman ecological impact has enormous evolutionary consequences ... and can greatly accelerate evolutionary change in the species around us. … [T]echnological impact has increased so markedly over the past few decades that humans may be the world's dominant evolutionary force" (2001, 1786).

It is important to understand that these technological advances in synthetic biology are not merely instrumental. Synthetic biology does not just reconfigure the biological sciences; the potential implications are far more profound. To begin with, biodiversity becomes a product of design choices and of industrial and political imperatives (security issues, for example), rather than evolutionary pressures. More broadly, the behavior and structure of biological systems increasingly become a function of human dynamics and systems, so that understanding biological systems increasingly requires an understanding of the relevant human systems. In short, biology increasingly becomes a cultural science. One important implication of this anthropogenic biology is that the contingency and lack of resilience that characterize human systems come to characterize biological systems. To take an obvious marketing example from conservation biology, in an arbitrary and profoundly cultural process some species are preserved because they are charismatic megafauna: pandas, tigers, or whales. Many, many others go extinct because they are only insects or plants or ugly or unknown; a few, like smallpox, because humans detest and fear them (with the important proviso that, in an age of biotech, national security and terrorism, extinction, at least for viruses and bacteria, is never forever).

These, then, are just examples of the anthropogenic – the human-made – Earth. It is important to understand that, although these are presented as separate examples, they are all coupled; indeed, this is a major source of the difficulty of dealing effectively with the issues they raise. Moreover, many of these systems are experiencing dramatic change as a result of accelerating human activity, especially since the Industrial Revolution. For example, if one normalizes economic activity to 100 in the year 1500, by 1990 global gross domestic product (GDP), a measure of economic activity, had exploded to over 11,600, while even per capita GDP grew from 100 to 942 over that period (McNeill 2000). Similarly, about ten million metric tons of coal were used annually in 1800; by 1900, this had grown to 1,000 MMT, and by 1990, less than a hundred years later, to 5,000 MMT. For petroleum, the equivalent numbers are 0 MMT in 1800, 20 MMT in 1900, and 3,000 MMT in 1990 (ibid.). Such growth across basic infrastructure technologies necessarily creates the large, integrated, human/natural/built systems that characterize the anthropogenic Earth (Grubler 1998; Allenby 2007b). But it is not just that our technologies construct a human Earth; it is far more complicated. For technologies are more powerful than we generally recognize, and those technologies are now not just ever-more powerful means to integrate previously natural systems into human systems but also to make the human itself a design space. Accordingly, we now turn to a brief discussion of technology.

Technology and Creation

Any meaningful discussion of technology in the Anthropocene must begin by making one critical point: technology is an integrated cultural process, not a collection of things (Bijker et al. 1997). This may be best illustrated by considering a technology system that is now taken for granted: the railroad. Today, it may be mundane; in the middle 1800s as it began its rapid expansion phase, the railroad was the most impressive piece of machinery most people ever saw. And it was more than just a huge engine and tracks across the continents: it was a sociocultural juggernaut. Among the changes the railroads brought in their wake were the following:

1. Operating a railroad required a uniform, precise system of time and, thus, was a powerful forcing function behind the coevolution of "industrial time" and its associated culture (Grubler 1998; Schivelbusch 1987);
2. Railroads also were a forcing function for, and coevolved with, national-scale communications systems (telegraph) (Schivelbusch 1987);
3. The scale and operational complexity of railroad firms was a forcing function for modern managerial capitalism (modern accounting, planning, and administration systems) (Rosenberg and Birdzell 1986; Freeman and Louca 2001);
4. Railroad firms were a major factor behind the development of modern capital and financial markets (railroad construction was the single most important stimulus to industrial growth in Western Europe by the 1840s) (Freeman and Louca 2001);
5. Railroads in the United States became a potent symbol of national power, and, more subtly, instantiated and validated the American integration of religion, morality, and technology (Marx 1964; Nye 1994);
6. Railroads played a major role in transforming landscapes at all scales: Chicago existed and structured the Midwest economically and environmentally because of railroads (Cronon 1991);
7. Like most major technological systems, railroads fundamentally changed American economic and power structures, restructuring the economy from local/regional business concentrations to trusts by creating the transportation infrastructure necessary to achieve scale economies of national markets (Marx 1964; Nye 1994);
8. Railroads played a major role in changing the underlying teleology of American culture from Jeffersonian agrarianism, an Edenic teleology, to a technology-driven New Jerusalem, a cultural schism that replays itself today in the continuing environmentalist challenge to technology (Nye 2003).

And railroads are only one example of what economic historians call "technology clusters" that power so-called long waves in economic and social history (Rosenberg and Birdzell 1986). Railroads and steam technology powered a wave from about 1840 to 1890; steel, heavy engineering. and electricity from about 1890 to 1930; the automobile, petroleum, and aircraft from about 1930 to 1990; the information cluster with its computerization of the economy from about 1990 to the present (Freeman and Louca 2001). While the dates are somewhat imprecise, the general idea of clusters of technology – which, it cannot be emphasized enough, always carry with them institutional, organizational, economic, cultural, and political changes – is a useful one. Thus, specialized professional managerial systems and associated "Taylorism" industrial-efficiency techniques characterized the heavy industry cluster, while a far more networked, flexible structure began to evolve during the information cluster. The automobile cluster not only reified mass production as the economic basis of modernity but created the idea of mass credit (after all, major capital purchases required some sort of credit system because the number of people who could pay cash up front for cars and other major purchases was too limited to support a mass market – it was to address this same dilemma that Sears developed the "lay-away" plan, which had the same practical effect).

In all these cases, it is not that the technology, arising out of nowhere, was the "cause" of the associated cultural, economic, technological, and institutional changes. Such "technological determinism," like other determinisms, dramatically and misleadingly oversimplifies the way such complex systems work. Rather, the technologies participated in a process of coevolution: railroads needed standard time systems, telegraphs, white-collar differentiation of labor, and efficient capital markets to operate and, in turn, encouraged the growth of those factors, which, in their turn, needed to be acceptable within the social and institutional contexts of the time. But using the technologies as an entry point to these self-referential and integrated constellations of institutional, social, and economic factors is useful for several reasons. Most importantly, many of the other dimensions are represented by particular disciplines: social institutions are studied by sociologists, economic systems are studied by economists, and political systems are studied by political scientists. Technology systems, however, are not studied by any specific discipline: engineers study artifacts and specific designs, and economists know that technology is there; but there is no discipline of technology systems per se. Thus, of all the aspects of the current discussion, technology systems are the most likely to be underestimated.

This is particularly unfortunate given the transformational power of technology systems, as the railroad example makes crystal clear. First, a technology of any significance will destabilize existing institutions, market arrangements, and power relationships and, thus, to some degree, cultural assumptions. Accordingly, it will be opposed by many (Nye 1994, 2003). Second, projecting the effects of technology systems before they are actually adopted is not just hard but, given the complexity of the systems, probably impossible. Thus, for example, the time structure that we moderns take for granted was not the time structure of prerailroad American agrarian society; it is a product of our technology. This raises a more subtle but equally important point: we are able to perceive our world and create our cultural constructs only through the lens that our technology provides (Allenby 2005).

The Five Horsemen

If the history of technological evolution is a warning, it is an inadequate one for the wave bearing down on us. Technological change, as suggested by the example of the railroads, is always potent, but now we have not just one or two enabling technologies undergoing rapid evolution, we have five: nanotechnology, biotechnology, robotics, information and communication technology, and applied cognitive science (NBRICT) (Garreau 2004; Kurzweil 2005). These technologies in some ways are the logical end of the chapter of human history that began with the Greeks. Nanotechnology extends human will and design to the atomic level and instantiates human domination over the material world (albeit at the high cost in energy that manipulating matter at that scale entails). As for biotechnology, J. R. McNeill, an environmental historian, notes that

> By the twentieth century, our numbers, our high-energy technologies, and our refined division of labor with its exchange economy made us capable of total transformation of any and all ecosystems. ... In the twentieth century we became what most cultures long imagined us to be: lords of the biosphere. (2000, 193-94)

ICT gives us the ability to create virtual worlds at will and facilitates a migration of functionality to information rather than physical structures. Thus, money used to be coins and paper bills, themselves mere symbols of value, but now even that physical premise is gone. Money is electrons somewhere in cyberspace, and financial instruments have become so mathematical that no one can figure out anymore which shell the risk is hidden under (Allenby 2012). Meaning in an information dense world has become contingent on belief, reinforced worldviews, and noise level, which is why Fox News and blogs proliferate and, to a large degree, can ring-fence their readership into self-reinforcing islands of belief that become strongly resistant to factual challenge.

Consider for a brief moment some of the implications of the NBRIC wave in just one area, human biology and cognition, as an example of some of the possibilities. At one extreme, some predict the achievement of "functional human immortality" within fifty years, either as a result of continuing advances in biotechnology, or as information and communication technology (ICT) and computational power enable downloading of human consciousness into information networks (Kurzweil 2005; De Grey and Rae 2007). This latter should not, however, be confused with the growing power of human/Internet cognitive networks, such as the off-loading of substantial memory function to search engines. Such developments, which are already well underway, arguably give rise to such a different form of extended cognition that it might be considered the first varietal of posthuman humanity. One may, of course, argue over what, exactly, constitutes a "human varietal," but that such developments mark significant changes in cognitive capability across the system as a whole, and increasingly differentiate populations with access to, and adept with, such human/technology networks from those that lack such capabilities, is clear.

Predictions of "functional human immortality" are viewed by most experts as highly unlikely, but there is a growing consensus that substantial extensions of average life spans, with a high quality of life, are achievable in the next few decades. For example, the IEEE *Spectrum*, a mainstream technical journal, ran a series of articles in 2004 on engineering and aging, which concluded that using "engineered negligible senescence" to control aging will allow average ages of well over 100 within a few decades. What is interesting, of course, is that, even though the scientists and technologists are perceiving such possibilities as age extension as increasingly probable, those in other areas of science – and in policy and in the environmental and sustainability communities – remain unaware of these possibilities, despite their obviously challenging implications (for pension and old-age systems and material and energy consumption patterns, for example).

Equally challenging from a technological perspective, as opposed to the cultural construct of transhumanism, is that it is becoming apparent that not just the Earth but the human is in the process of becoming a human-design project and that substantial changes in what it means to be human are probably inevitable (although specifics are unpredictable). N. Katherine Hayles, for example, in her aptly named book *How We Became Posthuman* (1999) traces the evolution of the posthuman through the concepts of homeostasis, then reflexivity, then, finally, virtuality. While Hayles is cautious about the implications of this ongoing and accelerating process, some foresee enormous potential: Roco and Bainbridge in an NSF report titled *Converging Technologies for Improving Human Performance*, for example, conclude, "With proper attention to ethical issues and societal needs, converging technologies could achieve a tremendous improvement in human abilities, societal outcomes, the nations's productivity, and the quality of life" (2003, ix).They continue:

> Examples of payoffs may include improving work efficiency and learning, enhancing individual sensory and cognitive capabilities, revolutionary changes in healthcare, improving both individual and group creativity, highly effective communication techniques including brain-to-

> brain interaction, perfecting human – machine interfaces including neuromorphic engineering, sustainable and "intelligent" environments including neuro-ergonomics, enhancing human capabilities for defense purposes, reaching sustainable development using NBIC tools, and ameliorating the physical and cognitive decline that is common to the aging mind. (Ibid.)

Effects of technological convergence on the human are only one small area of research and speculation; similar suites of possible scenarios are being developed in many other areas. It is obviously premature to regard most of these predictions as anything more than possible outcomes. Indeed, much of the thinking of technological futures is marked by a strong tendency to focus on a particular aspect of a technology or its implementation, implicitly holding other social, technological, or environmental systems fixed. This almost automatically assures that the scenarios are implausible because technological change, especially at this fundamental level and across virtually the entire technology salient, is integrated with most other human systems; and under such conditions, they too will be evolving and contingent. Additionally, except for the easy cases where particular applications of these core technologies are already in the process of being commercialized, it is very difficult to determine how probable even the most outré scenarios might be. The line between science fiction and tomorrow's headlines has seldom been quite so blurred, in part because technologies frequently tend to follow cultural precedents, which are often established in science fiction. Thus, for example, the structure of virtual realities shows a strong resemblance to the work of writers such as William Gibson and Neal Stephenson; accordingly, not only is it hard to tell the difference between fiction and soon-to-be fact, but the latter is constructed by the former.

This discussion illustrates four critical points regarding technology and the human. Most importantly, perhaps, technological change is not an isolated event. Rather, it represents movements toward new, locally stable, Earth-systems states (Allenby 2007a). These states integrate natural, environmental, cultural, theological, institutional, financial, managerial, technological, built and human dimensions, and even construct our sense of time. Technologies do not define these integrated Earth-system states, except by convenience, but technological evolution can destabilize existing clusters and create conditions leading to the evolution of new ones. These general characteristics of technological evolution are more foundational when the system being engineered, directly or indirectly, is the human (direct human engineering might be, for example, the use of genetic engineering to address conditions such as retinitis pigmentosa, a retinal disease; indirect human engineering might be, for example, the evolution of Google™ as a substitute and enhancement for internal-memory function).

Moreover, technology is the means by which humans have expressed their will to power. This is not just an academic observation. Cultures that develop technology and, importantly, create frameworks within which it can react upon itself and so accelerate its own evolution gain cognitive power over competitors. Because technologies create such powerful comparative advantages between cultures, those cultures that attempt to block technology will, all things beng equal, eventually be dominated by those that embrace it. Thus, it is likely that technological evolution will be difficult, if not impossible, to stop, as some argue. Whether and how it can be moderated in the age of global elites becomes an important research question.

Third, when, as today, the rate of technological change is already rapid and, in fact, accelerating dramatically, it has the effect of stretching the bimodal distribution between those who constitute the global elite and who, primarily through education and culture, are able to prosper under such conditions and those who are left behind. The latter have a strong tendency to seek stability in outmoded ideologies and fundamentalist movements. These movements are desperate responses to a world that, for such individuals, has become irrational, and, as it destabilizes patterns of belief and behavior, they invest these responses with meaning, profoundly challenging and frequently evil. Such movements need not be religious in nature; some environmentalist and political movements are superficially secular but represent the same revolt against change and complexity (e.g., the Tea Party movement in the U.S. or some of the anti-GMO campaigns in Europe).

Finally, although it is hard to judge events that are still unfolding, there nonetheless is reasonable support for the conclusion that current technological evolution is unprecedented. Previous technology clusters revolved around one or perhaps two evolving technologies – say, rails and steam or automobiles and petroleum. The constellation of nanotechnology, biotechnology, robotics, ICT, and cognitive science, however, marks a culmination of sorts of traditional technological evolution, for, among other things, it extends control of materials to the atomic scale and lays the groundwork for the complete integration of the human and the technological. The Earth, biology, and indeed even the human itself become design spaces and in doing so, render contingent virtually all of what has heretofore been understood to be fixed.

The Undermining of the Enlightenment

To summarize where we are at this point: the integrated cluster of technology that is rapidly beginning to redefine our world – NBRIC – is both providing the scientific and technological basis for dramatically accelerating physical, psychological, and social changes to the human, while at the same time rendering obsolete the mental models and cultural constructs through which we attempt to understand that process – most importantly including transhumanism itself.

In particular, we face radically increasing complexity of at least four different kinds: (a) static complexity (increasing numbers of components, stakeholders, interactions among different infrastructure, and linkages among them, for example); (b) dynamic complexity (as these factors interact in new and unanticipated ways, especially given the fundamentally changing nature of ICT systems); (c) "wicked" complexity (arising from the need to engineer and manage integrated human/natural/built systems increasingly displaying the reflexivity and intentionality of human systems and institutions); and (d) scale, as we realize we must begin to design, engineer, and manage integrated human/natural/built Earth systems at not just national but regional and global scales (Allenby 2007b; Allenby and Sarewitz 2011). This complexity has already had profound institutional implications in our era: Marxism in the Soviet Union collapsed not from external conquest but rather because the centralized economic model adopted by large Marxist societies simply became incapable of managing the complexity inherent in a modern industrial economy. More personally for many of us, the complexity in which we are now all embedded is eroding the unitary sense of self that was one of the principle gifts of the Enlightenment: not only are we fragmenting our memory across various Internet systems, but as we build avatars that represent different aspects of our personalities to play in different virtual realities, we create a multidimensional self that would have been simply impossible a hundred years ago in a small-town environment. Thus does the complexity that makes the human a design space at the same time invalidate the framework that we have previously associated with the human. The mental model of the human expressed in concepts such as the Great Chain of Being and the Enlightenment focus on the individual has not been displaced by an alternative formulation; rather it has been rendered obsolete by accelerating complexity that such concepts helped to create but are now unable to frame.

An important element of this complexity is that it confirms an unavoidable relationship between observer, frame of reference, and derivation of partial and contingent truth from underlying complex systems. Consider a simple example. If I am interested in the rates of crime in Phoenix, I am also implicitly defining the urban system by its political boundaries. If, on the other hand, I am interested in water and Phoenix, I am implicitly defining the system as including the Colorado River basin, not to mention American water law, patterns of tourism that make golf courses popular in Scottsdale, and xeriscaping initiatives. Yet in both cases, the relevant marker is "Phoenix." What is happening, simply, is that my query to the system calls forth from an underlying complex noumenal world a particular network that is responsive to my query (in Kantian terms, the query acts to define an appropriate phenomenal structure from a complex pattern of "things in themselves" that is not directly accessible). In short, complex urban systems can be thought of as interconnected, evolving networks of networks, covering not just the familiar subjects of urban engineering – built environments and infrastructure – but less physical ones such as technology states, lifestyles, cultural constructs, economic evolution, and the like. Thus, while it is true that Chicago is a collection of buildings, roads, stores, and so forth, it is also true that Chicago is the mechanism by which much of the American Midwest was commodified (Cronon 1991). The networks that are of interest in a particular situation will generally be determined not by the system being evaluated but by the particular questions being asked about it. There is a similarity to quantum mechanics here: what you perceive when you look at the system is determined by the purpose for which you are observing it. The system itself always remains more complex than you are able to capture at any one time. And the important corollary is that a complex system can only be defined in terms of the reasons for which a definition is desired. The query identifies the particular networks of the system that are relevant, and they, in turn, define the boundaries of the system for the purpose of the inquiry.

This reflexivity complicates any discussion of a complex system, of course, and reduces the value of standardized or ideological approaches. Equally important, these integrated systems are completely built by humans, but their dynamics and evolutionary paths are not planned, nor determined, by humans, and their effects ripple broadly across many human, natural, and built systems at many scales. They are thus excellent examples of systems that, like the Internet, are completely anthropogenic but are not understandable or transparent. When we design the human, to paraphrase Marx, humans will make themselves, but they will not make themselves just as they please, for our understanding and the complex nature of reality are not congruent but coupled weakly through our queries to the latter.

The accelerating evolution of technology systems, especially ICT, combined with the postmodern fragmenting of time, space, and culture, dramatically decreases the stability of all cultural constructs (Allenby 2006). In the current era, this has two profound effects: it renders not just the social and cultural landscapes that we look out on more unstable, but it renders that which looks out – the self and our individuality – more contingent as well. The dramatic increase of fundamentalism across most belief systems and in most societies reflects, in part, an effort to create a stable ground; it is an effort that will fail, at least for the elite for whom a form of transhumanism is already a reality. Marx's prediction – or curse, depending on your viewpoint – comes true: all that is solid melts into air.

An important dimension of transhumanism as a cultural construct is the implication, often expressed by those attempting to restrict humanenhancement technologies, that it represents some sort of victory of technology over the human, as if each were a separate domain. The Enlightenment romantics had their Frankenstein model, and it remains powerful today (as in Greenpeace's Frankenfood PR campaign). If history is any guide, this is at best a temporary opposition. Thus, the dialectic process does not end with technology opposing the human, not that the human and the technological will clash, and one will emerge victorious; rather, what is already happening is that the two are merging and continue to drive each other's evolution, and consequent integration, in an ongoing dialectic. This does not mean profound changes will not occur, especially in older concepts of what constitutes "the human." Nor does it mean that differing human varietals representing idiosyncratic weightings of different technologies with different human subpopulations will not evolve – as, indeed, the "digital natives" that are comfortably embedded in their ICT networks may already be. But one only need look at the popularity of cosmetic plastic surgery or the speed with which social-network technologies have been adapted to understand that integration of technology is not just ongoing but far more the rule than the exception.

It is important to note that one important implication of this discussion is that what we are seeing now is not fundamentally new, in that humans have always been integrating with their technologies. Thus, in 2003, the philosopher Andy Clark published *Natural-Born Cyborgs*, in which he argued that humans had always been cyborgs. In fact, he and others claim that our major competitive advantage as a species lies in our brain's unique and innate ability to couple to external social, economic, information, and technological systems in such a way as to evolve distributed cognitive networks. Clark is one of a growing number of scholars arguing that, looking at transhuman as the integration of technology and the human, it is not that we will become transhuman but that we already are. To this, one must add the important observation that rate of change of fundamental systems is an important independent variable and that what differentiates the current era from earlier periods is arguably the speed at which new technologies become integrated with the human, in a context of much greater complexity and reflexivity. Thus, the important characteristic of the modern age is not that integration occurs but that it is occurring at rates that create complexity, contingency, and unpredictability to which many individuals, and virtually all institutions and societies, are unable to adapt. A difference in degree, in other words, has grown to be a difference in kind.

Many groups, from deep greens (ideological environmentalists) to Marxists to religious conservatives opposing modernity, cling to ideologies and older worldviews implying necessary and foundational conflict between the human and technology, in the shape of the transhuman, for obvious reasons. It engages their base; it turns complex questions of fact into simplistic black-and-white scenarios; and, in many cases, it both reflects and validates their partial or even complete rejection of modernity. But ideological approaches of all kinds are particularly problematic at the dawn of the anthropogenic world, which as we have seen is characterized by exceedingly rapid and profound change in fundamental relationships and systems, involving natural, built, and human systems of extraordinary static and dynamic complexity. In such a context, there are four aspects of ideology that render it especially dysfunctional. First, any ideology is necessarily a simplification of reality; in fact, that is usually an important part of its mass appeal. Second, the elements and structure of this simplification necessarily lie in the past, not the future, and thus embed assumptions and implications that are necessarily increasingly anachronistic in a period of rapid and discontinuous change. Third, ideology creates an "ends justify the means" mentality; almost by definition the power of the Idea trumps the messy and contingent real world (Conquest 2000). Thus, it is characteristic of many ideologies that they posit a vision of utopia, the achievement of which is worth the sacrifices, usually imposed by the ideological group on othes – think of Marxism or of the poverty in this country because of our powerful antitax ideology or the tens of thousands of people who have died from malaria in developing countries because environmentalists blocked access to DDT. Regarding potential changes to the human, ideology can lead some opponents to glorify suffering and denigrate modern medicine – almost always imposing the costs of their beliefs on other, conveniently impersonalized, groups. Finally, as part of the elevation of the Idea over the real, ideology also cuts off information transfer and dialogue and is profoundly antidemocratic, anti-intellectual, and antirational (although, ironically, ideologies are creatures of the intelligentsia). It is not, then, just that ideologies are generally bad, although many of them seem to be in application, as any familiarity with the twentieth century would confirm (Conquest 2000); rather, it is that ideologies are *especially* bad in a period of rapid, discontinuous, and fundamental change at a global, multicultural scale. Because ideologies, with a quasi-rational and thus Enlightenment mien, have over time become a convenient way of simplifying a complex environment, their failure not just in practice but in principle is a further weakening of the original Enlightenment project.

The railroad example warns that foundational institutional and even cultural shifts are likely with sufficiently potent technological systems. In the case of NBRIC, for example, one might hypothesize that perhaps the changes we are currently beginning to experience mark, in fact, the end of the great Enlightenment project of radical democratic power. To begin with, it is clear that the rates of change we are now experiencing have already created a fundamentalist backlash that is increasingly potent around the world. This is occurring in virtually all major religions, as well as those belief systems – environmentalism, sustainability – that for many people, especially in secular societies, now begin to serve theological purposes. This is not random opposition to modernity but generated by the fact that, as rates of technological change accelerate, increasing numbers of people in every society are disenfranchised. They are incapable of keeping pace with continuing change, unable to integrate into the information webs that increasingly define human cognition, and aghast at the changes in lifestyle, traditional natural systems, income distribution, relative power relationships, and changes in sexual and family roles and structures that have resulted. And, importantly, these groups have not yet understood the degree to which their fundamental values are rendered contingent by that self-same progress. Thus, accelerating technological change can only increase opposition to itself, yet it is an important component of technological dominance. For those for whom Enlightenment representative democracy is an important value, then, technological evolution, especially as it affects the human, creates a difficult conundrum, for the more it succeeds, the more it creates an activist opposition that hobbles it in democratic cultures, giving the advantage to cultures where the elite, who benefit from technological evolution generally and advanced human enhancements specifically, are able to exercise control. Thus, what has been a world marked by intranational patterns of inequality may increasingly become a world where a global elite skilled in navigating complex and information-dense environments dominates, and more and more others sink into a global proletariat.

The political implications of the human as design do not just suggest the undermining of democratic structures as authoritarian societies become increasingly competent because of greater willingness to support technological change regardless of the cost. There is an obvious and dangerous destabilizing effect associated with foundational technological changes in general, and those affecting the human in particular. Most importantly, perhaps, the evolution of human technological competency such that virtually the entire material world (nanotechnology), including the biological world (biotechnology), is potentially subject to human design clearly challenges cultural assumptions about appropriate boundaries between the sacred and the human. This is particularly true for those for whom "nature" has become the repository of the Sacred, a reflection of the romantic project to protect God from science by shifting the Sacred to the wilderness. This is, indeed, an important foundational belief for many environmentalists, ranging from English royalty who perceive biotechnology as blasphemous because it is "playing God," to environmental writers such as McKibben, who implicitly frames technological and cultural evolution in Nitzschean terms when he first places God in "nature" and then bemoans the human impacts on the latter:

> Wild nature, then, has been a way to recognize God [of the Christian tradition] and to talk about who He is. How could it be otherwise? What else is, or was, beyond human reach? In what other sphere could a deity operate freely? (1989, 77)

More specifically, technological evolution, by making the human contingent (indeed, a reflexive design space, as humans and their institutions begin designing humans at the molecular to the cognitive network scale), is the final rejection of the roles assigned to deity, human, and beast in many religious traditions (as in the Christian Great Chain of Being). This does not, in itself, imply a necessary theological conflict, for rebalancing theological interpretation and scientific advance has in some ways been the critical discourse of the last several centuries, and authorities dating back to St. Augustine offer the applicable guidance (the necessarily unitary truth of science and theology under an omniscient God). Consider, for example, Pope John Paul II's comments in the encyclical letter *Fides et ratio*:

> Faith and reason are like two wings on which the human spirit rises to the contemplation of truth. … [T]he two modes of knowledge lead to truth in all its fullness. The unity of truth is a fundamental premise of human reasoning, as the principle of non-contradiction makes clear. … Both the light of reason and the light of faith come from God … hence there can be no contradiction between them. … It is an illusion to think that faith, tied to weak reasoning, might be more penetrating; on the contrary, faith then runs the grave risk of withering into myth or superstition. (1998, introduction and ¶¶ 34, 43, 48)

It can be argued, therefore, that current technologically driven changes to the human are only another step in redistributing responsibility between categories. But this is a theological argument, and the most active conflicts in religion today are not theological but social and more specifically class, as those who are increasingly powerless in a technological, information-dense (and, hence, free-market) environment, whether because of lack of education or cultural weaknesses in such a competition, strike back through fundamentalism. As these groups begin to understand that those aspects of the human they consider sacred are already being changed by human intent and design and that technological evolution generally and human enhancement specifically are strongly correlated with cultural and economic power, the reaction that has started will intensify, perhaps dramatically. It bears remembering that the invention of printing enabled the spread of literacy and democratization of the Bible, and thence was the technological foundation required for the Reformation – and the result was 450 years of religious conflict across all of Europe.

Personal Authenticity and the Reinvention of the Enlightenment

If my musings are correct, then, the cultural construct of transhumanism; the physical, psychological, and social changes to the human; and the broader technological wave of which these are indicators constitute a period of unprecedented and fundamental physical, emotional, psychological, and cultural change. What it means to be human is in play, in ways that it has never been before – and, importantly, in ways that undermine most of the mental models, cultural constructs, and institutional systems we have created to structure our relationships with our Selves, our institutions, our politics, and our conceptualization of our role in the universe and relationship to our deities. We and our world are contingent in a way that, despite the massive changes we have experienced in past waves of technology, we have never been before. Clearly, we will need to reconstruct our world on the run, as it were, and a necessary part of that project will be to reconstruct ourselves as contingent but grounded beings. To that challenge, then, let us turn.

Begin by observing that complexity and radical contingency have undermined the Enlightenment as it is now constructed and as it now underpins global culture. In some ways, this is desirable, as it opens new option spaces for continued evolution of cultures, the species, and individuals. Moreover, this is only an extension of the dynamic that has always characterized the Enlightenment and, arguably, must characterize any cultural system that successfully evolves. Thus, the Enlightenment as global culture has succeeded, ironically, because it uniquely carries within it the seeds of its own negation as a uniquely "true" or "valid" culture. Indeed, the strongest critics of the Enlightenment have been internal, from Jean-Jacques Rousseau (whose criticism has become internalized to much of the environmental discourse) to Karl Marx to the postmodernists of all stripes. Thus, thinkers from Richard Rorty to Theodor Adorno have emphasized two paradoxical observations:

1. Only a structure which, like the European Enlightenment, contained its own critique and negation within itself could possibly become the basis for a globalized cultural framework in a multicultural world; and
2. The Enlightenment framework succeeds only to the extent it continues to negate itself as a unique source of "truth." In these cases, the Enlightenment tradition has not only been the source of the negation but has itself been transformed, transcended, and made more universal and encompassing by the dialectic generated by the negation. This dialectical process, perhaps most closely associated with Marx and G.W.F. Hegel, is itself an important and self-conscious facet of the Enlightenment; in fact, much romantic thought, with the important exception of Rousseau, saw the dialectic as the process by which human progress toward a reintegrated high civilization (in religious terms, recovery from the Fall, which was itself seen as introduced by intellectualization) occurred.

As the original Enlightenment evolved through modernity, the relatively integral worldview it entailed shattered against the increasing complexity of the anthropogenic systems that it enabled. This is not a choice; this is our current reality.

Accordingly, we must transcend – not deny or oversimplify, but internalize and transcend – that complexity anew. The Enlightenment as explicit framing has been transcended yet again by the Enlightenment as process. And, as the framing of transhumanism demonstrates, perhaps the lynchpin at issue in the transhumanism debates and the technological evolution that continues even as we argue is the individual. Thus, it is fitting that I end with observations on the individual, for it is there that the first and most difficult demands of this age of radical change fall. Current comfortable whimsies, simplifications, and romantic ideologies fail in the face of a complexity that they have contributed to but are unable to comprehend. Moreover, each individual is, as a matter of existence, defined in contingent and idiosyncratic terms, inherently limited in perceptual capabilities and characterized by imperfect rationality. Nonetheless, we have created this world together and have reached the stage where we must now demand a reconstruction of personal authenticity. Let me then close by attempting to identify at least some characteristics associated with the authenticity that the rise of the human as design space, and the current state of the anthropogenic Earth, calls forth:

1. Following the existentialist formulation (and, for that matter, going back to Socrates's injunction to "know thyself"), an authenticity necessary for our times will require as a first element a recognition and acceptance of the world as it is, not as various ideologies would wish it to be.
2. This, in turn, implies acceptance of the human condition, in that the anthropogenic Earth requires each person to accept the validity of his or her condition and cognitive networks for him- or herself, while simultaneously recognizing them as contingent and stochastic in a world characterized by mutually exclusive but equally valid ontologies.
3. It also requires acceptance of the epistemological and existential implications of complex adaptive systems, in that any perceptual or cognitive network, or understanding of a complex system, is created by the query posed to the system and thus embodies unavoidable reflexivity between the system and the cognitive network and implies the contingency and incompleteness of any particular perspective on a complex adaptive system.
4. Given proposition 3, authenticity demands that we must have the integrity to create appropriate queries, since they will structure the cognitive networks within which we operate. Substituting wistful fantasies for honest query and thus construction of our local realities, or game-playing the query process to create ideologically predetermined local realities, must be rejected as profoundly inauthentic.
5. Authenticity requires that we accept the condition that meaning, truth, and values do not arise from first principles but are functions of network state and, thus, are contingent and continually regenerated in a reflexive dialogue

between cognitive systems posing queries to, and thus generating configurations of, external complex adaptive systems.

6. Following propositions 4 and 5, authenticity requires accepting as the human condition the challenge that, which you most believe, you must most distrust. Meaning, and truth arise from the dialectical process of their continued rejection. By the time you are comfortable with your understanding, you are to that same degree inauthentic.
7. Authenticity requires accepting rationality as partial and constructed, an interplay between different and contingent ontologies and partial structures of underlying complex adaptive systems, congealed intentionality and cognition (one way of defining technology and technological artifacts), and institutional and network dynamics. A similar stance must be taken toward institutions or, indeed, any cognitive network. In doing so, however, the mistake of slipping into a solipsistic relativism must be avoided, for that goes too far and becomes its own form of inauthenticity.
8. As a reflection of the increasing human role in, and responsibility for, integrated human/built/natural Earth systems, authenticity requires thoughtful rejection of ideologies and frameworks characteristic of the first Enlightenment and active movement toward reinvention of the Enlightenment for a profoundly multicultural, and much more complex, world: "thoughtful," for out of the first Enlightenment must be created a second that embodies the best elements of the first while enabling responses to new conditions, but there must also be rejection of those elements that now constitute cultural or temporal imperialism or are too simplistic for the systems that characterize the Anthropocene.
9. Finally, authenticity requires understanding that the individual is a contingent framework that has worked well in the past but is increasingly dysfunctional in a complex world characterized by cognitive networks extending across technological, biological, and human systems, and the evolution of human variants, already well underway. Thus, authenticity demands acceptance of cognition as increasingly involving production of emergent systems characteristics at levels higher than the individual.
10. This authenticity does not reject theology but redistributes domains between the theological and the human in ways that culturally may be very difficult for many individuals to accept. The strength to accept such shifts, while at the same time not succumbing to mere relativism, is an important element of the authenticity required.

Conclusion

With knowledge of the anthropogenic Earth and the human as explicit design space comes an existential crisis as the honest perception demanded by authenticity reveals a chaotic, unpredictable, highly problematic planet in the throes of anthropogenic change, with a complexity that neither existing intellectual tools nor perhaps language itself is adequate to address. Each individual is profoundly ignorant and strives hard to remain ignorant even of his or her ignorance; naiveté and willful perceptual and intellectual blindness become comfortable characteristics of discourse. The result is a fleeing into ideology, random myths, and stories, the creation of mental models that simplify reality into manageable fantasy, and reduce perception until it no longer threatens. This is understandable, but it is cowardice; it is bad faith; it is profoundly inauthentic. It is a flight from freedom, from responsibility, from integrity. As Jean-Paul Sartre said in the context of the individual, "Man is condemned to be free." And this is a far more daunting challenge in the context of an anthropogenic world that, having created, we now want to pretend not to see. For now this freedom, from whence rises moral obligation, is neither comfortable nor, sometimes, even bearable. But it is the freedom demanded by the historical moment, and it is nondelegable.

> He, only, merits freedom and existence
> Who wins them every day anew.
> J. W. Goethe, *Faust* [1833]

References

Abrams, Meyer H. 1971. *Natural Supernaturalism: Tradition and Revolution in Romantic Literature.* New York: W.W. Norton & Company.

Allenby, Braden R. 2005. *Reconstructing Earth.* Washington, DC: Island Press.

–. 2006. The *real* death of environmentalism. *Environmental Quality Management* 16 (1): 1-10.

–. 2007a. From Human to Transhuman: Technology and the Reconstruction of the World. Templeton Research lecture, Arizona State University, Tempe, Arizona, October 22.

–. 2007b. Earth systems engineering and management: A manifesto. *Environmental Science & Technology* 41 (23): 7960-66.

–. 2012. *The Theory and Practice of Sustainable Engineering.* Upper Saddle River, NJ: Pearson/Prentice-Hall.

Allenby, Brad R., and Daniel Sarewitz. 2011. *The Techno-Human Condition.* Cambridge, MA: MIT Press.

Bijker, Wiebe E., Thomas P. Hughes, and Trevor Pinch, eds. 1997. *The Social Construction of Technological Systems*. Cambridge, MA: MIT Press.

Check, Erika. 2005. Designs on life. *Nature* 438: 417-18.

Clark, Andy. 2003. *Natural-Born Cyborgs: Minds, Technologies, and the Future of Human Intelligence*. Oxford: Oxford University Press.

Conquest, Robert. 2000. *Reflections on a Ravaged Century*. New York: W.W. Norton & Company.

Cronon, William. 1991. *Nature's Metropolis: Chicago and the Great West*. New York: W. W. Norton and Company.

De Grey, Aubrey, and Michael Rae. 2007. *Ending Aging: The Rejuvenation Breakthroughs That Could Reverse Human Aging in Our Lifetime*. New York: St. Martin's Press.

Editorial. 2003. Welcome to the anthropocene. *Nature* 424: 709.

Erickson, Clark L. 2000. An artificial landscape-scale fishery in the Bolivian Amazon. *Nature* 408: 190-93.

Ferber, Dan. 2004. Microbes made to order. *Science* 303: 158-61.

Freeman, Chris, and Francisco Louca. 2001. *As Time Goes By: From the Industrial Revolutions to the Information Revolution*. Oxford: Oxford University Press.

Gallagher, Richard, and Betsy Carpenter. 1997. Human-dominated ecosystems: Introduction. *Science* 277: 485.

Garreau, Joel. 2004. *Radical Evolution*. New York: Doubleday.

Grubler, Arnulf. 1998. *Technology and Global Change*. Cambridge: Cambridge University Press.

Hayles, N. Katherine. 1999. *How We Became Posthuman*. Chicago: University of Chicago Press.

IEEE *Spectrum*. 2004. Engineering and aging. *Spectrum* 41 (9): 10, 31-35.

Kaiser, Jocelyn. 1999. Stemming the tide of invading species. *Science* 285: 1836-41.

Kurzweil, Ray. 2005. *The Singularity Is Near*. New York: Viking.

Mann, Charles C. 2008. Ancient earthmovers of the Amazon. *Science* 321: 1148-52.

Marx, Leo. 1964. *The Machine in the Garden: Technology and the Pastoral Ideal in America*. Oxford: Oxford University Press.

McKibben, William. 1989. *The End of Nature*. New York: Random House.

McNeill, John. R. 2000. *Something New under the Sun*. New York: W.W. Norton & Co.

Nye, David E. 1994. *American Technological Sublime*. Cambridge, MA: MIT Press.

–. 2003. *America as Second Creation: Technology and Narratives of New Beginning*. Cambridge, MA: MIT Press.

Office of the Pope. 1998. *Fides et ratio*. Pope John Paul II encyclical letter: www.vatican.va/holy_father/john_paul_ii/encyclicals/documents/hf_jp-ii_enc_15101998_fides-et-ratio_en.html, accessed July 18, 2011.

Palumbi, Stephen R. 2001. Humans as the world's greatest evolutionary force. *Science* 293: 1786-90.

Redman, Charles L. 1999. *Human Impact on Ancient Environments*. Tucson: University of Arizona Press.

Roco, Mihail C., and William S. Bainbridge, eds. 2003. *Converging Technologies for Improving Human Performance*. Dordrecht: Kluwer Academic Publishers.

Rosenberg, Nathan, and L. E. Birdzell Jr. 1986. *How the West Grew Rich: The Economic Transformation of the Industrial World*. New York: Basic Books.

Schivelbusch, Wolfgang. 1987. *The Railway Journey: The Industrialization of Time and Space in the Nineteenth Century*. Berkeley: University of California Press.

Smil, Vaclav. 1997. *Cycles of Life: Civilization and the Biosphere*. New York: Scientific American Library.

Thomas, William L., Jr., ed. 1956. *Man's Role in Changing the Face of the Earth*. Chicago: University of Chicago Press.

Turner, B. L., W. C. Clark, R. W. Kates, J. F. Richards, et al., eds. 1990. *The Earth as Transformed by Human Action*. Cambridge: Cambridge University Press.

Is Transhumanism Scientifically Plausible? Posthuman Predictions and the Human Predicament

William J. Grassie

The debate about transhumanism frequently revolves around whether such a vision is desirable or detestable but typically glosses over the question of whether it is actually feasible. The plausibility of the transhumanist vision is a scientific question, not an ethical or aesthetic one. Can we realistically expect the creation of superintelligent machines, enhanced brains, and immortal bodies? Can we realistically anticipate the supersession of the human by some kind of superhuman, spiritual artificial intelligence? If we extrapolate the technological advances of the last century into the future, then we are in for some big changes in the coming decades. But is such an extrapolation really appropriate? We can imagine such possibilities, but that does not mean they are credible. Both sides of the transhumanism debate seem to assume the technological feasibility of some of these bold predictions – it is only a matter of applied effort or the prevention thereof. The scientific claims of transhumanism, however, need to be examined critically because some of these technoscientific prophecies may not be plausible. Of course, our ability to predict the future is always limited. The sciences involved in transhumanism are also incredibly complicated. The point of this essay is to raise some scientific doubts about our posthuman future.

In this chapter, I will argue, first, that the idea of controlling or designing a posthuman future flies in the face of past evolutionary and cultural history. It is an evolutionary truism that change is the only constant. Based on past experience, we can anticipate dramatic changes in the future evolution of life on the planet. This means also dramatic changes for our species and its distinct modes of cultural and technological evolution. This elemental evolutionary insight runs amok of both the transhumanists and the bioconservatives because, in either case, we should not assume that we will control the selective environment at some future date decades, centuries, or millennia hence.[1]

Second, I will argue that we face epistemic limits to technoscience that will mitigate against consciously achieving the otherwise laudable, largely humanist goals advocated by transhumanists. Here I will discuss the limitations of compu-

---

1 For advocates of transhumanism, see Salvalescu and Bostrum 2009; Bostrom 2003; Kurzweil 2005; Stock 1993; and Bailey 2005. For critics of transhumanism, also known as bioconservatives, see Fukuyama 2002; Kass 2002. For a point-counterpoint exploration of issues around transhumanism, see Hansell and Grassie 2011.

tation, chaos and complexity theories, and the misuse of metaphors in science, all with an eye to seeing some possible technoscientific limitations to the transhumanist vision.

Third, I will argue that we are already "posthuman" in a profound sense, more so in the twentieth century than in ten thousand years of prior human civilization. This recognition, however, should give us pause to reject both utopic and dystopic predictions of transhumanists and bioconservatives. Our posthuman predicament is simply that we have exponentially more power and more knowledge than our ancestors could have possibly imagined but no real control and no real predictive capacities on the evolutionary scale of transformation in which we are currently involved.

In making this argument, I propose to sidestep the question of whether the transhumanist vision is desirable. If my argument is correct, then we will be saved from confronting these possibilities by the complexity and ambiguity inherent in technoscience and evolution. These emerging limitations, however, are not necessarily something to be celebrated, as I will attempt to illuminate in a closing discussion on the collapse of the "Precautionary Principle" in contemporary ethics. If my argument is correct, then transhumanism is more about our recent past than the near future.

Designer Evolution

"Designer evolution" (Young 2005) is perhaps an oxymoron. Natural selection edits phenotypic variations based on their adaptive utility in specific contexts. On an evolutionary time scale, the species itself has little or no control over the context of selection. It matters not whether the variations are random or intentional, natural or artifactual: the utility of any phenotypic trait is "decided" post hoc based on whether the variations promote survival leading to reproduction in some future context.[2]

The species, as individuals or as a population, cannot anticipate in advance what the selective environment in the future will actually be. Past performance is no guarantee of future returns. The selective environment is normally thought of as stable (tropical rain forest), seasonally variable over a long time frame (temperate zones), or highly variable episodically over a long time frame (drought and monsoon patterns). In the short term, we can assume stable patterns in different

2 There is, of course, a vast literature on evolutionary theory. In this respect, I am especially influenced by systems theory and developmental biology. See, for instance, Gilbert and Epel, 2009; D. Depew and Weber 1996; Wesson 1991; Oyama 1985, 2000; Margulis 1998; Margulis and Sagan, 2002.

bioregions. If we take a long-term view of evolution, however, then the backdrop of life on Earth is highly variable, dramatically changing climatic and environmental conditions. These have often involved catastrophic climate change, as occurred sixty-five million years ago with the extinction of the dinosaurs due to an Earth-impact event. During the Pleistocene, the last 2.5 million years of evolution, Earth has been visited by as many as forty ice ages, each dramatically reshaping ecosystems and selective environments (Gibbard and van Kolfschoten 2005). Living in New York City, I like to remind myself that not so long ago Manhattan was under a thousand feet of moving ice and probably will be again someday.

Humans, perhaps more than any other species, have excelled in niche creation, also known as the Baldwin Effect (Depew and Weber 2003). We have phenotypic plasticity in the form of technological and cultural innovations that have made it possible for our species to inhabit almost every bioregion of the world. We are the only large mammal to do so. While a sudden, catastrophic climate change would no doubt cause a massive die-off of humans due to agricultural failures and economic collapse, there is no reason to assume that our species would actually go extinct. Humans at the species level would presumably be better positioned to adapt to these new environmental conditions than most other large flora and fauna on the planet, but this does not mean we can predict such events, nor how major environmental transformations would change the selective pressures on future humans. Remember also that selection for humans, and we may presume also for transhumans, involves not simply natural environments but also extremely complex social, political, economic, and cultural environments (Grassie 2009a).

While I posit a significant ontological break between biological evolution and cultural evolution, this distinction does not change the logic of selection (Grassie 2004, 2010). Cultural evolution occurs in a Lamarckian pattern, more so than Darwinian, because acquired characteristics can be passed on more or less directly to future generations through collective learning. Lamarckian processes can generate variations much faster than random genetic drift, but this does not eliminate selection on the back end of those variations.[3]

Based on past performance, we should anticipate dramatic climate changes at some point in our future, as well as other potentially catastrophic events. What we cannot predict is how our complex global civilization will adapt to these traumas, if and when they occur. In the end, the resulting social, political, and economic instability may be more dangerous to humans than the natural catastrophe itself. Our complex cultural adaptations are also inherently unpredictable. Humans on

3 There is a vast literature on cultural evolution and great debates within this domain about the extent to which Darwinian processes can account for cultural evolution. See, for instance, Boyd and Richerson 1985, 2005, 2006; Cartwright 2000; McNeill and McNeill 2003; Christian 2004.

an individual level have absolutely no way to prepare effectively for widely divergent future scenarios, even though we are blessed with incredible cognitive and behavioral plasticity.

How, for instance, in 1937, would one living in central Europe have best prepared for the advent of World War II? In hindsight, it is easy to make judgments about relative risks and safety. Living at the time, however, one would not have known the extent of the danger; when and where best to flee, if that were an option; and what skills and resources best to cultivate to maximize one's prospects for survival and reproduction. How, today for that matter, would one best prepare for the possible advent of global warming and a rise in ocean levels, if indeed these are realistic dangers? It is hard to design one's life in the event of extreme and unpredictable future scenarios.

Of course, science and engineering require a lot of designing. Professionals are trained over many years to employ the tools of physics, chemistry, and biology. When it comes to building and flying an airplane, designing and programming an iPad, or performing heart surgery, there is very little room for error. We should be appropriately mesmerized by the wonders of human agriculture, architecture, science, medicine, engineering, and technology, and the rapid growth of these domains in the last century. It would be wrong to assume, however, that we at the species level can actually control the selective environment in the same way that we engineer the International Space Station.

Human activity on the planet, especially as empowered by technoscience, certainly changes the natural and cultural context of selection for our own and other species, but the changes that matter are expressions of distributed cultural, political, and economic choices, as well as diverse environmental factors (Kelly 1994). It was not the invention of the automobile that mattered as much as the circuitous process over a century in which the automobile replicated and evolved to become ubiquitous in the world today. The automobile as a "natural kind" is not as much a designed object as an evolved artifact. In what sense could Karl Benz have anticipated or predicted the evolution of his 1885 Motorwagen into today's Mercedes-Benz S400 Hybrid Sedan? Nor could Henry Ford have predicted the modern highway system when he invented his gasoline-engine powered Quadricycle in 1896, itself another step in the evolution of Benz's Motorwagen. The evolution of the automobile is a complex, distributed history that involved lots of designs, innovations, and variations that survived and reproduced, albeit with humans as symbionts in their replication. Artifacts evolve and so do the humans who create them.

When we want to talk about evolution, and transhumanism must be assessed on an evolutionary time scale, then engineering is not the right metaphor. Charles Darwin, of course, is famous for employing the metaphor of laissez-faire economics in his *Origin of Species*. "The whole economy of nature" was not a command economy but a complex, distributed system. Perhaps we can detect an "Invisible Hand" working in the evolutionary and technological markets of human evolution.[4] Perhaps this Invisible Hand will lead us to some transhumanist utopia. Our niche creation efforts, however well intended and well informed, cannot predetermine the relevant phenotypic, cultural, and technological traits that will ensure survival and reproduction in unknown and unknowable future environments, not ten years or ten thousand years hence.

I have come to believe that there is an Invisible Hand working through and with the evolution of the universe and human history. I believe this on two accounts. First, I think it is a plausible, indeed probable, reading of the history of the universe, the planet, and our species based on overall trends. Second, I think that a belief in transcendence is functionally adaptive for our species and for me personally. I certainly cannot prove the existence of this Invisible Hand. Nor do I think we should necessarily equate this complex, distributed system with our tradition's inherited understanding of God, by whatever name, though there are certainly some interesting questions there to be explored. I am content to leave this as a somewhat vague teleology, cajoling the universe and us toward greater complexity and self-creative possibilities (Grassie 2010).[5]

Critical for the moral and aesthetic debates between transhumanists and bio-conservatives are whether this Invisible Hand includes some empirically based norms conducive to successful evolution and then which group's ideology better embodies these general norms. This, of course, is a philosophical and ideological debate about norms and values, more than a scientific debate about the future trajectory of technoscience. I would argue that the past history of technoscience is consistent with this reading of our evolutionary history. Whether we are for or against the transhumanist vision of the future, we need to ground these preferences in some interpretation of evolutionary history, if they are to be realistic and compelling. Note that the "Is" and the "Ought" are inextricably interwoven, as our desires and doings literally change reality.[6]

---

4 See, for instance, Kelly 1994; Beinhocker 2006. The idea of a progressive incarnation of God in history was advocated by G.W.F. Hegel 1977 [1807] and taken up again in an evolutionary guise by Alfred North Whitehead 1978 [1929], 1967 [1933] and by Teilhard de Chardin1999 [1955]. See also Haught 2000.

5 I develop these ideas in *The New Sciences of Religion* (2010). I am drawing on both economic theory (Beinhocker 2006) as well as Whitehead's process philosophy (Whitehead 1978 [1929]) and Teilhard's evolutionary theology (Teilhard de Chardin 1999 [1955]) as interpreted by Berry and Swimme (1992) and others.

6 The "Is/Ought" distinction was first posed as such by Moore (1903). Many consider this formulation inadequate. See, for instance, Wilson (1998). Transhumanism frames the problem in a new way, because what *is* the case is increasingly transformed by what we think *ought* to be the case. See my discussion of Lamarckian cultural evolution.

The larger point is that we can no more predict our future evolution than an economist can predict short-term or long-term market trends. We cannot design a transhumanist evolutionary future any more than we can design an economy to grow forever annually at 4 percent. Designer evolution is, therefore, an oxymoron, but this is hardly a validation of bioconservativism. Transhumanism may not be realistic, but it reframes the question in the appropriate context. We live at an extraordinary moment in the natural history of our planet and the cultural evolution of our species. We have every reason to expect dramatic changes in the next hundred years, though little basis on which to claim optimism or pessimism in the short term.

Epistemic Limits and Category Mistakes

Another set of technical problems with the transhumanist vision of designer evolution deals with emerging epistemic limits in technoscience about what we can know and control. In this section, I will take Ray Kurzweil's book *The Singularity Is Near* (2005) as a case study because it provides a useful overview of multiple developments in genomics, nanotechnology, robotics, and artificial intelligence that all have implications for transhumanism.

Kurzweil proposes a "Law of Accelerating Returns" woven into the fabric of the universe, the evolution of biological complexity, the development of human culture, and the trajectory of technological innovation. What this means is that we are surfing a wave of exponential growth, although our minds and cultures are oriented toward linear processes and gradual changes. The "magic" of exponentiality is that innovations begin slowly at first and then progress into a steep, accelerating curve. Kurzweil argues that, sometime around 2045, the trajectory of technological innovation will lead to a "Singularity" in which some kind of "post-biological" civilization will "take off" (Kurzweil 2005).

In his book and lectures, Kurzweil discusses a number of logarithmic plots of technological innovation (i.e., linear representations of exponential trends): Mass Use of Inventions (50); Dynamic RAM in computers (57); Average Transistor Price (59); DNA Sequencing Cost (73); Internet Data Traffic (80); Decreasing Size of Mechanical Devices (82); Per-Capita GDP (99); and Noninvasive Brain Scanning (159), to name a few examples. Taken separately and together, these trends are very impressive. If these trajectories continue, as Kurzweil and others argue they will, then humanity is riding a very big wave of technological innovation in multiple and interrelated fields of science and engineering (GNR plus AGI). Within ten-to-twenty years, we should have a pretty good assessment of whether this really is an evolutionary tsunami. And if we make it to 2045 without crashing, the world will certainly be significantly, perhaps singularly different.

Critic Jaron Lanier refers to this fixation on the exponentials as "the fetishizing of Moore's Law" and argues that the difficulty of writing software will thwart these hyperbolic predictions (Lanier 2000). Sun Microsystem founder Bill Joy wrote an impassioned plea for restraint in a now infamous *WIRED* cover story titled "Why the Future Doesn't Need Us?" (Joy 1999). Far from a utopia, Joy worries that the GNR revolution was a misanthropic nightmare leading to the extinction of our species. Others wonder whether the supersession of our species by immortal and superintelligent postbiological entities would be such a bad thing (Houellebecq 2000). Kurzweil knows his critics and addresses each of their points to varying degrees of satisfaction in his lectures and in his book. Let's review some of the most salient arguments presented by Singularity skeptics, because, as we will learn, the implications for transhumanism are also singularly significant.

The first problem in these Singularity predictions lies in the very nature of computation. There are known limits to computation. Computer scientists know that sometimes even very simple problems cannot be solved by the very nature of the problem. As David Harel at the Weizmann Institute of Science explains in his book *Computers Ltd.: What They Really Can't Do*,

> [W]e shall see interesting and important problems for which there simply are no algorithms, and it doesn't matter how smart we are, or how sophisticated and powerful our computers, our software, our programming languages and our algorithmic methods . . .
>
> These facts have deep philosophical implications, not only on the limits of machines like computers, but also on our own limits as beings with finite mass. Even if we were given unlimited amounts of pencil and paper, and unlimited lifespan, there would be well defined problems we could not solve. It is also important to stress that this is not just about computing, by brain or by machine. It is a fact about knowing. In a strong sense, what we can compute is what we are able to figure out by careful step-by-step processes from what we already know. The limits of computation are the limits of knowledge. (2000, 27-28)

This is a very technical discussion in computer science, but the short of it is that many problems simply do not compute (Barrow 1999).

There are also other theoretical and practical limits to computation. These are called intractable problems because they "require hopelessly large amounts of time even for relatively small inputs" (Harel 2000, 79). Computer encryption depends on this second fact. It may be that the genome, in dynamic relationship with proteins and its environment, is in some sense "encrypted" (Gilbert and Epel 2009). It may be that the mind–brain is similarly "encrypted" (Grassie 2009b; Penrose 1989, 1994), in which case we will never be able fully to understand, let alone reliably control, life and mind, no matter how exponentially our scientific knowledge grows or how fast technological know-how accelerates.

The second problem that could scuttle the hopes and dreams of the prophets of transhumanism is the nature of chaos and complexity (Gleick 1987). This is both a computational problem and a biological and engineering problem. When you design a program or model a complex natural phenomena with too many feedback loops and too many input variables and parameters, you quickly meet the proverbial "butterfly effect" in which minor variations in initial conditions can ripple through the system with widely variable, unpredictable, and unintended results. Complex distributed systems can be incredibly resilient, true; but they can also be incredibly fragile. It is hard to know in advance. While some complex systems can be represented mathematically with simple reiterative formula (Wolfram 2002), it is a big leap of faith to think that all chaotic and complex systems can be thus represented, understood, and controlled. This, then, is the "useless arithmetic" problem (Pilkey and Pilkey-Jarvis 2007; Grassie 2007). For better or worse, the same principles apply to other complex distributed systems. The genome (which requires also proteomics, developmental biology, and a whole lot more) and the mind–brain (which requires bodies, nature, cultures, and a whole lot more) strike me as likely candidates for irreducible complexity. Instead of an exponential explosion in technoscience, we should more likely anticipate asymptotic limits to many sciences in the twenty-first century, limits set by chaos, complexity, and computational finitude as determined by the real complexity of natural entities that we hope to understand and reengineer (Gleick 1987; Kelly 1994; Castellani and Hafferty 2009; Castellani 2009; Grassie 1997).

The third problem has to do with the challenges of writing software. Jaron Lanier lays out this argument in his essay "One Half of a Manifesto" with the subtitle "Why Stupid Software Will Save the Future from Neo-Darwinian Machines":

> This breathtaking vista [the Singularity] must be starkly contrasted with the Great Shame of computer science, which is that we don't seem to be able to write software much better as computers get much faster. … If anything, there's a reverse Moore's law observable in software. (Lanier 1999)

Lanier discusses software "brittleness," "legacy code," "lock-in," and "other perversions" that work counter to the logic of Kurzweil's exponential vision. It turns out there is also an exponential growth curve in programming and IT support jobs, as more and more talent and hours are drawn into managing, debugging, translating incompatible databases, and protecting our exponentially better, cheaper, and more-connected computers. This exponential countertrend suggests that humanity will become "a planet of help desks" long before the Singularity.

Fourth, when computer programs are designed to simulate natural processes, for instance, the human brain, you get layers of abstraction from the real thing. Science works best by simplifying and isolating processes, but that does not mean that reality is actually simple, isolatable, or adequately represented in this manner. In addition to the "useless arithmetic" problem, we have a problem of representation, which in this case may be too simplistic and too abstracted from reality. Alfred North Whitehead warns of "the fallacy of misplaced concreteness" (1967 [1925], 51) and the imperative to "seek simplicity and distrust it" (2010 [1920], 163). The map is not the terrain, and the details that matter depend on the context and cannot always be known in advance. It seems to me that the transhumanist prophets have underestimated both these problems.

The fifth problem is the fallacy of exponential logic. It is hard to imagine any Earth-bound natural process, especially at the scale of humans and human technologies that can grow exponentially forever. Whether it is a pair of aphids on potted plants in my office or the rapid growth in the Chinese economy, nothing can grow exponentially for all that long on the relevant time scale without running into some stark limitations. We have lived through an extraordinary century of exponential growth-population, economic growth, energy consumption, water usage, mining, manufacturing, domesticated plants and animals, technological and scientific advances, publishing and media. How long can this continue? Instead of an exponential explosion into the new age of spiritual machines, we are more likely to have an economic and environmental implosion (McNeill 2000). The actual history of civilizations and the evolution of life involve periods of collapse disrupting the overall trend toward complexification. I will return to this problem below.

One rough measure of complexity is energy-density flow. Astronomer Eric Chaisson has estimated the comparative energy-density flow of different entities in the universe, measured as the amount of free energy flowing through a system in respect to its mass over time, in this case measured as erg per seconds per grams (erg s^{-1} g^{-1}). Earth's climasphere, which consists of the atmosphere and oceans, has roughly a hundred times the energy-density flow of a typical star or galaxy. Through photosynthesis, plants achieve an energy-density flow roughly a thousand times more than that of a star. The human body is sustained by a daily food intake resulting in an energy-density flow about twenty thousand times more than that of a typical star. Remember that we are comparing the ratio of energy consumed to mass of the objects. So here is another way to think of this. If a human body could be scaled up to the mass of our sun, it would be twenty thousand times more luminous (assuming it could obtain enough food energy). The human brain, which consumes about 20 percent of our energy intake while constituting about 2 percent of our body weight, has an energy-density flow 150,000 times that of a typical star.[7] And finally, modern human civilization has

7 Energy-density flow is only indicative of complexity as we see in comparing the brain to the kidneys. A pair of kidneys weighs about one-fourth as much as the brain but consume roughly the same amount of energy as the brain as measured by oxygen consumption rates. We need to combine the concept of energy-density flow with some understanding of informational complexity in order to develop a useful scale of complexity. There is no universal, cross-disciplinary definition of information within the sciences.

an energy-density ratio some five hundred thousand times that of a typical star. Energy-density flows turn out to be a useful way to think about emergent complexity but also about the exponential trajectory of energy consumption in Kurzweil's nanobot postbiological, transhuman complexity (Chaisson 2001, 139; Chaisson 2006, 293-96; Christian 2004).

There is an important caveat to the fallacy of exponential logic because disembodied information, if such a thing exists, can conceivably grow exponentially forever. Information, in this view, would not be subject to the Second Law of Thermodynamics and the limitations of space-time and matter-energy. We do not, however, have an adequate definition of information (or complexity) across different scientific disciplines. We do not really know what disembodied information would really mean except as some Platonic mystification. It may be that computer scientists, mathematicians, and theoretical physicists are prone to such disembodied mystifications, more so than, say, chemists, geologists, and physicians, a thought that leads to the next point.

Metaphors matter in science. An apt metaphor can lead to interesting insights. The misinterpretation of a metaphor can lead as well to major category mistakes. Certainly, the real revolution in science in the last thirty years has been the advent of ever-more powerful and less expensive computer technology. We can now collect and analyze large datasets, create new models and simulations, build new tools, and conduct research and collaboration over the Internet. This has been a Kuhnian revolution in science, a paradigm shift not just in one discipline but in all the sciences, as well as in practically every other aspect of human life. The metaphors of computer science have now been adopted in diverse disciplines from psychology to economics, from cell biology to cosmology. A metaphor is a comparison of two unlike entities. Metaphors can be symbolically profound but are never literally true. Metaphors enrich language and thought, but if we become literal fundamentalists, we are sadly and sometimes tragically mistaken.

So, my sixth point is to deconstruct the metaphors on which artificial intelligence, life-extension technology, nanotechnology, robotics, and genomics are all based – the idea that life and mind are machines that can be reverse-engineered. Human engineering is pretty fantastic stuff, but I doubt whether anything that humans have ever designed approaches the biochemical complexity of a single cell. Let me quote Bill Bryson's description of a simple prokaryotic cell from his book *A Short History of Nearly Everything*:

> Blown up to a scale at which atoms were about the size of peas, a cell would be a sphere roughly half a mile across, and supported by a complex framework of girders called the cytoskelton. Within it, millions upon millions of objects – some the size of basketballs, others the size of cars – would whiz about like bullets. There wouldn't be a place you could stand without being pummeled and ripped thousands of times every second from every direction.

> Even for its full-time occupants the inside of a cell is a hazardous place. Each strand of DNA is on average attacked or damaged once every 8.4 seconds – ten thousand times in a day – by chemicals and other agents that whack into or carelessly slice through it, and each of these wounds must be swiftly stitched up if the cell is not to perish.
>
> The proteins are especially lively, spinning, pulsating and flying into each other up to a billion times a second. Enzymes, themselves a type of protein, dash everywhere, performing up to a thousand tasks a second. Like greatly speeded-up worker ants, they busily build and rebuild molecules, hauling a piece off this one, adding a piece to that one. Some monitor passing proteins and mark with a chemical those that are irreparably damaged or flawed. Once so selected, the doomed proteins proceed to a structure called a proteasome, where they are stripped down and their components used to build new proteins. Some types of protein exist for less than half an hour; others survive for weeks. But all lead existences that are inconceivably frenzied. (Bryson 2005, 477-78)

Bryson's vivid trope for describing the trillions of biochemical reactions per second in a simple prokaryotic cell does not even begin to approach the real nanotech-level, informational, and developmental complexity of this smallest unit of life. A typical such cell contains twenty thousand different types of proteins, each with capacities to fold and unfold in specific context to accomplish specific tasks. A small cell contains perhaps one hundred million protein molecules. The adult human body contains some ten trillion (10^{13}) large eukaryotic cells. All these cells began as a single fertilized egg in your mother's womb, a single cell with twenty-three chromosomes, some seventy thousand genes, and three billion base pairs, a single cell that replicated, initially exponentially, and along the way differentiated into 210 tissue types in their proper organs performing their proper function.

Can a computer model the complexity inside a single cell, let alone the complexity of the entire brain of some hundred billion neurons (10^{11}) connected together in a tangled web of over one hundred trillion synaptic connections (10^{14})? What details are we necessarily going to exclude from these models? If we follow Bryson's lead and blow an entire human brain up to a scale where each atom would be the size of a pea, then suddenly the only other human creation that might compare to the informational complexity of the brain would be the entire global economy shrunk to the size of a brain. Nobody designed and nobody controls the global economy, even though we try to influence it as best we can as differentially empowered participants with different interests, motivations, and expectations.

But wait! A disembodied brain is a useless mush of gray matter. For a human brain to realize its extraordinary abilities requires in its ontogeny and phylogeny an entire body and an evolved history. A brain requires a network of nerves and a metabolism. It requires vocal cords and oppositional thumbs. The brain must evolve and develop in natural environments rich in semiotic and semantic meanings. It requires the nurture of families, communities, and civilizations from which it acquires language, tools, and purpose (Deacon 1997; Donald 1991). The brain, much like the genome, does absolutely nothing by itself. When separated from this messy matrix of embodied relationships – top-down, bottom-up, side-to-side – the brain really has no capacities at all, computational or otherwise.

In a profound ontological sense, the human body-brain-mind-spirit is an emergent phenomenon in which the whole is "exponentially" more than the sum of its parts. Different levels of analysis are necessary for different kinds of scientific and philosophical questions that we might ask about body-brain-mind-spirit. Reductionistic approaches to the neurosciences and artificial intelligence can quickly become category mistakes, as silly as trying to use particle physics to interpret a novel, evolutionary psychology to ascertain the truth-value of physics, or life-extension technology to realize the meaning of life. Metaphors matter. It is time to jettison the machine metaphor that dominates much of the transhumanist, singularitian, and extopian vision.

I have nothing in principle against scientists pushing the envelope up to and if possible beyond the asymptotes: trying to reduce complex problems into more manageable levels, building all kinds of models and simulations, trying to enhance and extend human health and well-being, as well as that of other species and our environments, building ever-more intelligent, efficient, and useful prosthetic devices, machines that change what we know, how we live, and in a profound sense also who we are. By all means, push the envelope! I think society should spend more resources, not fewer on these issues, including educating children and adults alike about this remarkable cosmic, chemical, geological, biological, cultural, and technological evolutionary adventure in which we are now so consequentially participating. My hope, however, is that by doing so, our species and science itself will become less hyperbolic and more humble, more appreciative in a religious sense that nature, including our own embodied human nature, turns out to be fantastically super.

The values articulated by transhumanism favor more life, abundantly lived, perhaps even altruistically shared, so there is not much to criticize in these conventionally humanist values whose origins we can trace back to religious cultures. Dig a bit deeper, and we will discover that bioconservatives and transhumanists are both motivated by a very similar set of humanist values. When they disagree, it is about how those values are ranked and distributed, how costs and benefits are assessed, and how they calculate optimism and pessimism about humanity, science, economics, and the environment. The real complexity of the universe and the human person means that our future calculations of optimism versus pessimism, costs versus benefits, humanist values versus other humanist values will always be at best informed intuitions and at worst wishful thinking.

Our Posthuman Past

Scientists are now referring to the contemporary moment in the evolution of life as the Anthropocene, an era in evolution when humans dominate Earth processes (Zalasiewicz et al. 2008). It did not happen overnight. Indeed, one can say that it really began with the advent of agriculture some ten thousand years ago. Of course, ten thousand years is but an instant in the deep time of evolution, which makes the dramatic changes over the last century all the more remarkable and worrisome. Certainly, the rate of change over the last few decades has greatly intensified, so much so that much of the technology that we take for granted today would seem like magic to our ancestors even a hundred years past.

The point of this discussion is to suggest that, in a profound sense, we are already transhumans, more posthuman now in the first decade of the twenty-first century than in all the millennia of prior human civilization. This recognition, however, should give us pause to reject both utopic and dystopic predictions of transhumanists and bioconservatives. Our posthuman predicament is that we have exponentially more power and more knowledge than our ancestors could have possibly imagined, but no real control or real predictive capabilities on the evolutionary scale of transformation in which we are currently involved. It would also seem that we do not possess any greater capacity for ethical judgment and moral living.

Humans evolve and exist in a dynamic relationship with the rest of nature. In spite of our impressive cognitive and technological abilities, we remain fundamentally biological creatures. Our genetic disposition, psychological temperament, and life trajectory as individuals have barely changed over the millennia. As evolved mammals, we are dependent on biological processes to sustain our individual and collective lives. The capacity of our species to change the environment has increased dramatically over our evolutionary history, so much so that the only comparable event in evolution may have been the invention of photosynthesis some two billion years ago.[8] We see this certainly in the history of

8 In the Paleoproterozoic, photosynthesizing cynobacteria radically changed the atmosphere of the Earth, drawing carbon dioxide out of the atmosphere and releasing oxygen. The content of oxygen went from an estimated 2 percent to 20 percent, thus creating the largest pollution crisis ever visited upon the planet. There were two consequences. First, oxygen is a radical element that reacts with other elements and molecules, i.e., oxidization. Oxygen attacked the membranes of the mostly anaerobic life on the planet at that time, thus causing a huge die-off of bacterial life. Second, photosynthesis caused the reduction of carbon dioxide and other greenhouse gases in the atmosphere, resulting in a cooling of the Earth and a massive Ice Age, in which the only liquid surface water was in equatorial regions. Humans are the first species since these photosynthesizing bacteria radically to change the atmosphere of Earth and to also cause a mass extinction of other species. Photosynthesis provided a new trajectory for evolutionary complexification. It may also be that human cultural evolution, which includes our technoscientific evolution, now provides the new trajectory for future evolution of our species and the planet, one that will begin with an epic crisis perhaps comparable to what happened two billion years ago.

agriculture, which has resculpted ecologies and supported a growing human population. Physical anthropologists discovered that agriculture also changes our genetic makeup. There is a dynamic relationship between our biology and our culture, encoded in our genetic and neural evolution but increasingly also projected outward onto the environment, which we harness and transform to our perceived benefit. The selective environment is changed by us and thus will change us as well. This is the magic of coevolution (Durham 1992).

In the twentieth century, there was a dramatic intensification of human editing of natural environments. We see this in the realms of mining, construction, energy consumption, forestry, trade, travel, communications, and agriculture. J. R. McNeill provides a matter-of-fact overview of these changes in his book *Something New under the Sun* (2000), bringing together diverse data-sources to tell the history of the biosphere, all increasingly and profoundly transformed by the human spheres of activity on the planet.

Human population has increased four-fold between 1890 and 1990. The total urban population of the world increased thirteen-fold in the same time period. Today, there are over six billion humans on the planet, and while birth rates are declining in most regions, we can still expect growth over the next few decades (McNeill 2000, 360-61).

Sustenance for this growth in human population required increased food production and energy consumption, as well as new systems for distributing clean water, sanitation, and the containment and cure of diseases. McNeill calculates that the world economy grew fourteen-fold in the period 1890-1990, while industrial output grew forty-fold, all fueled by a sixteen-fold increase in energy use and a nine-fold increase in water consumption. The domestic-cattle population grew four-fold in this period, and the domestic-pig population by nine-fold. Land under cultivation doubled in this time frame, while forest area decreased by 20 percent. Marine fish catch increased thirty-five-fold in the last century and is now in radical decline save for a dramatic increase in fish farming (McNeill 2000, 360-61).

Demographers cited by McNeill estimate that about eighty billion hominids have lived in the past four million years, for a total of 2.16 trillion years of human life lived on the planet. So while the twentieth century represents only one hundred out of the four million years of hominid evolution, it has hosted 20 percent of all human-years lived. Certainly, this was a prodigious century by any measure (McNeill 2000, 9).

To this we add the many transformations in science and technology that have become part of our daily lives. Transformations in medicine, computers, entertainment, communication, transportation, manufacturing, agriculture, and energy are so dramatic in this hundred-year time horizon that it boggles the mind. The ubiquity of these new technologies – for instance, the "simple" cell phone –

makes it difficult to remember the time when these technologies did not exist. We take these changes for granted, as if our generation were the norm.

In order to capture the magnitude of these changes, it might be better already to employ the terminology of *transhuman* or *posthuman* to describe our current hominid condition, rather than some future possibility. Perhaps by recognizing the many ways that we are already transformed humans, we will gain a better perspective on history and ourselves. Perhaps by calling ourselves posthumans, we can begin to see the many ways that our human nature is a moving target in an accelerating evolutionary drama.

Traditional ethics would evoke the precautionary principle: do no harm. If there is a chance that our technological and cultural evolution will cause harm, then we should desist. Genetically modified organisms or self-reproducing nanotechnology, for instance, might get out of control and cause irreparable damage to ecosystems; ergo, we should not pursue such technologies. That is the logic of "do no harm" frequently evoked in medical ethics. We should also remind ourselves of the concept of opportunity costs typically evoked in economics. Not pursuing nanotechnology, genomics, robotics, artificial intelligence, and life-extension technologies is an opportunity cost and could conceivably make it impossible to feed the world, reduce cropland, restore ecosystems, solve the energy crisis, or cure the next pandemic. We do not know. We cannot see beyond the horizons of complexity, but it might help if we could better interpret the changes that we have witnessed in the recent past. In that respect, it would be better to understand ourselves as already transformed humans. We are already cyborgs. We are already posthumans. Some decades ago we entered the age of transhumanism. That, I believe, is a more plausible interpretation of the science and our history than some religious, philosophical, genetic, or evolutionary essentialization of a fixed "human nature."

Conclusion

In the critical analyses of the science of transhumanism, we were "saved" from that future by the nature of evolution, the bite of complexity, and the fallacy of misplaced concreteness. This, however, is not something we should necessarily be celebrating with a sigh of relief because, without dramatic technological innovation, we may be in big trouble. We are not saved from our posthuman past because, in a very real sense, we have long since crossed this important threshold in the evolution of our species and the planet.

Do no harm is all fine and well as long as there are no opportunity costs that offset our inaction. So we put our faith in some future; we invest in some vision, perhaps with a hope that this unfolding drama is guided by an Invisible Hand. Optimism is never simply rational. The future is never simply empirical.

What we should remember, however, is that religions, cultures, and ideologies are all part of a complex distributive normative system that shapes our collective lives. It is not just the free markets of evolution, economies, and technologies that should concern us. Human values and beliefs are also part of the equation. Ideas matter. If the past is any guide to our future, then ideologies will be more dangerous to our species than technologies. It is perhaps appropriate that we debate the ideologies of transhumanism, rather than the technology itself, because the ideologies change us even before the science and technology have been invented. Bioconservative ideologies, of course, require a similar critique.

There is no reason necessarily to privilege this moment in natural history and cultural evolution. In that sense, transhumanists have more appropriately framed the question and challenges for the twenty-first century and beyond. Strict environmental or cultural preservationism would freeze history in principle and in practice would not work. Evolution is not static. Both transhumanists and bioconservatives adopt a sometimes naïve understanding of technological progress and evolutionary change. Here, however, I think the skepticism of the bioconservatives is a necessary antidote to the technoscientific optimism of the transhumanists.

My hope is that humans will be more like gifted artists in our future evolution, taking the materials at hand, the more-than-human realms of nature, and transforming them with our science, technology, and culture to create something more beautiful. To do so, we will need to reread the books of revelation and the new books of nature, creating a dialectic between our cultural and biological inheritances. To this we add our hopes for a better future, an Earth that is safer and healthier, which probably means not changing quite as rapidly as it has in the recent past and prudentially preserving intact natural environments as best as we are able. We may hope that there is an Invisible Hand working through the distributed systems of natural history and cultural evolution, but we will not know.

Again, I challenge the scientists to push the envelope as far as possible. We have an obligation to help and heal, to minimize suffering, to be all we can be as individuals, as a species, and as an interdependent community of many species on a planet, which will be the only home for future evolution for the foreseeable future. We could do, however, with less hype, more critical realism, more straightforward science, and certainly more humility. Perhaps in the end we can both humanize the transhumanists and transform the humans into something altogether better for the planet and ourselves.

References

Bailey, Ronald. 2005. *Liberation Biology: The Scientific and Moral Case for the Biotech Revolution*. New York: Prometheus Books.

Barrow, John D. 1999. *Impossibility: The Limits of Science and the Science of Limits*. New York: Oxford University Press.

Beinhocker, Eric D. 2006. *The Origin of Wealth: Evolution, Complexity, and the Radical Remaking of Economics*. Cambridge: Harvard Business Press.

Berry, Thomas, and Brian Swimme. 1992. *The Universe Story: From the Primordial Flaring Forth to the Ecozoic Era*. San Francisco: Harper.

Bostrom, Nick. 2003. The Transhumanist FAQ: A General Introduction 2.1: http://humandefinition.blogspot.com/2009/10/transhumanist-faq.html, accessed July 20, 2011.

Boyd, Robert, and Peter J. Richerson. 1985. *Culture and the Evolutionary Process*. Chicago: University of Chicago Press.

–. 2005. *The Origin and Evolution of Cultures*. New York: Oxford University Press.

–. 2006. *Not by Genes Alone: How Culture Transformed Human Evolution*. Chicago: University of Chicago Press.

Bryson, Bill. 2005. *A Short History of Nearly Everything: Special Illustrated Edition*. New York: Broadway Books.

Cartwright, John. 2000. *Evolution and Human Behavior: Darwinian Perspectives on Human Nature*. New York: Palgrave.

Castellani, Brian. 2009. Map of Complexity Science: http://www.art-science factory.com/complexity-map_feb09.html, accessed July 20, 2011.

Castellani, Brian, and Frederic W. Hafferty. 2009. *Sociology and Complexity Science: A New Field of Inquiry*. Berlin: Springer Verlag.

Chaisson, Eric. 2001. *Cosmic Evolution: The Rise of Complexity in Nature*. Cambridge, MA: Harvard University Press.

–. 2006. *Epic of Evolution: Seven Ages of the Cosmos*. New York: Columbia University Press.

Christian, David. 2004. *Maps of Time: An Introduction to Big History*. Berkeley: University of California Press.

Deacon, Terrence W. 1997. *The Symolic Species: The Co-Evolution of Language and the Brain*. New York: Norton.

Depew, David J., and Bruce M. Weber. 1996. *Darwinism Evolving: Systems Dynamics and the Genealogy of Natural Selection*. Cambridge, MA: MIT Press.

–. eds. 2003. *Evolution and Learning: The Baldwin Effects Reconsidered*. Cambridge, MA: MIT Press.

Donald, Merlin. 1991. *Origins of the Modern Mind: Three Stages in the Evolution of Culture and Cognition*. Cambridge, MA: Harvard University Press.

Durham, William H. 1992. *Coevolution: Genes, Culture, and Human Diversity*. Stanford: Stanford University Press.

Fukuyama, Francis. 2002. *Our Posthuman Future: Consequences of the Biotechnology Revolution*. New York: Picador.

Gibbard, P., and T. van Kolfschoten. 2005. The Pleistocene and Holocene epochs. In *A Geological Time Scale 2004*, edited by F. M. Gradstein, J. G. Ogg, and A. G. Smith, 441-52. New York: Cambridge University Press.

Gilbert, Scott F., and David Epel. 2009. *Ecological Developmental Biology: Integrating Epigenetics, Medicine, and Evolution*. Sunderland, MA: Sinauer Associates.

Gleick, James. 1987. *Chaos: Making a New Science*. New York: Penguin.

Grassie, William J. 1997. Wired for the future: Kevin Kelly's techno-utopia. *Terra Nova: Nature and Culture* 2 (4): 91-101.

–. 2004. Biocultural evolution in the 21st century: The evolutionary role of religion. *Metanexus Global Spiral*: http://www.metanexus.net/magazine/tabid/68/id/8779/Default.aspx, accessed July 20, 2011.

–. 2007. Useless arithmetic and inconvenient truths: A review. *Metanexus Global Spiral*: http://www.metanexus.net/Magazine/tabid/68/id/9854/Default.aspx, accessed July 20, 2011.

–. 2009a. A thought experiment: Envisioning a civilization recovery plan. *Metanexus Global Spiral*: http://www.metanexus.net/magazine/tabid/68/id/10943/Default.aspx, accessed July 20, 2011

–. 2009b. Post-Darwinism: The new synthesis. *Metanexus Global Spiral*: http://www.grassie.net/articles/2009_postdarwinism.html, accessed July 20, 2011.

–. 2010. *The New Sciences of Religion: Exploring Spirituality from the Outside In and Bottom Up*. New York: Palgrave Macmillan.

Hansell, Gregory, and William J. Grassie, eds. 2011. *H± Transhumanism and Its Critics*. Philadelphia: Metanexus Institute.

Harel, David. 2000. *Computers Ltd.: What They Really Can't Do*. New York: Oxford University Press.

Haught, John. 2000. *God after Darwin: A Theology of Evolution*. Boulder, CO: Westview.

Hegel, G.W.F. 1977 [1807]. *The Phenomenology of Spirit*. Translated by A. V. Miller. Oxford: Clarendon Press.

Houellebecq, Michel. 2000. *The Elementary Particle*. Translated by F. Wynne. New York: Alfred Knopf.

Joy, Bill. 1999. Why the future doesn't need us. *WIRED* 8 (4): http://www.wired.com/wired/archive/8.04/joy.html, accessed July 20, 2011.

Kass, Leon. 2002. *Life, Liberty, and the Defense of Dignity: The Challenge for Bioethics*. San Francisco: Encounter Books.

Kelly, Kevin. 1994. *Out of Control: The New Biology of Machines, Social Systems, and the Economic World*. New York: Addison-Wesley.

Kurzweil, Ray. 2005. *The Singularity Is Near: When Humans Transcend Biology*. New York: Penguin Books.

Lanier, Jaron. 2000. One-half of a manifesto: Why stupid software will save the future from neo-Darwinian machines. *WIRED* 8 (12): http://www.wired.com/wired/archive/8.12/lanier.html, accessed July 20, 2011.

Margulis, Lynn. 1998. *Symbiotic Planet: A New Look at Evolution*. New York: Basic Books.

Margulis, Lynn, and Dorian Sagan. 2002. *Acquiring Genomes: A Theory of the Origins of Species*. New York: Basic Books.

McNeill, J. Robert. 2000. *Something New under the Sun: An Environmental History of the Twentieth-Century World*. New York: W.W. Norton and Company.

McNeill, J. Robert, and McNeill, William H. 2003. *The Human Web: A Bird's-Eye View of World History*. New York: W.W. Norton.

Moore, George E. 1989 [1903]. *Principia Ethica*. Cambridge: Cambridge University Press.

Oyama, Susan. 1985. *The Ontogeny of Information*. New York: Cambridge University Press.

–. 2000. *Evolution's Eye: A Systems View of the Biology-Culture Divide*. Durham, NC: Duke University Press.

Penrose, Roger. 1989. *The Emperor's New Mind: Cencerning Computers, Minds and the Laws of Physic*. New York: Oxford University Press.

–. 1994. *Shadows of the Mind: A Search for the Missing Science of Consciousness*. New York: Oxford University Press.

Pilkey, Orrin H., and Linda Pilkey-Jarvis. 2007. *Useless Arithmetic: Why Environmental Scientists Can't Predict the Future*. New York: Columbia University Press.

Savulescu, Julian, and Nick Bostrom, eds. 2009. *Human Enhancement*. New York: Oxford University Press.

Stock, Gregory. 1993. *Metaman: The Making of Humans and Machines into a Global Superorganism*. New York: Simon and Schuster.

Teilhard, Pierre de Cardin. 1999 [1955]. *The Human Phenomenon*. Translated by S. Appleton-Weber. Portland, OR: Sussex Academic Press.

Wesson, Robert. 1991. *Beyond Natural Selection*. Cambridge, MA: MIT Press.

Whitehead, Alfred North. 2010 [1920]. *The Concept of Nature*. Cambridge: Cambridge University Press.
–. 1967 [1925]. *Science and the Modern World.* New York: Free Press.
–. 1978 [1929]. *Process and Reality*. New York: Free Press.
–. 1967 [1933]. *Adventures of Ideas*. New York: Free Press.
Wilson, Edward O. 1998. *Consilience: The Unity of Knowledge*. New York: Knopf.
Wolfram, Stephen. 2002. *A New Kind of Science*. Champaign, IL: Wolfram Media.
Young, Simon. 2005. *Designer Evolution: A Transhumanist Manifesto*. Amherst, NY: Prometheus Books.
Zalasiewicz, Jan, et al. 2008. Are we now living in the Anthropocene? *GSA Today* 18 (2), 4-8: http://www.geosociety.org/gsatoday/archive/18/2/pdf/i1052-5173-18-2-4.pdf, accessed July 20, 2011.

Select Bibliography

Agar, Nicholas. 2004. *Liberal Eugenics: In Defence of Human Enhancement*. Oxford: Blackwell.

Allenby, Braden, and Daniel Sarewitz. 2011. *The Techno-Human Condition*. Cambridge, MA: MIT Press.

Arthur, W. Brian. 2009. *The Nature of Technology: What It Is and How It Evolves*. New York: Free Press

Badmington, Neil, ed. 2000. *Posthumanism*. New York: Palgrave.

Bailey, Ronald. 2005. *Liberation Biology: The Scientific and Moral Case for the Biotech Revolution.* Amherst, NY: Prometheus Books.

Baily, Harold W., and Timothy K. Casey, eds. 2005. *Is Human Nature Obsolete? Genetics, Bioengineering and the Future of the Human Condition*. Cambridge, MA, and London: MIT Press

Bainbridge, William Sims. 2007. *Across the Secular Abyss*. Lanham, MD: Lexington Books.

Bainbridge, William Sims, and Mihail C. Roco, eds. 2006a. *Managing Nano-Bio-Info-Cogno Innovations: Converging Technologies in Society*. Dordrecht: Springer.

–. eds. 2006b. *Progress in Convergence: Technologies for Human Wellbeing*. Boston: Blackwell (on behalf of the New York Academy of Sciences).

Bernal, John Desmond. 1969 [1929]. *The World, the Flesh and the Devil: An Enquiry into the Future of the Three Enemies of the Rational Soul*. Bloomington: Indiana University Press.

Bostrom, Nick. 2005. A history of transhumanist thought. *Journal of Evolution and Technology* 14 (2): http://jetpress.org/volume14/bostrom.pdf, accessed July 12, 2011.

Clark, Andy. 2003. *Natural-Born Cyborgs: Minds, Technologies, and the Future of Human Intelligence.* Oxford and New York: Oxford University Press.

Fukuyama, Francis. 2002. *Our Posthuman Future: Consequences of the Biotechnology Revolution*. New York: Picador Books.

Garreau, Joel. 2004. *Radical Evolution: The Promise and Peril of Enhancing Our Minds, Our Bodies, and What It Means to Be Humans.* New York: Doubleday.

Gillett, Grant. 2008. *Subjectivity and Being Somebody: Human Identity and Neuroethics*. Exeter, UK: Imprint Academic.

Glannon, Walter. 2002. *The Mental Basis of Responsibility*. Aldershot, UK: Ashgate.

–. 2006. *Bioethics and the Brain*. New York: Oxford University Press.

Gordijn, Bert, and Ruth Chadwick, eds. 2008. *Medical Enhancement and Posthumanity*. Amsterdam: Springer.

Haldane, J.B.S. 1924. *Daedalus: or Science and the Future*. New York: E.P. Dutton & Co.

Hansell, Gregory R., and William J. Grassie, eds. 2011. *H+ Transhumanism and Its Critics*. Philadelphia: Metanexus Institute.

Harris, John. 1992. *Wonderwoman and Superman: The Ethics of Human Biotechnology*. Oxford: Oxford University Press.

–. 2007. *Enhancing Evolution: The Ethical Case for Making Better People*. Princeton, NJ: Princeton University Press.

Hayles, N. Katherine. 1999. *How We Became Posthuman: Virtual Bodies in Cybernetics, Literature, and Informatics*. Chicago: University of Chicago Press.

Hefner, Philip. 2003. *Technology and Human Becoming*. Minneapolis, MN: Fortress.

Hughes, James. 2002. The politics of transhumanism. Version 2.0. Paper presented at the 2001 Annual Meeting of the Society for Social Studies of Science, Cambridge, MA: http://www.changesurfer.com/Acad/TranshumPolitics.htm, accessed July 13, 2011.

–. 2004. *Citizen Cyborg: Why Democratic Societies Must Respond to the Redesigned Human of the Future*. Boulder, CO: Westview Press.

Huxley, Julian. 1927. *Religion without Revelation*. New York: Harper and Brothers.

Jonas, Hans. 1984. *The Imperative of Responsibility: In Search of an Ethics for the Technological Age*. Chicago: University of Chicago Press.

Kass, Leon. 2002. *Life, Liberty, and the Defense of Dignity: The Challenge for Bioethics*. San Francisco: Encounter Books.

Kass, Leon, Elizabeth H. Blackburn, Rebecca S. Dresser, Daniel W. Foster, et al. 2003. *Beyond Therapy: Biotechnology and the Pursuit of Happiness*. New York: Harper Perennial.

Kurzweil, Ray. 2005. *The Singularity Is Near: When Humans Transcend Biology*. New York: Viking.

Maher, Derek F., and Calvin Mercer, eds. 2009. *Religion and the Implications of Radical Life Extension*. New York: Palgrave Macmillan.

McKibben, Bill. 2003. *Enough: Staying Human in an Engineered Age*. New York: Henry Holt & Co.

Mehlman, Maxwell J. 2003. *Wondergenes: Genetic Enhancement and the Future of Society*. Bloomington: Indiana University Press.

–. 2009. *The Price of Perfection: Individualism and Society in the Era of Biomedical Enhancement*. Baltimore, MD: Johns Hopkins University Press.

Minsky, Marvin. 2006. *The Emotion Machine: Commonsense Thinking, Artificial Intelligence, and the Future of the Human Mind*. New York: Simon & Schuster.

Moravec, Hans. 1999. *Robot: Mere Machine to Transcendent Mind*. New York: Oxford University Press.

More, Max. 2004. Extropian Principles 3.0, http://www.maxmore.com/extprn3.htm, accessed July 31, 2011.

Olshansky, S. Jay, and Bruce A. Carnes. 2001. *The Quest for Immortality: Science at the Frontiers of Aging*. New York: W.W. Norton.

Pinker, Steven. 2002. *The Blank Slate: The Modern Denial of Human Nature*. New York: Penguin.

Parfit, Derek. 1987. *Reasons and Persons*. Oxford: Oxford University Press.

Roco, Mihail C., and William Sims Bainbridge, eds. 2002. *Converging Technologies for Improvement of Human Performance: Nanotechnology, Biotechnology, Information Technology and Cognitive Science*. Dordrecht and Boston: Kluwer Academic Publishers.

Roco, Mihail C., and Carlo D. Montemagno, eds. 2004. *The Coevolution of Human Potential and Converging Technologies*. Annals of the New York Academy of Sciences 1013. New York: New York Academy of Sciences.

Rose, Steven. 2005. *The Future of the Brain: The Promise and Perils of Tomorrow's Neuroscience*. New York: Oxford University Press.

Royal Society and the Royal Academy of Engineering. 2004. *Nanoscience and Nanotechnologies: Opportunities and Uncertainties*. London: Royal Society and Royal Academy of Engineering.

Sandel, Michael. 2007. *The Case against Perfection: Ethics in the Age of Genetic Engineering*. Cambridge, MA: The Belknap Press of Harvard University Press.

Savulescu, Julian, and Nick Bostrom, eds. 2009. *Human Enhancement*. New York: Oxford University Press.

Scanlon, Thomas. 1998. *What We Owe to Each Other*. Cambridge, MA: Harvard University Press.

Seidensticker, Bob. 2006. *Futurehype: The Myths of Technology Change*. San Francisco: Berrett-Koehler Publishers.

Stock, Gregory. 1993. *Metaman: The Making of Humans and Machines into a Global Superorganism*. New York: Simon and Schuster.
–. 2002. *Redesigning Humans: Our Inevitable Genetic Future*. Boston: Houghton Mifflin.
Tipler, Frank J. 1994. *The Physics of Immortality: Modern Cosmology, God and the Resurrection of the Dead*. New York: Doubleday.
–. 2007. *The Physics of Christianity*. New York: Doubleday.
Waters, Brent. 2006. *From Human to Posthuman: Christian Theology and Technology in a Postmodern World*. Burlington, VT: Ashgate Publishing.
Wolfe, Cary. 2009. *What is Posthumanism?* Minneapolis: University of Minnesota Press.
Young, Simon. 2006. *Designer Evolution: A Transhumanist Manifesto*. New York: Prometheus Books.

Web Sites

Global Spiral: http://www.metanexus.net/Magazine/
Humanity+: http://humanityplus.org/
Journal of Evolution and Technology: http://jetpress.org/
Metanexus Institute: http://www.metanexus.net/
Nick Bostrom: http://www.nickbostrom.com/

List of Contributors

Braden Allenby (J.D. University of Virginia, 1978; Ph.D. Rutgers University, 1992) is Lincoln Professor of Engineering and Ethics and professor of civil and environmental engineering in the Department of Civil and Environmental Engineering in the Ira Fulton Schools of Engineering at Arizona State University, Tempe. Allenby also holds a faculty appointment in the Sandra Day O'Connor College of Law. His research interests are in Earth systems engineering and management; industrial ecology science; and technology policy. He is the author of *Industrial Ecology* (2006) and *Reconstructing Earth: Technology and Environment in the Age of the Humans* (2005). A Templeton Fellow at ASU (2007-8), Allenby is coauthor (with Daniel Sarewitz) of the *Post-Human Condition* (2011).

Daniel Barben (Ph.D. University of Potsdam, Germany, 1995) is professor at the Institute of Political Science at RWTH Aachen University. Since April 2010, he holds the first chair of futures research in Germany. Formerly an associate research professor at the Consortium for Science, Policy & Outcomes at Arizona State University, Barben's main research interests are in social and political studies of emerging technologies; globalization, transnationality, and democracy; and the environment. His most recent scholarship has focused on acceptance politics and public understanding of science and technology, as discussed in *Public Understanding of Science* (2010) and in the *Encyclopedia of Nanoscience and Society* (2010).

Linell E. Cady (Th.D. Harvard University, 1981) is the Franca G. Oreffice Dean's Distinguished Professor of Religious Studies in the School of Historical, Philosophical and Religious Studies and the director of the Center for the Study of Religion and Conflict at Arizona State University, Tempe. She writes on the relationship of religion and the public/private boundary, with primary attention to the American context. Her current scholarship focuses on the constructions of religions and the secular and their bearing on the place of religion in public life within modern pluralistic societies. She is the author of *Religion, Theology and American Public Life* (1993) and coeditor of *Comparative Secularisms in a Golden Age* (2010) and of *Religion and Conflict in South and Southeast Asia: Disrupting Violence* (2006). Cady founded and coedited of the daily online magazine Religion Dispatches.

Eugene Clay (Ph.D. University of Chicago, 1989) is associate professor of religious studies in the School of Historical, Philosophical and Religious Studies at Arizona State University, Tempe. His research interests are in Eastern Orthodox Christianity and Russian religious history. Clay explores the variety and vitality of the Christian traditions in Russia and concentrates especially on the Russian Orthodox Church and those movements that broke away from it. He is the coeditor of *Centers and Peripheries in the Christian West* (2011), and his essays have been published in *Church History*, *Russian History*, *Cahiers du monde russe*, and several Russian scholarly journals.

Jerry Coursen (Ph.D. University of Arizona, 1978) is senior lecturer of biomedical engineering in the School of Biological and Health Systems Engineering in the Ira Fulton Schools of Engineering at Arizona State University, Tempe. Coursen's research activities have been primarily in neuroscience and complexity theory. He is also interested in focusing on curriculum development for the education of bioengineers in all areas of practical medicine. He has published in *Anatomical Record.*

Michael M. Crow (Ph.D. Syracuse University, 1985) is president of Arizona State University and professor in the School of Public Affairs, College of Public Programs. A fellow of the National Academy of Public Administration, President Crow writes on technology transfer; science and technology policy; and the practice and theory of public policy. He is the author of *Limited by Design: R & D Laboratories in the United States* (1998), a coauthor of *Synthetic Fuels: Technology Development in the United States: A Retrospective Assessment* (1988), and coeditor of *Strategic Management of Industrial R & D* (1984) and *High Sulfur Exports: An International Analysis* (1983). President Crow serves on the board of directors of the Stardust Foundation and the National Association of State Universities and Land-Grant Colleges (NASULGC) and is the chair of the Pacific 10-Conference. His speeches and essays on science and technology policy are widely disseminated.

Walter Glannon (Ph.D. Yale University, 1995) is associate professor of philosophy and holds the Canada Research Chair in Biomedical Ethics and Ethical Theory at the University of Calgary. He is the author of many professional papers, as well as six books, including *Bioethics and the Brain* (2006), *Biomedical Ethics* (2004), *The Mental Basis of Responsibility* (2002), and *Genes and Future People: Philosophical Issues in Human Genetics* (2001). Glannon's essays on biomedical ethics and ethical theory have appeared in the *Journal of Medical Ethics*, *Cambridge Quarterly of Healthcare Ethics*, *Bioethics*, and *Neuroethics*, and other distinguished venues.

William J. Grassie (Ph.D. Temple University, 1994) is the founder of the Metanexus Institute located in Bryn Mawr, Pennsylvania, and serves as a senior contributing editor of the institute's online publication *The Global Spiral*. The Metanexus Institute promotes the transdisciplinary approach to research and education about the most profound questions of nature, culture, and the human person. Grassie is the author of *The New Sciences of Religion: Exploring Spirituality from the Outside In and Bottom Up* (2010) and *Politics by Other Means: Science and Religion in the 21st Century* (2010) and coeditor of *H+: Transhumanism and Its Critics* (2011).

Brian Gratton (Ph.D. Boston University, 1980) is professor of history in the School of Historical, Philosophical and Religious Studies at Arizona State University, Tempe. Gratton studies immigration, ethnicity, and immigration policy in the United States, Latin America, and Europe, and also Mexican American geography and settlement and family demography. His book *Old Age and the Search for Security* (1994) focused on social security, retirement, and the circumstances of the American elderly. He currently writes on immigration and migration, particularly among Hispanics. His essays on ethnicity and immigration in the U.S., Ecuador, and Europe have appeared in the *Journal of American Ethnic History*, *Professional Geographer*, *The Journal of Ethnic and Migration Studies*, *Historical Statistics of the United States*, and the *Journal of Interdisciplinary History*.

Steven A. Hoffman (Ph.D. University of Colorado, 1975) is associate professor of immunology in the School of Life Sciences at Arizona State University, Tempe. Hoffman's research focuses on the interactions and relations between mind, brain, and the immune system. This includes biomedical research into how the immune system can lead to neuropsychiatric manifestations. Recent publications on immune function and disease include "Intrathecal Antibodies and Brain Damage in Lupus-Prone MRL Mice" with M. Stanojcic, G. Loheswaran, L. Xu, and B. Sakic in *Brain, Behavior, and Immunity* (2010); and "Circulating Brain-Reactive Autoantibodies and Behavioral Deficits in the MRL Model of CNS Lupus" with S. Williams and B. Sakic in the *Journal of Neuroimmunology* (2010).

Alexandra López (J.D. University of Puerto Rico, 2006) is currently an adjunct professor at the University of Puerto Rico School of Law, where she teaches courses and seminars on the ethical and legal aspects of biotechnology and nanotechnology. While completing requirements for the J.D. degree from the University of Puerto Rico School of Law, López coedited the *University of Puerto Rico Law Review* (volume 74). Currently, she works as a judicial clerk for the Supreme Court of Puerto Rico and completed an LL.M. degree in biotechnology and genomics from Arizona State University.

Farzad Mahootian (Ph.D. Fordham University, 1990) is on the faculty in the College of Arts and Science, New York University. He is a former lecturer in the School of Letters and Sciences, Arizona State University, Phoenix. Mahootian's research interests include philosophy of science; philosophy of chemistry; process philosophy; science and values; science and religion; environmental philosophy; and Islamic and non-Western philosophies. He recently published "Cosmology without Finality" in the *Astronomical Society of the Pacific Conference Series* CS413 (2009); "Complementary Frameworks of Scientific Inquiry: Hypothetico-deductive, Hypothetico-inductive, and Observational-inductive" in *World Futures: The Journal of General Evolution* (2009); and "Self-Limitation in Science, Philosophy and Religion," in the online journal *Global Spiral*.

Gary E. Marchant (Ph.D. University of British Columbia, 1986; J.D. Harvard University, 1990) is the Lincoln Professor of Emerging Technologies, Law and Ethics at the Sandra Day O'Connor College of Law at Arizona State University, Tempe. He is also a professor in the School of Life Sciences and executive director of the ASU Center for Law, Science and Innovation. Professor Marchant's research interests include environmental law; risk assessment and management; genetics and the law; biotechnology law; food and drug law; legal aspects of nanotechnology; and law, science, and technology. Marchant is coauthor of *Arbitrary and Capricious: The Precautionary Principle in the European Union Courts* (2004) and coeditor of *Genomics and Environmental Regulation: Science, Ethics, and Law* (2008).

Joan L. McGregor (Ph.D. University of Arizona, 1985) is professor of philosophy in the School of Historical, Philosophical and Religious Studies at Arizona State University, Tempe. Professor McGregor's research focuses on moral and legal philosophy. In bioethics, she works on sustainability questions generated from the ethics of emerging technologies, nanotechnology, biotechnology, information technology and cognitive science (NBIC); and in bio-medical ethics, she questions the subtle influences that affect individuals' choices and what should be done to militate against the forces that can undermine voluntariness. She is the author of *What Is Rape? On Acquaintance Rape and Taking Women's Consent Seriously* (2005), and her essays have appeared in *The American Journal of Bioethics, Medicine and Law Journal, Health Policy, Journal of Intensive Care Medicine*, and *Journal of Law, Medicine and Ethics*, among other distinguished venues.

Kenneth L. Mossman (Ph.D. University of Tennessee, 1973) is professor of health physics in the School of Life Sciences and an affiliated faculty member of the Center for Law, Science and Innovation in the Sandra Day O'Connor College of Law, Arizona State University, Tempe. He is also an administrative judge (technical) of the Atomic Safety and Licensing Board, U.S. Nuclear Regulatory Commission. Professor Mossman is a fellow of the American Association for the Advancement of Science and a Guggenheim fellow. Mossman works in the general areas of public health and science-informed public policy, with specific interests in cancer causation, radiological risk assessment, and risk management. He is the author, with William Mills, of *The Biological Basis of Radiation Protection Practice* (1992); *Arbitrary and Capricious: The Precautionary Principle in the European Union Courts* (2004), with Gary Marchant; and *Radiation Risks in Perspective* (2007).

Craig T. Nagoshi (Ph.D. University of Hawaii, 1984) is associate professor in the Department of Psychology, Arizona State University, Tempe. Nagoshi's research interests include social and cognitive predictors of college-student alcohol use/abuse; effects of religiosity/spirituality on psychological functioning; and psychological components of gender roles and gender identity. Recent scholarship includes "Effects of Gender, Status, and Mating Cues on Expected Aggressive Responses," with H. Terrell and J. Patock-Peckham in *Aggressive Behavior* (2009); and "Gender Differences in Aggression: The Role of Status and Personality in Competitive Interactions," with H. Terrell and E. Hill in *Sex Roles* (2008).

Julie L. Nagoshi is currently a Ph.D. student in social work at Arizona State University. Her research focuses on lesbian, gay, bisexual, and transgender (LGBT) issues and topics. Specifically, Nagoshi explores the comparison of gender roles, gender identity, and sexual orientation. She is coauthor with Katherine Adams, Heather Terrell, Eric Hill, Stephan/ie Brzuzy, and Craig Nagoshi of "Gender Differences in Correlates of Homophobia and Transphobia," published in *Sex Roles* (2010); and coauthor with Stephan/ie Brzuzy of "Transgender Theory: Embodying Research and Practice", published in *Affilia* (2010).

Barry G. Ritchie (Ph.D. University of South Carolina, 1979) is professor of physics at Arizona State University, Tempe. Ritchie has served on technical advisory panels at Los Alamos National Laboratory and at the Thomas Jefferson National Accelerator Facility (Jefferson Lab). He and a large group of collaborators study the structure of the protons and neutrons that make up atomic nuclei through experiments at international particle-accelerator facilities. Recent papers include "Beam Spin Asymmetries in Deeply Virtual Compton Scattering (DVCS) with CLAS at 4.8 GeV" in *Physical Review C* (2009); and "Electroproduction of p pi(+)pi(-) off Protons at 0.2 < Q(2) < 0.6 GeV2 and 1.3 < W < 1.57 GeV with the CLAS Detector" in *Physical Review C* (2009). He is the coeditor of *Hadronic Probes and Nuclear Interactions* (1985).

Norbert M. Samuelson (Ph.D. Indiana University, 1970) is Harold and Jean Grossman Professor of Jewish Studies in the School of Historical, Philosophical and Religious Studies at Arizona State University, Tempe. Samuelson's research interests include the history of Western philosophy; Jewish philosophy; philosophy and religion; philosophy and science; the Jewish Aristotelians, with an emphasis on Gersonides; and twentieth-century philosophy, with an emphasis on Alfred North Whitehead and Franz Rosenzweig. Among his works on Judaism and science are *Jewish Faith and Modern Science: On the Death and Rebirth of Jewish Philosophy* (2009); *Revelation and the God of Israel* (2002); and *Judaism and the Doctrine of Creation* (1994). His books on Jewish philosophy include *Jewish Philosophy: An Historical Introduction* (2003); *A User's Guide to Franz Rosenzweig's Star of Redemption* (1999); and *An Introduction to Modern Jewish Philosophy* (1989).

Hava Tirosh-Samuelson (Ph.D. Hebrew University of Jerusalem, 1978) is professor of history in the School of Historical, Philosophical and Religious Studies at Arizona State University, Tempe. She is the director of the Center for Jewish Studies and the Irving and Miriam Lowe Professor of Modern Judaism. Tirosh-Samuelson writes on Jewish intellectual history with a focus on philosophy and mysticism in premodern Judaism, feminist theory, Judaism and ecology, and Judaism and science. She was the principal investigator of a large grant from the Metanexus Institute for the project "Facing the Challenges of Transhumanism: Religion, Science and Technology" that led to this volume. She is the author of the award-winning *Between Worlds: The Life and Thought of Rabbi David ben Judah Messer Leon* (1991) and of *Happiness in Premodern Judaism: Virtue, Knowledge and Well-Being* (2003). She is the editor of *Judaism and Ecology: Created World and Revealed Word* (2002) and *Women and Gender in Jewish Philosophy* (2004), and coeditor of *The Legacy of Hans Jonas: Judaism and the Phenomenon of Life* (2008).

Steven M. Wasserstrom (Ph.D. University of Toronto, 1985) is Moe and Izetta Tonkon Professor of Judaic Studies and Humanities in the Department of Religion at Reed College in Portland, Oregon. His areas of expertise are Judaic and Islamic studies, and he writes extensively on theories of religion. He is the author of the award-winning book *Between Muslim and Jew: The Problem of Symbiosis* (1995) and *Religion after Religion: Gershom Scholem, Mircea Eliade and Henry Corbin at Eranos* (1999).

Quentin Wheeler (Ph.D. Ohio State University, 1980) holds the Virginia M. Ullman Chair in Natural History in the School of Life Sciences and was formerly the Vice President and Dean of the College of Liberal Arts and Sciences at Arizona State University. His research interests include the morphology, taxonomy, and phylogeny of beetles, systematic biology theory, and the role of taxonomy in biodiversity. Wheeler is a fellow of the American Association for the Advancement of Science, Linnean Society of London and Royal Entomological Society. He is the author of *The Revision of the Genera of Lymexylidae (Coleoptrea Cucujiformia)* (1986) and *Slime-Mold Beetles of the Genus Agathidium Panzer in North and Central America* (2005). He is the editor of *The New Taxonomy* (2008) and co-editor of *Special Concepts and Phylogenetic Theory: A Debate* (2000) and *Fungus-Insect Relationships: Perspectives in Ecology and Evolution* (1984).

Michael J. White (Ph.D. University of California-San Diego, 1974) is professor of philosophy in the School of Life Sciences and an affiliated faculty member in the School of Historical, Philosophical and Religious Studies at Arizona State University, Tempe. He also holds a part-time faculty appointment in the Sandra Day O'Connor College of Law. White works in the areas of history of philosophy, science, and mathematics (especially during Greek and Roman antiquity and the seventeenth and eighteenth centuries), formal logic, and political philosophy and jurisprudence. His publications include *Political Philosophy: An Historical Introduction* (2003); *Partisan Or Neutral? The Futility of Public Political Theory* (1997); *The Continuous and the Discrete: Ancient Physical Theories from a Contemporary Perspective* (1992); and *Agency and Integrality: Philosophical Themes in the Ancient Discussions of Determinism and Response* (1985).

Index

D

F

H

I

J

K

N

O

P

Q

R

S

T

U

V

W

X

Y

Z

BEYOND HUMANISM: TRANS- AND POSTHUMANISM
JENSEITS DES HUMANISMUS: TRANS- UND POSTHUMANISMUS

Edited by / Herausgegeben von Stefan Lorenz Sorgner

Vol./Bd. 1 Robert Ranisch / Stefan Lorenz Sorgner (Eds.): Post- and Transhumanism. An Introduction. *In preparation.*

Vol./Bd. 2 Stephen R. L. Clark: Philosophical Futures. 2011.

Vol./Bd. 3 Hava Tirosh-Samuelson / Kenneth L. Mossman (eds.): Building Better Humans? Refocusing the Debate on Transhumanism. 2012.

www.peterlang.de